GALLOWAY'S BOOK ON RUNNING has sold over 400,000 copies since it was first published in 1984, and is known among runners as the finest work ever published on the art and science of running. Jeff Galloway is a world-class runner who decided back in the '80s that his mission in life was to teach others how to run, and in so doing, make fitness a permanent part of their lives.

The original book featured training programs for 10K races and marathons. Since he recently wrote an entire book devoted to marathons, Jeff decided to remove marathon training from *Galloway's Book on Running*, and include the very popular 5K and half-marathon distances, along with the 10K.

WHAT'S NEW IN THE 2ND EDITION:

- 5K and half-marathon training programs
- Less focus on pulse-checking as a component of training
- Walk break concept introduced for all race distances
- Much more information on training in the extremes of hot and cold weather
- A new chapter on motivation and mental training
- The most current information on nutrition
- More in-depth analysis of injuries and their treatment, such as heel problems like plantar fasciitis and heel spurs, and a special report on iliotibial band injuries
- A greater focus on the particular needs of the older runner, with an emphasis on fat burning, and the importance of rest

***Galloway's Book on Running* is a must-read for runners of all levels.**

It's the definitive general guide to running, and in addition, has training programs for three races. It shows novices how to get started and stick with it. It also has serious training advice for competitive racers. It will get you moving and keep you motivated to make running your secret to good health for the rest of your life!

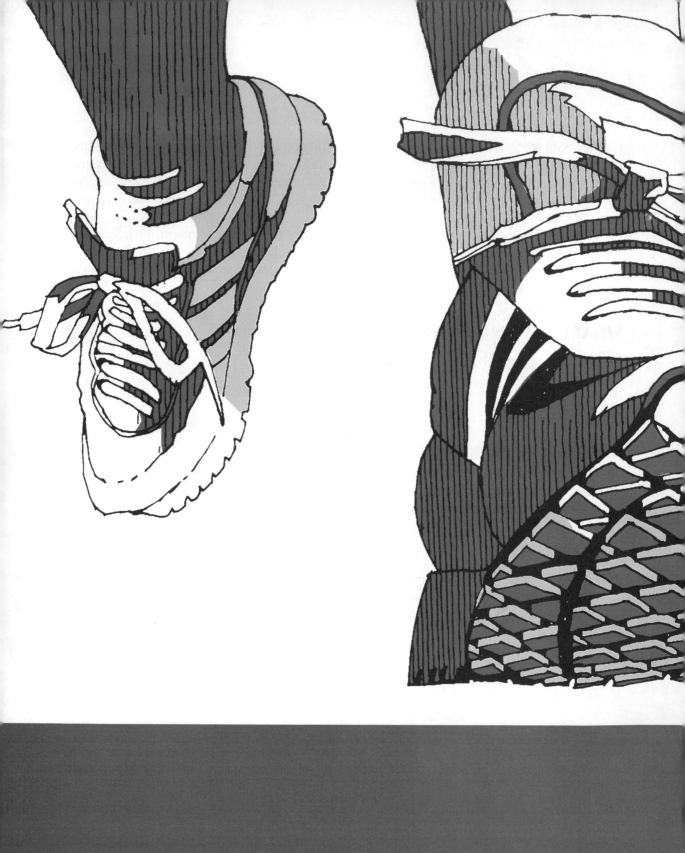

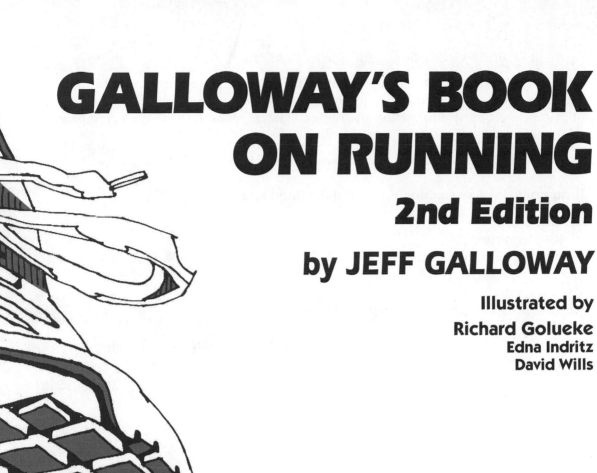

GALLOWAY'S BOOK ON RUNNING

2nd Edition

by JEFF GALLOWAY

Illustrated by

Richard Golueke
Edna Indritz
David Wills

Shelter Publications
Bolinas, California, U.S.A.

Distributed in the United States and Canada by Publishers Group West.

Library of Congress Cataloging-in-Publication Data

Galloway, Jeff, 1945–
    [Book on running]
    Galloway's book on running / by Jeff Galloway ; illustrated by Richard Golueke, Edna Indritz, and David Wills.—Rev. ed.
        p.   cm.
    Includes bibliographical references and index.
    ISBN 0-936070-27-7 (pbk.)
    1. Running.   1. Running—Training.   I. Title: Book on running.   I. Title.
    GV1061 .G34 2002
    796.42—dc21   2002001558

7 6 5 4 3 2 1—08 07 06 05 04 03 02
(Lowest digits indicate number and year of latest printing.)

Printed in the United States of America

Additional copies of this book may be purchased at your favorite bookstore or by sending $14.95 plus $4.50 shipping and handling charges to:

Shelter Publications, Inc.
P. O. Box 279
Bolinas, California 94924
415-868-0280
E-mail: shelter@shelterpub.com
Orders, toll-free: 1-800-307-0131

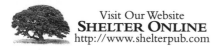

Visit Our Website
SHELTER ONLINE
http://www.shelterpub.com

CONTENTS

Injuries

Food

Shoes

Start to Finish

Appendices

INTRODUCTION

IT WAS 1973. A beautiful September dawn was breaking over the Cascade Mountain Range as I left the city limits of Eugene Oregon, and headed east, racing through the early morning mist in an old Volvo sedan. My reliable car cruised along in fourth, but my mind shifted into neutral: it was time for reflection. What had I been doing the past seven years?

I guess I was the running equivalent of a ski bum, working for college degrees in history and social studies during the school year, and following the racing circuit each summer. I'd had some wonderful times those summers—rich and varied experiences. I'd made lots of friends, shared the joys and agonies of racing with other competitors, traveled abroad, and seen practically every state in the Union.

One summer I'd been to Russia as a member of the U.S. National Track and Field Team. At a track meet in Minsk, a crowd of 50,000 cheered only for their countrymen; victorious Americans were met with stony silence. No Holiday Inns awaited us in Dakar; we stayed in grass huts. Temperatures in this town on the west coast of Africa were so high that officials handed us water-filled sponges as we ran. In Morocco we ran a cross-country race on a horse track with a detour in the middle through a mud hole.

Another summer I bought a Eurail pass and traveled from one end of Europe to the other. I once ran an afternoon race in Luxembourg, then caught the midnight train to Torino, Italy, for a race the next day. Ah, the resiliency of youth!

In 1972 I'd realized my life's dream: making the U.S. Olympic Team. I'd also set an American record in the 10-mile. I felt happy about these achievements. But that was then. Now, though, rolling across Oklahoma, I realized I had to begin thinking about the future. I'd finished graduate school and had my teaching credentials, but after one year of teaching fourth grade in Raleigh, North Carolina, I missed the excitement of traveling and running. Yet I knew I couldn't keep driving around the country in an old car forever.

Driving through the gently rolling terrain of Kansas I thought of recent runs with my friend Steve Prefontaine, who was preparing himself to be the best 5000-meter runner in the world by the Montreal Olympics in three years. One of my best friends, Geoff Hollister, had just started full-time work for a struggling company called Nike. I wondered if they would still be in business in 1976. But passing through the Ozark foothills I thought about what a great thing Geoff was doing: building a company that promotes health and fitness products.

By the time I got to Nashville, I knew what I was going to do. With my eyes fixed on the road and a cup of coffee in hand, I dreamed of a running store stocked with the best gear, staffed by runners trained in the science of fitting shoes. Then I imagined a summer camp in the mountains where people could vacation and run with some of the world's best coaches. I could still be a teacher, I decided, but not one sitting in front of a row of desks.

The idea seemed timely, for something new seemed to be happening with running. New faces were starting to appear on the roads. The serious and often eccentric competitors were still out there of course, but now people of all ages, shapes and abilities seemed to be trickling out into the streets, sidewalks and parks. The vitality of regular endurance running was not only personally addictive, but socially contagious.

There was also a growing sense of communication among runners. People compared notes and traded tips. Runners began asking me questions and I enjoyed trying to work out creative solutions to their problems. It seemed that what I'd learned on the racing circuit could be helpful and instructive to everyday runners.

After arriving home, I found a store with the cheapest rent in Tallahassee — $125 a month. It was hardly in a prime location: a suburban neighborhood next to a beauty parlor, with no walk-by traffic. I withdrew my life's savings of $4000, borrowed $2000 from my grandmother and started learning the rudiments of running a retail business. At first we had no credit rating and very few equipment or clothing manufacturers would sell to us. The only shoe suppliers that would set up accounts for us were a warehouse operation with left-over Converse high-tops. Since no one knew the store was there, and no one walked by, I printed up flyers and handed them out to students as I ran through nearby college campuses. Somehow we survived these growing pains, and after a year and a half, moved to Atlanta.

By 1976 the running boom was on, and business started picking up. By 1978 we were firmly established. Now, over 20 years later, my two Phidippides stores are breaking sales records every year, my Galloway Running Clubs are in over 30 cities, and our summer running camps are in full swing. I've been able to make a career out of running—the dream has become a reality.

Business has its rewards, but it's the teaching that brings me the most satisfaction. I'm now back on the road (about a third of the time), conducting clinics and seminars, talking to beginners and veterans, to large groups and small.

This book was put together from hundreds of these experiences. I've learned firsthand about the problems of everyday runners, and the patterns of stress and rest that improve fitness while minimizing injury or fatigue. When we stay within the boundaries, the natural rewards we get from running make it one of the most pleasurable experiences in life.

There's much more to running than competition. Although a good deal of what follows will help runners go faster, the same principles—mileage programs, a running log, good form, hill training, walk breaks, stretching, strength exercises—apply to runners of all levels and with varying objectives. You may be just starting to run. If so, this book will help get you started comfortably and with confidence. If you've been running for a while, you'll learn how to make running more enjoyable, to better prepare for races, and to avoid stress-related injuries. Veteran competitors will find new ideas on racing strategy and improving future performance. Whatever your level or goals, you want to run intelligently, stay healthy and strong, keep your weight down, run with good form, avoid injuries, and have fun.

There's a great deal of information in this book, but only one message: *You can do it!* We find ourselves on this earth with a generous supply of hopes, abilities and expectations. Many people live out their lives without discovering how to rise above obstacles and enjoy the immense satisfaction and exhilaration of improving. With determination, patience and persistence, you can mold yourself into a runner and, in the process, have a more healthy and productive life.

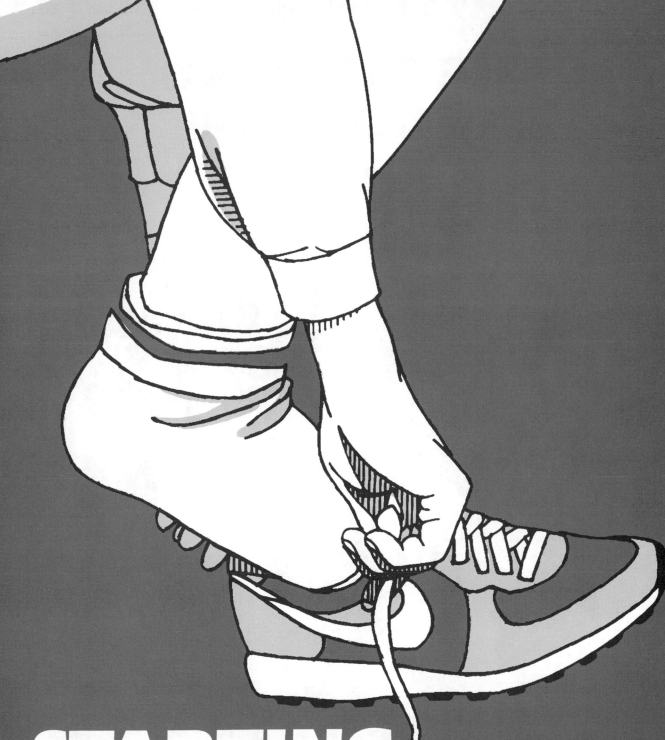

STARTING

1 THE RUNNING REVOLUTION

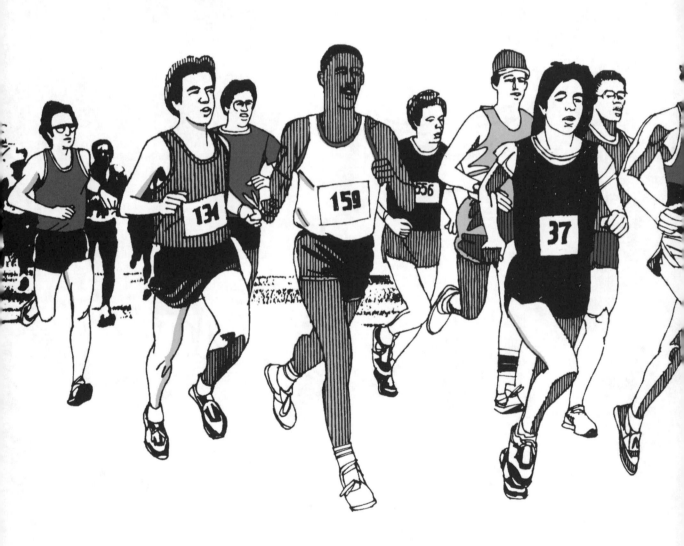

RUNNING IS NOTHING NEW. Our ancient ancestors had to walk and run to survive. The ancient Greeks had foot races at least as early as 776 B.C., the year of the first Olympics. The famous runner Phidippides, in 490 B.C., covered 300 miles in four days to solicit help from neighboring Sparta against the imminent invasion of Athens. In pre-industrial England, *footmen* were sent running ahead of horse-drawn carriages to warn their lords of danger. To this day, the Tarahumara Indians of northwestern Mexico compete in foot races and cover 150–200 miles a day—kicking a ball along the way. Running is a natural activity for humans. The sport of running has existed for centuries, from informal tests of ego and will, to high school track meets, to the Olympic games, but only recently have people from all walks of life taken to the roads en masse.

While runners tend to be optimistic, even the most positive running fan couldn't have predicted the wild increase in our activity. I've personally worked with over 100,000 average citizens who've discovered that the attitude boost and relaxation of a daily run makes them feel better, and enjoy life more. Those who run sensibly, about three times a week, don't quit because they feel so good!

The reasons for running are diverse: to lose weight, become fit, feel good, reduce stress, compete, or share the experience with others. It may also have something to do with the advanced state of technology. Most work formerly done by hand is now done by machines. While our distant ancestors led physically active lives, covering long distances to gather roots, nuts and grains or to pursue game; while our grandparents or great-grandparents tilled the fields for food and handcrafted everyday necessities, we now find ourselves in a largely sedentary economy.

In increasing numbers, people are seeking to regain the health, fitness, and leanness that was once natural to our physically active predecessors. A new spirit seems to have arisen. Perhaps when a society attains a high level of industrial and technological efficiency, those people who have long neglected their physical nature react and begin seeking ways to reestablish harmony between body, mind, and spirit.

I was running before it caught on in America. Then in the late '60s I began to see a trickle of other runners out on the roads I once ran alone. By the early '70s, there were more and now, millions are out running regularly. It seemed to have been a natural evolution, but in retrospect I can pinpoint a few key people who helped propel running into the revolution we now see in our towns and cities: three teachers —Arthur Lydiard, Bill Bowerman, and Dr. Kenneth Cooper; and four runners— Amby Burfoot, Frank Shorter, Bill Rodgers, and Joan Benoit Samuelson. There were many others, of course, but these seven were catalysts, reflecting and magnifying the spirit of the times. They were at the right places, at the right times, with the right inspiration for the new outlook that was crucial to the birth of fitness running.

Running in New Zealand. In the 1940s, Arthur Lydiard, a former rugby player, now overweight and working on the line at a New Zealand shoe factory, decided he had to make a change in his own life. Playing rugby weekends had done nothing to deflate the spare tire around his middle, so he decided he'd try to run off the excess weight. But watching the local runners of the day was discouraging. They sped around and around the track at full speed until they collapsed. "No pain, no gain" was the philosophy of the day.

Arthur wanted to get in shape, but not that way. Instead, he took to the open New Zealand roads and embarked on a conditioning program of long, slow runs. Over the months he lost weight. Over the years he became addicted to running and discovered a long-hidden competitive spirit. He began to wonder how he might fare in a marathon and soon Lydiard the jogger became Lydiard the racer. He eventually came to represent New Zealand in the 1951 Commonwealth Games.

A few local youngsters had begun running with Lydiard and eventually they asked if he'd be their coach. Lydiard agreed and developed his own program—emphasizing long, slow runs—into a sequence of running workouts for his students. In the 1960 Rome Olympics, three of these neighborhood kids—Peter Snell, Murray Halberg and Barry Magee—won distance running medals. Lydiard became an acclaimed public figure and a national hero.

You might say Lydiard invented jogging. After the Olympics, he was frequently invited to speak to groups of sedentary men and women in their 30s, 40s and beyond. The people he talked to began to sense that they, like the formerly overweight rugby player, could run gently and improve their physical condition. Running not only could take off the weight, but

could be fun. Lydiard transformed the public's image of running from an intense, tedious, painful activity into a social, civilized component of the active New Zealand lifestyle. The credibility of the Olympic medals gave Lydiard a platform from which to reach millions. He got them out of their chairs and onto the roads in the early '60s, and the underground running movement began.

Jogging in America. Bill Bowerman is one of the most successful track coaches in the United States, but his role in bringing jogging to America is of even greater importance. In the winter of 1962, shortly after his University of Oregon four-mile relay team broke the world record, an invitation came for a match race with the team from New Zealand, the previous world recordholders. Bowerman and his team were the guests of Arthur Lydiard.

"The first Sunday I was down there," Bowerman recalled in Bill Dellenger's book, *The Running Experience*, "Lydiard asked me if I wanted to go out for a run with a local jogging club. I was used to going out and walking 55 yards, jogging 55 yards, going about a quarter of a mile and figuring I had done quite a bit. . . . We went out and met a couple hundred people in a park—men, women, children, all ages and sizes. I was still full of breakfast as Lydiard pointed toward a hill in the distance and said we were going to run to Two Pine Knoll. It looked about 1½ miles away. We took off and it wasn't too bad for about ½ mile, and then we started up this hill. God, the only thing that kept me alive was the hope that I'd die. I moved right to the back of the group and an old fellow, I suppose he was around 70 years old, moved back with me and said, 'I see you're having trouble.' I didn't say anything . . . because I couldn't. So we turned around and got back about the same time the people did who had covered the whole distance."

Bowerman, then 50, spent six weeks in New Zealand and ran every day. He lost nearly ten pounds and reduced his waistline by four inches. By the time he returned to Oregon, he had learned to jog—slowly and comfortably. As soon as he arrived home, he got a call from Jerry Uhrhammer, a sportswriter from the *Eugene Register-Guard*. Uhrhammer wanted to know how the team had run, but Bowerman was much more excited about what he'd learned about jogging. Uhrhammer, who later became a jogger after open-heart surgery, published several articles based on Bowerman's revelations. Bowerman began staging Sunday morning runs and Uhrhammer publicized them.

Interest in the Sunday runs grew and Bowerman was asked to hold classes and clinics for neighborhood groups in Eugene. He did so, using some of his great Oregon distance runners as instructors. Before long Bowerman was overwhelmed with requests for information on this new phenomenon, so in 1966 he wrote a 20-page pamphlet—*Jogging*—with a Eugene cardiologist, Dr. Waldo Harris. The following year he published an expanded version of *Jogging*, which eventually sold over a million copies. The seeds of the jogging movement had been firmly planted in American soil.

Aerobics for Fitness. By 1960, more Americans were dying of heart disease than any other malady. A generation of Americans had leaped too quickly into the "good life."

People worked relatively hard until the mid-1940s. Finances kept meat consumption down and vegetable consumption up. Postwar prosperity, however, ushered in more leisure time, sedentary jobs and the funds to buy meat, cream, butter. . . . The rate of heart disease climbed rapidly.

The Air Force became concerned when its pilots started dying of heart failure, often bringing multi-million-dollar planes down with them. Air Force officials showed great interest when one of their young doctors, Kenneth Cooper, suggested a study to see if exercise could influence the risk factors in heart disease.

Cooper had been doing his medical residency in Boston when Bill Bowerman returned from New Zealand. A high school and college track star (he ran a 4:18 mile), Cooper had high blood pressure and had gained 40 pounds after medical school and internship. One day, as he recalls, he decided to go water skiing. Having been an expert skier in his youth, he " . . . put on a slalom ski, told the driver to accelerate immediately to almost 30 miles per hour, and prepared to have a great time, just like in the old days.

"But I was in for a surprise. Within three to four minutes I was totally exhausted, and I suddenly began to feel nauseated and weak. I told the boat driver to stop and get me back to land as quickly as possible. For the next 30 minutes, as I lay nauseated, in agony on the shore, my head was spinning and I honestly couldn't put a series of logical thoughts together."

This experience had the same effect on Cooper that the Sunday New Zealand run had on Bill Bowerman, He embarked upon an exercise and diet program that brought his weight down from 210 to 170 and reduced his body fat from 30% to 14%. His enthusiasm about exercise and the heart disease factor in airplane crashes convinced the Air Force brass of the value of his proposed testing program. The results of his studies were published in the landmark book *Aerobics*.

Cooper's book was a popular explanation of the facts that were beginning to pile up —that the good life would be cut short by poor eating habits, and that exercise could overcome many of the risk factors. Americans were receptive to these ideas. What good was a fine home, family and income without the good health to enjoy them?

Cooper's aim was to counteract the great lethargy and inactivity of most Americans by demonstrating the benefits of regular exercise. Most important, he showed how to do it. His point system gave even out-of-shape beginners a guide to exercise.

The Final Push by Runners. Just as the Olympic medals provided the fuel for Lydiard's fitness wildfire in New Zealand, Olympic success by Americans showed fellow countrymen that they, too, could be distance runners. Prior to the 1964 Tokyo Olympics, there had been only one gold medal won by an American distance runner since 1908: Horace Ashenfelter in the 1952 steeplechase.

All this changed in the Tokyo Olympics when Billy Mills, a complete unknown, upset Australian star Ron Clarke and Tunisian Mohamed Gammoudi to win the 10,000 meters. Four days later, American Bob Schul won the gold medal in the 5000 meters and one second back, in third place,

was Bill Dellenger, a 30-year-old high school track coach from Springfield, Oregon.

After years of small fields, the number of entries in major U.S. road races began to increase. In 1964 the Boston Marathon, the country's oldest road race, topped 300 entries for the first time. In 1967, it went to 479; in 1970, 1150. San Francisco's Bay to Breakers showed a similar growth. From a field of 15 in 1963, there were 124 the following year, 1241 in 1969 and 75,000 in 1984!

Although there were more racers each year, Americans had still not won the country's most important marathon— Boston—since 1957, when a schoolteacher from Groton, Connecticut named John J. Kelley broke the course record. After Kelley's victory, the Finns and Japanese dominated the event until 1968 when another New Englander, also from Groton and coached by Kelley, won. The now historic victory by my college roommate, Amby Burfoot inspired thousands of recreational runners to take up the burgeoning sport.

Then, in the early 1970s, Frank Shorter, a Yale graduate and law student, developed into a national-class distance runner while a former track star in Oregon —Kenny Moore—moved off the track onto the roads and finished second in the 1970 Fukoka Marathon.

In 1971, both Shorter and Moore qualified for the Pan Am Games Marathon, which Shorter went on to win. Kenny Moore was a writer and went to work for *Sports Illustrated*. He wrote some inspiring accounts of world-class running that appealed to millions of readers.

The force of the American fitness revolution was magnified in 1972 at the Munich Olympics by ABC Sports, which selected the marathon as one of their feature events. That Shorter beat one of the greatest fields ever assembled by more than two minutes was final confirmation that Americans could indeed be successful distance athletes.

Further proof was provided a few years later when Bill Rodgers surprised everyone by winning the 1975 Boston Marathon. He went on to win it in 1978, 1979 and 1980. The likeable Rodgers had a young kid-like energy and openness so different from the cocky professional athletes of the day. He was accessible to the countless fans who lined up after the races to talk to him and he seldom refused an autograph.

Joanie Benoit competed hard in everything she did as a child in Maine, taking up running to get back in shape after a ski injury. According to her coaches, she didn't win every race she entered, but gave everything she had in workouts and races. This got her into trouble several times, producing at least six surgeries. Less than three weeks before the 1984 Olympic marathon trials, Joanie injured her knee so badly that surgery was necessary. She not only qualified for the Olympic Team in Los Angeles, but won the first ever Olympic marathon for women. Today, Joan Benoit Samuelson is a devoted mother who still runs more than an hour a day.

Just as Lydiard, Bowerman, and Cooper were teachers who awakened an interest in the benefits of regular exercise, so Burfoot, Shorter, Rodgers, and Samuelson (all from the "baby boom" generation) provided inspiration at key times to the country's growing group of runners. Americans knew that physical activity was the secret to their future health, and that running, for many, was the common denominator.

2 THE FIVE STAGES OF A RUNNER

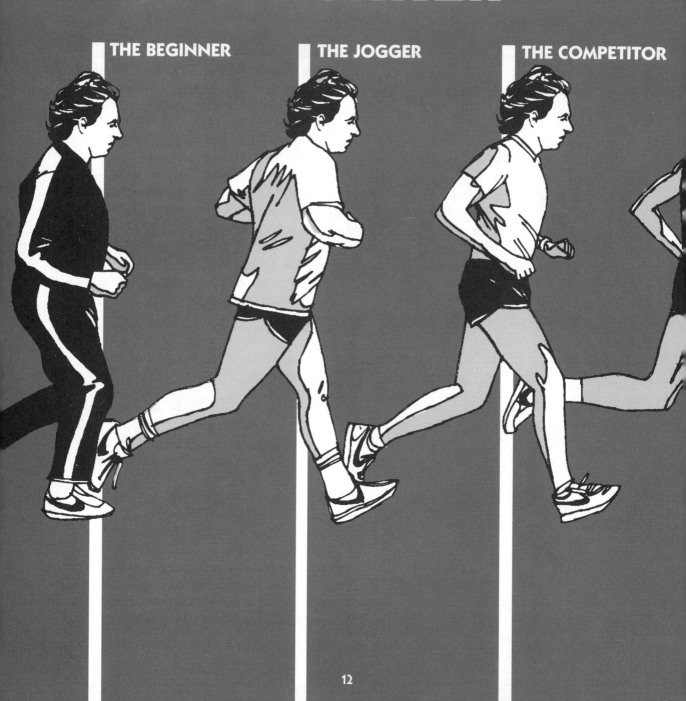

THE BEGINNER   THE JOGGER   THE COMPETITOR

THE ATHLETE
THE RUNNER

I STARTED RUNNING when I was 13. I was immediately intoxicated with a beginner's enthusiasm: the very special thrill of exertion, and a feeling that my body had vast capabilities. Of course, I tried to use all of my youthful but untrained muscle energy on that first run and then had to hobble around for a week, almost too sore to move.

But once the soreness diminished I was back out there, running again. I was hooked. As in any skill or craft, there were various stages of involvement, competence and enjoyment. Now that I've been running for over 40 years, and have spent a great deal of time helping others weave running into their lives, I see a similar pattern of evolution in just about all runners.

Progress is a process in which you balance learning and maturing, as you gain knowledge of yourself. When your running goes smoothly, one stage leads logically to the next. But real growth in running occurs when you pull yourself out of the motivational dumps, learn from your mistakes, try a few new things, and suddenly find yourself looking at running in a different way.

Only a few runners seek Olympic gold, but anyone can finish every run feeling like a champion. While you may not go through all five stages, understanding the experiences that are possible along the way will help you to minimize the pitfalls and maximize the gains of your running future.

THE BEGINNER
Stage One — Making the Break

Every beginning is precarious. There you are, perched on the edge of starting something entirely new, yet there are distractions, even criticisms, that cause detours and dead ends. You want to be more healthy and fit, but you may not realize how secure you've become in an inactive world. Each time you go out for a run you encounter a new side of yourself—one that must somehow be integrated into your daily life.

There is usually a struggle within and without. The old lifestyle is there and offers security. When the energy of "beginning" wears off, it's harder to motivate yourself to go out for that daily run. You'll face a lot of obstacles at first. It's all too easy to stop when the weather turns cold, when it rains or snows, or when you feel the aches and pains of starting. You haven't had to deal with these things before and the temptation to quit is strong.

Your running may also be threatening to your less active friends. Eventually you—the beginner—and your non-running friends work it out. The transition period, however, can be unstable and uncomfortable for both. If you falter, the old world—comfortable in many ways—is waiting for you to slip back in. If you're lucky enough to make new friends who share similar fitness goals (by joining a running group, for example), you'll probably find refuge in the "fit" world while you gain your "running security."

Social reinforcement makes it easier to establish the fitness habit. One good approach is to find a group that meets regularly. Or you can make a pact with a friend who drags you out on bad days and vice versa. Races and fun runs are great opportunities to meet people.

At times, you may not progress as fast as you expected. We Americans are traditionally hyperactive and impatient. When we plant a seed, we not only want it to grow, we want it to become a tree by next week. We want *results*. When you start, you want to see physical and psychological benefits. But if you push too hard, you can tire yourself out and end up quitting in frustration.

The seeds of exercise—if you don't crush them—will survive periods of moisture and drought. Just when they seem to be drying up, they will spring to life, rejuvenated, and propel you further down the road. Don't be discouraged, even if you've stopped. Tomorrow's another day. Many beginners stop and start again 10 or 15 times before they get the habit established.

Beginners who don't put pressure on themselves seem to have an easier time staying with it. If you simply walk/jog 30–40 minutes every other day, you'll find yourself gently swept along in a pattern of relaxation and good feeling. Your workout starts to become a special time for you.

As you make progress you find within yourself the strength and security to keep going. At first you're "just visiting" that special world when you go out for a run. But gradually you begin to change. You get used to the positive relaxed feeling. Your body starts cleaning itself up, establishing muscle tone, circulating blood and oxygen more vigorously. When you miss running on a scheduled day off, you're starting to become addicted. This is where the beginner becomes a jogger.

THE JOGGER
Stage Two—Entering the New World

The jogger feels secure with running. It may be hard to start each day's run but, unlike the beginner, you can identify with those who are truly addicted. You may be intimidated by the "high achievers"—competitors and marathoners—but you have begun to understand the benefits of fitness and made a significant break with the old, non-fit world. The jogger's runs are satisfying in themselves. There is almost always a "glow" at the end of the run, a reward for the effort. If you miss a run you may feel guilty—a rare experience for the beginner. Beginners often complain that they're bored while running, but joggers find this problem decreases and then disappears as their distances increase.

Rarely does a jogger have a plan or goal. Most run as a healthy diversion and don't feel the need to get anything more out of it. They just get out there when they can and do what they can. Those who *do* feel they need a plan often think they don't know enough to prepare one. They may pick up a few tips from a more experienced running friend or ideas from a running magazine. Unfortunately this often ends in frustration or injury because such plans are not based upon the jogger's own individual abilities and goals, but upon someone else's.

At first you probably needed a group or at least another person for motivation and direction. As a jogger you are a bit more independent. You'll prefer company to running alone, but you'll pick and choose your group with care. Most beginners seek anonymity within a group, while joggers often enjoy identification with a group.

As a beginner you may have attended a few fun runs or an occasional race. Joggers, however, mark the local 10K's on their calendars. These are motivational stepping stones to keep the daily runs on track. There will often be one major race in the jogger's schedule, like the Bay to Breakers, Peachtree Road Race, or the Corporate Challenge. Although you're not running competitively or for time improvement, a sense of competition may begin to develop. By piecing together a growing series of successful and non-threatening running experiences, you begin the transition into a more fit lifestyle.

There are always conditions—injury, a long stretch of bad weather, a partner dropping out—that may stop your running and force you to start over again as a beginner. When the year's big race is over, you may lose the motivation to keep going. A jogger will sometimes give up running completely, but usually will start again after an extended layoff.

THE COMPETITOR
Stage Three—When Competition Is the Main Driving Force

There is a competitive streak, sometimes hidden, in all of us. Among those who continue to run for two years or more, about 30% feel some of these urges. If kept under control, the competitive push can be a great motivator, stimulating you to train well and to push yourself further than you might have otherwise. Unfortunately, many competitors give a higher priority to the times, the age group awards, and the bragging rights, losing sight of the many other benefits of running.

You become a competitor when you start to plan your running around racing goals. It all starts innocently enough. After a few races you begin to wonder how fast you might run if you really trained. Before you know it you're caught in a compulsive drive to run faster at the expense of running enjoyment.

Not all joggers enter this stage. Many simply remain joggers, while a very few pass directly to the stage of "runner." If you do find yourself becoming obsessed with competition, however, here are some things you might expect:

Initially the competitive spirit is exciting and rewarding. You're running faster because of increased training. You read everything you can on training, stretching, nutrition, etc., and become somewhat of an expert on each. There are always new training techniques to try out and you give them all a whirl. (Only later do you realize that many of them are contradictory.)

But as the competitive drive grows, you start feeling insecure. You no longer value your daily runs for their own worth, but think only of how well they prepare you for races and better times. Missing a run seems to spell racing doom. You can almost feel the fat being deposited on your body and see the seconds you fought hard to erase ticking back on the clock. When you hear of a workout a friend has performed before achieving a personal record, you have to match it or die trying.

Occasionally you'll run alone, but often you'll seek out small groups of better runners to train with and find you're making every workout a race; you'll push the pace to "victory" or make others earn theirs. In the same way, every race becomes a challenge to a new personal record. You may begin to choose races for the ease of terrain and lack of quality competition. At some point, you're training so hard during the week that there is no bounce in your muscles or willpower to go faster in the races. Your times slow and your motivation begins to ebb.

Once the competitive spirit has taken over, you tend to lose sight of your limitations, and mistake fatigue for loss of motivation. Deciding to "break through" this mental weakness, a warped logic emerges: If a small mileage increase brought about a small improvement, you'll try large mileage increases to gain a large improvement. Although you've read many times about the need for rest, you feel that yours is a special case—you don't need as much recovery time as other mortals. For weeks you may feel tired most of the time, yet have trouble sleeping at night. You become irritable and make life difficult for your family and friends. Finally you push too far and break down with injury, sickness or fatigue, and you either can't or don't want to run.

At this point you may feel betrayed by your body. Here you are trying to mold it into greatness and it won't respond. You fail to realize the improvements you've made during the past months or year and only visualize your fitness slipping away, your goals going down the drain. Thinking that your body is tricking you (or that an injury layoff is a sign of weakness) you get back into training too soon. Trying to run through the problems only makes them worse and leads to new injuries, and you miss the very races you've pushed yourself so hard for. Competitors take prolonged rest breaks—because injury forces them to do so.

Still, when the frustration has passed (and the pounds have settled back on) you'll probably start running again. Hopefully you'll have learned a lesson. You'll "recycle" and work your way up the ladder again. When you've put competition into perspective you'll pass into the stage of "athlete," or even "runner." Competitors who move directly to the enjoyment of the runner category often realize that time goals, trophies, and age group awards are rewards for the ego. It's OK to enjoy these, in their place. But don't let the ego ruin the satisfaction and positive attitude gained from a run at any pace—even a very slow one.

There are some very positive lessons to be learned from competition, and fortunately not all competitors have to go to such extremes to learn them. Pushing through tiredness and discomfort in a race to a new personal record is not only rewarding in itself, but gives you an idea of what you can do in other areas of your life. Strengths we have never used lie buried in each of us. Being challenged to our limits through competition helps these surface. Competition can be the pathfinding mission which allows us to map our inner resources. At the same time, experiencing some frustration and pain can help us realize our limitations. By struggling we discover a bit more about the person inside us, and we learn from our mistakes and move on to new heights.

THE ATHLETE
Stage Four—Being the Best You Can Be

As an athlete, you find more meaning in the drive to fulfill your potential than in compulsively collecting times and trophies. You've finally got a handle on competition, and it's not the only motivation. Being an athlete is a state of mind which is not bound by age, performance, or place in the running pack.

For a competitor, victory and defeat are tied to performance. Times, flat courses, ideal conditions are all important. For the athlete, victory lies in the *quality* of effort. When you run close to your potential on a given day, it's a victory. You internalize competition and transcend it, knowing your limits and capabilities. You understand what's important and what you must do to accomplish it. As you compete, you breathe in the race, vaporize it, absorb what you need, and exhale the rest. Running becomes your own work of art and you produce the best expression you can, on that day.

Competitors search for races they can win. Athletes look for competition which can bring out the best in them, win or lose. Not intent on a higher ranking or better performance (from a flat, fast course, etc.) in itself, they thrive on a challenging race that is run in the best way possible—from the inside out—and they are, not incidentally, rewarded in the long run by faster times at all levels of performance. Yes, athletes are scattered throughout the spectrum of runners, including the back of the pack. They often choose smaller races over the big media events because they don't want to feel lost in the sea of humanity.

Gradual progress is more important to the athlete than a fast time in a given race. You now have an internal concept of what you can do. When progress slows or is blocked, you revise. With every run, your internal training computer is fed with good data that processes several possibilities. You know when to disregard a bad run and not get depressed.

Though you once may have been a competitor who read everything and tried most of it, as an athlete you now read only what has practical value. When problems arise you look for literature on the subject by authors you trust. Your reading ties into an overall plan. You're no longer sampling everyone's tips and tricks like treats out of the cookie jar.

Planning is important. Although you're flexible, you plot goals and races 6–9 months in advance. The athlete is capable of continuous re-evaluation, and may change goals from week to week. Plans are not always written; some athletes are so in tune with their bodies they can work from a mental notebook. Whether your plan is written or "programmed" you know where you're going. You may not know the exact vehicle you'll take, but you know you will arrive.

Like other humans, athletes are not perfectly consistent. Sometimes you'll slip back and become a competitor. After a series of successes, you may become dissatisfied with performances that fall short of your goals. Rather than evaluating, analyzing and readjusting, you may dwell upon the bad day, the slump, or the poor showing, and feel a sense of failure.

Great athletes at any level realize that "success" is in the eye of the performer. There can be success in every experience.

If you can seize upon the positive aspect of each experience you can string together a series of internal victories that form a pattern of progress.

Some athletes reach a level of achievement or satisfaction and retire from competition; a few even quit running entirely. Most choose a reduced level of racing activity, others maintain a fairly high yet sensible level. Many continue to grow and move into the final and most rewarding stage, the runner.

THE RUNNER
Stage Five — The Best of All Stages

The final stage of the running journey blends the best elements of all the previous stages. The runner balances the elements of fitness, competition, training and social life and blends running with the rest of his or her life. There may be times when the runner reverts to earlier stages — mature people in any field have this problem — but these are only passing bouts that are assimilated into the overall harmony. The runner is a happy person.

As a runner, the primary focus of your life is not running. It may be family, friends, work, and is often a blend of many things. Running is now a natural part of your daily program — as is eating, sleeping, or talking. You know you'll get in that daily run although you may not know when. When you do miss a run you aren't in agony. In fact, you don't miss many days over the span of a year, because you just feel better during and after every run.

If scientists announced tomorrow that running was harmful, you'd read the news with interest and go out on your daily run.

You know about the positive effects of exercise, but that alone doesn't get you out on the roads. You get so much satisfaction from the experience itself that running has become a necessary and stable part of your active lifestyle.

As a runner, you'll enjoy the companionship of running with others, but most of your running will be done alone. You appreciate the peace and inner reflection provided by the solitary run more than you did in the earlier stages.

Great satisfaction comes from being able to mold your body into what it is capable of doing. You enjoy the art of combining just the right amounts of strength, endurance, form, and performance training. A race can be the icing on the cake, the opportunity to pull out deep hidden strengths. Once you're in this frame of mind, the joy lies not in the race, but in the running.

Even though you may plan for occasional competition with the same care as a competitor, there is none of that fixated intensity. The race isn't sacred. If stresses or problems arise there are always other races.

Occasionally the runner is injured. This is usually due to reverting to one of the earlier stages in a workout or race. Now— through experience—you'll know the difference between a common ache and a problem and you'll back off at the first sign of the latter. You'll sacrifice workouts, races and time goals to heal an injury early and get back to 100% as soon as possible.

As a runner you experience the enjoyment of each stage and retain the best of each of them. You can relive the beginner's excitement in discovery, appreciate the jogger's balance of fitness and enthusiasm, share the competitor's ambition, and internalize the athlete's quest. Having consolidated and balanced all these stages, you enjoy the creative and positive aspects of each and let them enrich your running life.

3 GETTING STARTED

WE'VE ALL HEARD HORROR STORIES about the pain and agony of the first week of running. In fact, this is probably why so many people give it up soon after they start or say they're bored, or go on about how they hate running. They never get past that painful stage. It doesn't have to be that way.

Whether you're taking your first steps, are starting again for the twentieth time or are helping others who are beginners, this chapter will help you. Newton's Law applies: a body at rest tends to stay at rest.

Starting any new activity takes courage and strength. To cross from the known to the unknown requires a leap of faith. Newton's Law can be adapted to read: a body on the couch wants to stay on the couch. But once you get that body in motion, watch out! Due to the great attitude boost from a run, those who gradually introduce the body to running become runners. Whether you are a mentor for others or yourself, your greatest challenges will be motivation on the down days, and holding back on the exuberant ones.

If you start slowly, gradually increase the exertion through a series of small steps, and rest adequately throughout, you can improve your condition steadily with almost no risk of soreness or injury.

Set Aside 30 Minutes. The threshold to fitness is three 30-minute periods of endurance running (and walking) each week. Make an appointment with yourself. This is the time for *you*, a sacred half-hour. To take this time away from the rest of the world may seem difficult at first, but you can do it if you really want to. Once you habitually set this time aside, you're almost certain to gain fitness and lose weight. Effort, in a sense, is not as important as scheduling. If you get out there regularly, the results are practically guaranteed.

A Benign Addiction. By regularly exercising 30–40 minutes several times a week for about six months, runners (or walkers) seem to develop an addiction to the relaxed feeling that comes during and especially at the end of the run. It is suspected that this is caused by the beta endorphin hormones which lock into your mid-brain area and produce a subtle tranquilizing effect. The body and mind begin to anticipate this after-exercise effect and miss it when you don't exercise. The withdrawal symptoms vary: crankiness, tiredness, irritability, depression, etc. This natural reward will sustain you if you can just stick with your program for 3–6 months. It may not even take that long, but if it does, even a half-year isn't a big investment for improved health and fitness the rest of your life.

Don't Worry About Pulse Rate. Over the past 30 years the research on heart disease and long-term health continues to show that the prime indicator for lifestyle disease reduction and life extension is the number of calories burned per week. Whether you go fast or slow, whether you walk or run, you benefit more, health-wise, by covering more miles per week. So it's actually better to cover more ground by slowing down, and walking more, than by speeding up, tiring early, and having to stop.

What Benefit Does Running Give, Above Walking? Because running burns twice as many calories per mile as walking (100 calories/mile vs. 50 calories/mile) you can condense the time spent exercising by running. The greatest benefit, however, is in the increased feeling of well-being and relaxation which running bestows. Many studies have shown that runners have higher levels of the positive attitude traits, and very few negative attitude traits. Running changes us in a positive way.

The Merger of Walking and Running. It's better for all of us, even veterans, to include walk breaks in our runs. The reasons are explained fully in the Walk Break chapter. *(See p. 81.)* Beginners should understand clearly that there is no benefit from running continuously. By inserting walk breaks, as you need them, you can avoid excess fatigue, reduce or eliminate injury, and allow your body to adjust to the running motion gently.

FIVE STEPS TO GETTING STARTED

Start by Walking. Everyone needs to feel comfortable and successful right from the start. Begin by walking for 30 minutes. Keep doing this until it feels easy.

Walk Briskly. When normal walking becomes easy, walk briskly for 30 minutes. Many people will never want or need to go beyond a brisk walk, provided they can gain the feeling that they want from their exercise, but most walkers reach a point at which the walking doesn't provide the exhilaration they want and start to insert some segments of jogging.

Insert a Few "Jogs." When you are comfortable walking briskly and want to step up the pace, jog for 30–60 seconds after walking for 5 minutes. Complete your 30 minutes doing these insertions. After doing this for 2–3 weeks, if there are no problems, reduce the walking to 4 minutes for 2–3 weeks. Then you may move to 3–1 for 2–4 weeks, followed by 2–1, and then 1–1. If you need more than 3 weeks before reducing the walking, take it.

Increase the Running as Desired. Increase the running segments as you feel stronger, always avoiding discomfort. You may eventually fill in the 30 minutes with slow running—or you may keep your walking breaks. Most runners find, even after years of running, that their walk break frequency will vary from day to day. Some days, I will walk for 30–60 seconds every mile or two, and other days I won't need to walk more than every 9 minutes or so. When in doubt, walk more frequently—especially at the beginning of the run.

Step It Up. If you wish, increase the time to 40 minutes three times a week. Work up to 60 minutes for at least one of these weekly sessions to increase the cardiovascular, psychological, and fat-burning benefits.

Don't underestimate the effect of rewards. Small regular rewards for specific accomplishments will often spark interest when motivation is down. Promise yourself something—a dinner out, a new pair of shoes, a good book—for finishing each of the five steps above, for when you finally put in your first hour-long session, etc. If you feel "down," find yourself a positive experience, or see someone who will bring you up. Look for something good in every run.

When you're in shape, you begin to think differently about yourself and your life. It's always hard to shake off the sedentary lifestyle, and the adjustment period—once you do—is difficult. But if you make it through this period, an addiction often occurs which makes the activity self-sustaining. So *have faith!* Better times are coming. Be patient and enjoy yourself.

HELPING SOMEONE ELSE GET STARTED

Don't preach. If you've made a recent and powerful change in your health and lifestyle it's all too easy to get up on the soap box—the born-again runner. When you do it's going to turn others off, even cause a "backlash" against running. Motivation must come from within. Your friends and people you meet will know when their time has come. Trying to turn a non-physical friend on to running is like preaching to a stone.

Some "Do's" and "Don'ts" of Helping Someone Get Started

Do:

• Wait until the person asks for help or advice.

• Watch a fun run or race together; this is the best way to get a beginner excited.

• Show personal interest and listen well to your friend. Then offer advice based on his or her goals—not yours.

• Recommend some good reading material like—ahem!—this book.

Don't:

• Don't promise running will improve everything from sex to failing hair (at least not falling hair).

• Don't drag your prospect out on the roads like an animal with prey.

• Don't threaten instant cardiovascular doom if your friend doesn't start training tomorrow.

• Don't talk for more than four hours straight on the wonderful changes you've made through running.

The greatest problem for a beginner is "How do I get started and stick with it?" The answer must come from within, but you, as the advisor or coach, can help stage a series of successes to ensure continued progress.

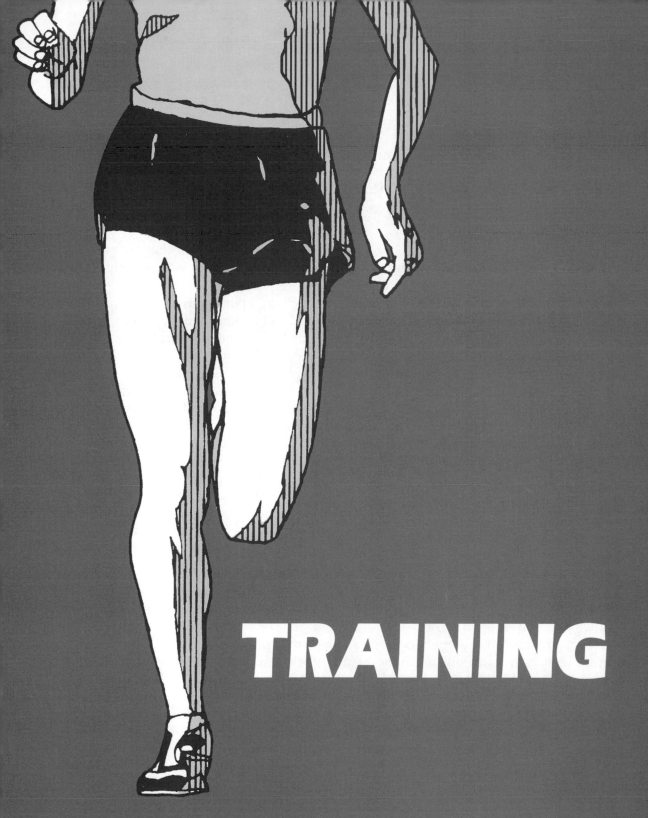

TRAINING

4
PHYSIOLOGY
WHAT HAPPENS INSIDE WHEN YOU RUN

THE BEST WAY to understand the training process is to look at the vital processes of the body—at least those that relate directly to running. If you understand some of your body's inner workings and are sensitive to its needs and states of tiredness, it can perform magnificently for you. Without such sensitivity you can too easily push yourself into pain or injury. It's often a series of small errors in training that leads to substantial injuries. With a little fine tuning, however, most of us can make our training safer and more productive.

Unity of Body and Mind. First, let's try to shed two or three thousand years of Western thinking—the idea that mind and body are separate entities, even adversaries. Westerners tend to think of the body as a slave, a chariot that can be driven and pushed at will. We often let our minds drive us toward goals, pushing to exhaustion or injury. Then we limp around in the aftermath, trying to re-establish communication.

In contrast, Eastern philosophy stresses unity of mind and body. Instead of a dichotomy, body and mind are a team communicating and working toward the same goal. Dr. E.C. Frederick, physiologist and author of *The Running Body*, illustrates the different approaches with a story about

the first two people to climb Mt. Everest, Sir Edmund Hillary and his Sherpa guide, Tensing Norgay.

When reporters asked how they made the difficult climb, Hillary replied that they had "... conquered the mountain"—it was an obstacle they had attacked and overcome. The Sherpa, who had lived on and in the shadow of the mountain all his life, said that he and the mountain had worked together to attain the peak.

Mountains can be climbed, miles run and goals attained when the mind and body work together. When the mind coaxes adaptations out of the body, steady progress can result. But the "macho" mind that forces its intentions upon a slave-like body will only reduce it to an injured slave.

The Most Important Training Principle. Most of us know that if we want to improve, we must stress ourselves in some of our training sessions. Exercise stresses the muscles, stimulating them to grow stronger and work more efficiently. Without enough rest after the stress, however, the muscles are driven to exhaustion or injury. Stress must be balanced by rest in sufficient quantity and quality for adequate growth.

Hard or long runs must always be followed by several easy days in which the pace or distance is reduced. In addition, you must build rest *weeks* into your program: every second or third week, you should automatically reduce total mileage. This gives your muscles the extra time to "catch up."

Improvement is based upon the quality of your speedwork and the length of your long run. By taking a day off and then running easily between these two "quality days" you will recover, rebuild stronger and reduce the chance of injury. Common mistakes that lead to injury are:

- Trying to attain a high mileage level week after week
- Running daily runs too fast
- Not enough rest

What Goes On Inside the Muscle. When most people think of a cell, they generally picture a round basic cell, surrounded by a membrane, with a nucleus at the center—like a bacteria or amoeba seen through a high school microscope. But there are hundreds of millions of cells in the human body, with a variety of functions and a diversity of shapes. The ones we are concerned with here—the skeletal muscle cells—are quite different from skin cells or those round, single-celled organisms studied for their simplicity.

A muscle cell is a fiber, composed of smaller and smaller units of fibers, and can run the entire length of the muscle. *(See drawing on next page.)* Picture a length of electrical conduit with bundles of wires inside—the muscle cell is like this. There is an external membrane, the *sarcolemma*, inside of which there are bundles *(myofibrils)*

of fibers. Also inside the muscle cell are the mitochondria, the "power plants" of the cell, which break down fuel (from food) into usable energy.

What Happens When the Muscle Is Overstressed. Muscles are generally capable of performing the amount of work they have been accustomed to during the previous 7–14 days. Your recent training has developed them to a certain fitness level. If you push beyond this level, you strain the horses that do the actual work—the individual muscle cells.

Cells pushed beyond their capacity are damaged with tears in the membranes. The mitochondria within the cells become swollen and glycogen, the fuel stored within the mitochondria, is often almost depleted.

Following is a brief description of some of the physiological aspects of two important rest principles. Then in Chapter 7, *Daily and Weekly Mileage Programs*, we'll look at the practical aspects of these short-term and long-term considerations.

The Easy Day (Short-Term). Research has shown it takes 48 hours to repair this stress-related damage. *With rest*, each overstressed cell is programmed to rebuild stronger when it is broken down, so it can handle a greater load next time. Cell walls become stronger as the membrane rebuilds a bit thicker. The mitochondria increase in size and number so they can process more energy. Vessels and arteries repair and strengthen, and over several months more capillaries are produced to better deliver nutrients and withdraw wastes. *(See Changes Inside the Muscle Cells, p. 55.)*

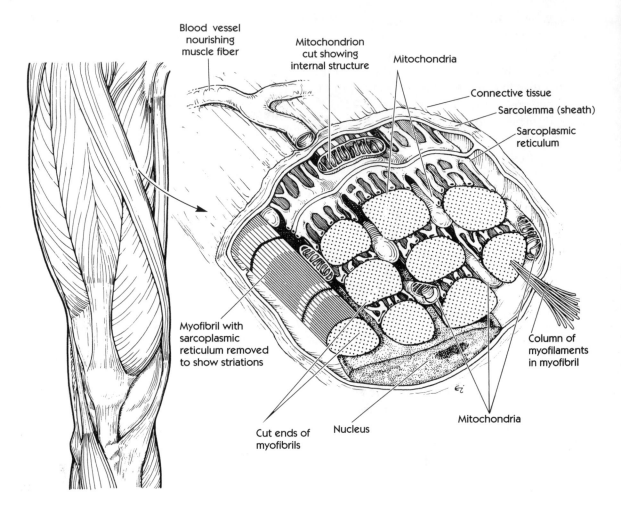

Cross-section of Single Muscle Cell

Magnified view of short segment of a single muscle fiber taken from the sartorious muscle of the leg. The sheath from the fiber has been cut away to show the internal structure. The mitochondria, the "power plants" of the cell, are shown in both intact and cut-away form.

You can see why it is important to give yourself 48 hours' rest in between stressful runs. Most runners recover much faster when they take a day off from running. Non-pounding cross training, however, encourages faster recovery than sedentary behavior. During a water-running workout, or a good walk, the blood vessels in the area dilate and allow more blood to flow into the stressed area—this is called *reactive hyperemia*. So cross training promotes better flow into the "beaten up" muscles, of restorative blood with oxygen, recovery nutrients, and more fuel. You can't push your training ahead and avoid the 48-hour rule without paying dearly. Maybe it won't happen right away, but eventually injury will result.

The Easy Week (Long-Term). The second important rest concept is that it takes about 21 days for muscles to adapt to the stress when you move into a new and more challenging training program. After about 11 days you'll feel stronger when the muscles have adapted to about half the stress. There is a strong temptation then to think you're ready to increase the stress again, but the body is not quite ready. After three weeks, the body has theoretically adapted and is ready for a new stress load.

I have found, however, that by *reducing* stress on the second or third week—cutting mileage by 30–50%, say—the body comes around quicker and is ready for new challenges. This allows for more of the ruptured fibers to be rebuilt and for the muscles to be rested and restocked for the next challenge. Again, as with the 48-hour rule, you may break this rule and get away with it for a while but you'll pay

later in tiredness and injury. You can push yourself too far for some time, but your body will ultimately protect itself by breaking down.

A more detailed explanation of the *Easy Day* and the *Easy Week* concepts follows on pp. 55–57, along with guidelines for putting these principles to work in your daily and weekly mileage programs and examples of the concepts in practice.

Aerobic/Anaerobic Exercise

Aerobic means "in the presence of oxygen." You are running aerobically when you run slowly and comfortably and do not exceed the pace or distance for which you have recently trained. Here your muscles are strong enough to carry the load and there is enough oxygen available from the blood stream. The few waste products that are produced are easily whisked away in the blood before building up and obstructing muscle function.

Anaerobic running is when you exceed the speed and/or distance for which you have trained. The muscles are pushed beyond their capacity and need more oxygen than the body can supply. For a limited period of time, muscles continue to function by utilizing chemical processes that free oxygen from within the muscle itself. The amount of oxygen available this way is quite limited, large amounts of waste build-up, and the muscles get tight and sore. You find yourself huffing and puffing, and slowing down. After the exercise is over, this oxygen must be "paid back" to the muscle (the "oxygen debt").

One of the main purposes of speedwork is to give you anaerobic experience in measured doses; if you follow it with sufficient rest, you'll train your body to deal with oxygen debt. *Anaerobic running is not necessary for health, only for improving speed.*

The Food-Into-Energy Cycle. When you eat carbohydrates (bread, fruit, starches, sugars, etc.), they are broken down into simple sugars, some of which is then recombined into glycogen and stored in the muscles as fuel. Glucose, lactose (milk sugar), and fructose (fruit sugar) are mono-saccharides and are converted into glycogen in one step. Sucrose (white sugar) is a di-saccharide and requires an additional step, using extra energy and slowing down the process.

After being absorbed through the walls of the stomach, glucose is transported by the blood throughout the system. Muscle cells absorb this energy source and store it as glycogen for use during exercise. Extra supplies are stored in the liver. When all storage areas are filled, glucose is converted to fat and stored as such.

For the first 10 minutes of aerobic exercise, the exercising muscles will use the most convenient energy source, the glycogen in the muscle cell, almost exclusively. Glycogen combines with oxygen from your blood to produce energy and several waste products, including lactic acid. As long as you are not exercising anaerobically (out of breath, etc.), the percentage of lactic acid will be relatively low and the blood can whisk it away.

After about 10 minutes of exercise, your body will start a transition to fat as a fuel source. It takes this long for the stored fat to release free fatty acids into the blood in sufficient numbers to satisfy the demands of so many hungry muscle cells. After about 30 minutes, fat becomes the primary fuel source, with a small "primer" of glycogen. (Just because you're burning fat doesn't mean you should be eating a lot of fat. Carbohydrates are the best source of energy; too much dietary fat can hamper your performance.)

A Physiological Look at "The Wall." Fat is a more abundant fuel than glycogen. Whereas glycogen stores are limited (normally about 20 miles' worth), even a skinny person has enough fat for about 600 miles. The trade-off for this long-range fuel is that fat can only be burned aerobically (in the presence of oxygen). As long as you run within the pace and at the distance you've been training for—you will burn mostly fat. When you run faster than you've trained, or farther, you overwhelm the muscles. They are forced beyond their capacity and cannot get enough oxygen. In this anaerobic situation, glycogen is burned, and large amounts of lactic acid and waste products pour into the muscles faster than they can be removed. This is what causes your muscles to get tight and *burn* and this is what causes you to slow down and hit "the wall." Once the muscles have shifted to glycogen, it's unlikely that they can shift back to fat. You'll be depleting your limited supply of glycogen very quickly.

One important objective of training is to teach the body to conserve glycogen and deal with lactic acid buildup. Your base period training *(see pp. 40–41)* will improve the blood's capacity to deliver oxygen and withdraw wastes. Speedwork and long runs gradually push back the point at which you start becoming anaerobic; they also teach you to deal with the discomfort and burden of lactic acid buildup without slowing down as much as before. When you have fine-tuned the muscles through speedwork, you will accumulate approximately the same amount of waste, but won't have to slow down as much because now you're used to the feeling.

The most effective way to conserve glycogen, and avoid hitting the wall, is to put walk breaks into your runs from the beginning, and to slow down the pace of your running. Think of this as an extended "warm up" in which you're fooling your "tiredness sensors." These conservative methods, which will be discussed later *(see p. 81)* reduce the fatigue, wear and tear so

much that you can get as far as 12 miles in a marathon with muscles that feel like you've just started.

By pushing too far beyond your current capabilities you can cause your body some serious damage. When you have run too far or too fast and have shifted to glycogen as a fuel source, you're on unstable ground in a long race. Glycogen is the only fuel used by the brain and the supply of this energy source is greatly limited. At critically low levels of glycogen, your body's survival defenses take over and reserve what's left for the brain. When the brain senses a low supply, it protects itself by making it difficult for you to concentrate on finishing the long event—or even telling you to quit. These are warning signs that should put you on alert.

WHAT YOU BURN WHEN YOU RUN

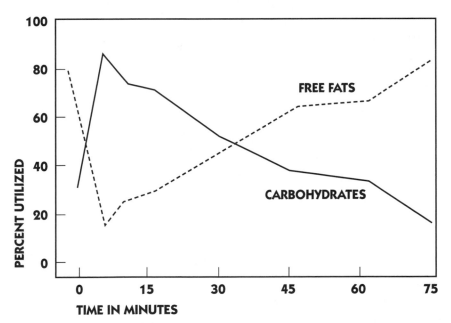

Estimate of energy derived from carbohydrates and fats in 75 minutes of running. Note that at 30 minutes you start burning more fats than carbohydrates. Adapted from A Scientific Approach to Distance Running *by David L. Costill.*

What's a working muscle to do? There's not enough oxygen to burn fat, and the glycogen supply has been stolen. Glycogen can be processed from fat, and from muscle protein. This is a very uncomfortable process and leaves a lot of waste—but it is done. When nearby fat stores are used up and the exercising muscle absolutely demands glycogen, exercising muscle tissue itself may be broken down. All of this can be avoided by conserving your resources from the beginning of a run.

Remember to take care of your body. An injured body cannot perform. Damaged, overstressed muscles cause you to miss training and retard progress. Stay within the bounds of the training you have done in the recent past and push only slightly beyond this once a week to improve speed and endurance.

Blood Chemistry. Our bodies were not intended to digest large amounts of fat. The marvelous instruments we've inherited from our ancient ancestors were designed for processing foods high in complex carbohydrates (grains, vegetables, fruits). Although small amounts of fat can be easily taken care of, the modern diet—rich in fried foods and red meat—overwhelms the body's fat-processing capacities. The walls of our circulatory and organ systems become coated with the excess of these fats, particularly if the arteries or heart passages are naturally narrow through heredity. This can lead to a variety of serious circulation problems, especially in the vessels that supply blood to the heart. Fats have also been linked to other serious diseases, such as cancer of the colon.

The Heart . . . and Its Supporting Cast. The heart is an endurance muscle, a pump that squeezes blood into the body every minute of every day. Like any muscle, it needs regular exercise or it will deteriorate. Working at a desk job, without any supplemental physical exercise, is not enough exertion to maintain the heart in healthy condition. Over time, deposits may build up in lazy heart arteries. The small and crucial passageways in this vital organ must be kept clean and functioning. Regular endurance exercise will accomplish this.

Exercising muscles are in a real sense small pumps that pull blood in from the heart and then push it back. The heart is forced to increase its pumping speed to send needed blood to the exercising muscle. The sustained increase in heart rate will keep this important muscle fit and lean.

Endurance exercise also increases the number of capillaries and promotes a better flow of nutrients to the cells and a better withdrawal of wastes. When you exercise regularly, your body increases its production of blood and your blood volume increases, so more blood is available to the exercising cells. The sustained pressure during several months of long runs forces little tongues of capillaries into the muscle cells. The result is a greater flow of oxygen to a greater number of cells all over the body, helping them work to capacity. The heart muscle becomes stronger, is given an extra infusion of oxygen, and is regularly cleaned.

As the heart gets stronger, it sends a greater flow of blood throughout the body with each stroke. With fewer squeezes, the "fit" heart will accomplish more work, and your resting pulse rate will go down. Well

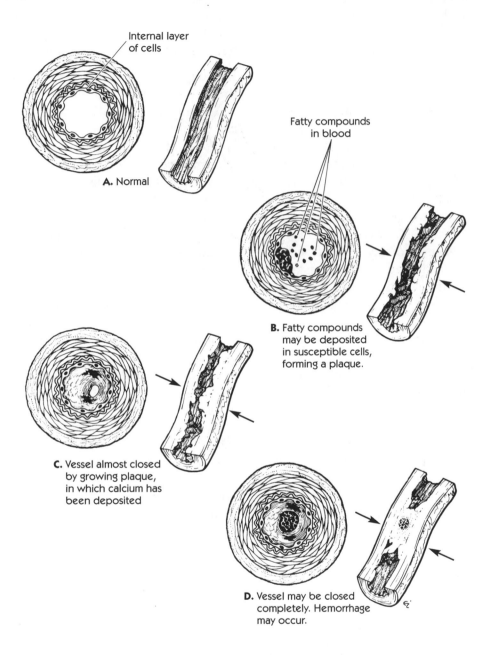

Internal layer
of cells

A. Normal

Fatty compounds
in blood

B. Fatty compounds
may be deposited
in susceptible cells,
forming a plaque.

C. Vessel almost closed
by growing plaque,
in which calcium has
been deposited

D. Vessel may be closed
completely. Hemorrhage
may occur.

Inside look at heart disease. *Shown here are a normal artery and three stages of progressive closure from an excess of fats in the diet.*

conditioned leg muscle cells help the heart significantly by "pushing" the "used" blood back to the heart.

See pp. 46–49 for an explanation of monitoring your heart rate as a guide to workout performance.

Fast-Twitch/Slow-Twitch/Intermediate-Twitch. Some people are born to run faster, and others farther. If you could look inside your muscle cells you could tell whether you were designed to run sprints or distance events. If you have a high percentage of fast-twitch muscle fibers, you have a tendency to run fast. These sugar-burning muscle cells fire quickly and powerfully, burn fuel quickly and are not resistant to fatigue. In contrast, slow-twitch fibers burn fat, can be trained to fire repeatedly for a long time, and resist fatigue.

Sports scientists can determine an individual's percentage of fast- or slow-twitch muscle fiber by injecting a needle into the muscle and withdrawing a small sample to examine under a microscope. It is a relatively simple procedure, but a bit painful and usually done only for research studies. Runners with a predominance of slow-twitch muscles (I have 97%) must abandon hope for success in the 100-meter race. Speedy runners, however, can train their fast-twitch muscles to become fat burners and act as slow-twitch fibers.

In recent years, scientists have discovered a third type of muscle fiber: intermediate-twitch. They have a mixture of the characteristics of fast-twitch and slow-twitch.

The Lungs. When you breathe, air enters through your mouth and/or nose and then travels through the back of your throat (the *pharynx*) and your windpipe (the *trachea*). At its lower end the trachea branches out to form the *bronchi*, one of which enters each lung. These then subdivide and eventually lead to several hundred million air sacs—the *alveoli*—that accomplish the exchange of gases: oxygen in, carbon dioxide out.

Exercise puts the lungs under greater pressure to perform. More alveoli are involved in the process of gaseous exchange and their ability to perform this task rapidly and efficiently is improved. Continued smoking and prolonged exposure to air pollution can significantly reduce the ability of the alveoli to accomplish this exchange and diminish the capacity of whole sections of the lungs to function. Fortunately exercise, running in particular, can help reverse this process and over time enable the tissue to regain its functional ability (unless the smoking and air pollution have destroyed the walls of the alveoli themselves, as in emphysema).

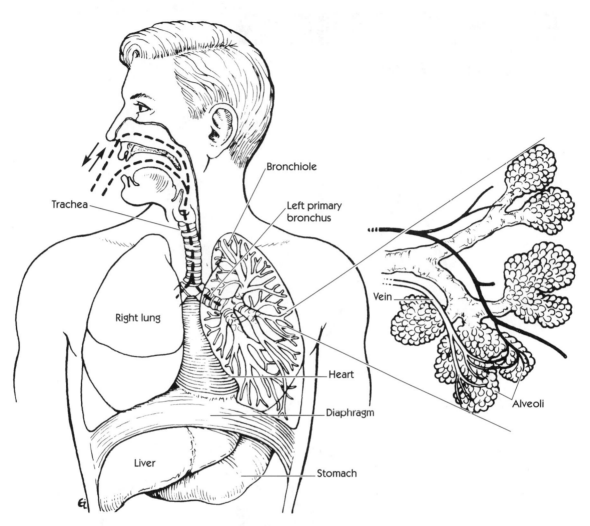

Air is exchanged through the nose and/or mouth. Air enters the lungs via the trachea, which branches to form the bronchi, which in turn branch, tree-like, to form smaller subdivisions, the bronchioles. Here a terminal bronchiole is enlarged to illustrate the air sacs (alveoli), in which exchange of gases takes place between air and blood.

5 PLANNING

WHERE TO START

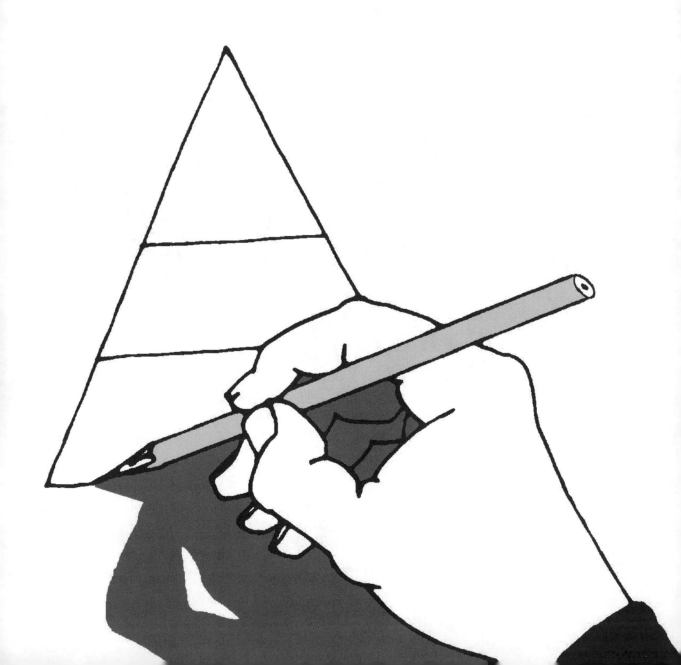

SOME YEARS BACK, I got a call from Marlene Cimons, a runner and a staff writer for the *Los Angeles Times*. I'd met Marlene earlier at the Boston Marathon and she'd been interested in my new approach to training. "Do you think I could improve my marathon time of 3:53?" she asked.

I asked a few questions about her background and then said I could practically guarantee better performance if she followed some different training principles. Marlene was eager to give it a try, so I set up a running program for her. We agreed we'd talk on the phone every few weeks so I could monitor how things were going and recommend any necessary adjustments.

As she got into her new routine, she decided it might make a good story for her paper. Would this new approach—planning her training in advance and emphasizing long, slow runs—lead to better performance? She sent away for an application to the Nike-Oregon Track Club Marathon in Eugene, Oregon, that fall and I agreed to run with her in the race, to keep her on pace and provide psychological support.

Marlene followed the major points of the training program, but one thing she had trouble with, and that we argued over, was the long run. She got up to 20 miles and didn't want to run farther. (The program recommends that you work your way up to running at least the race distance before the race, so your body is prepared for the strain.) She had a mental block, based on painful experiences "crashing" each time she'd gone 20 miles, either in practice or racing. She was afraid she'd hurt herself before the race.

I explained Arthur Lydiard's theory of long, relaxed running. I told her to go slow, to stop and walk when tired, but to be sure to go *farther* than the race *before* the race. This way she shouldn't hit "the wall" she so dreaded. I also pointed out how this principle of easy long runs had not only been used by Lydiard's Olympic champions, but now by neighborhood runners throughout the country to run (and finish) marathons.

I finally convinced Marlene to continue her long runs and to build up to 26 miles. We met in Eugene that September and Marlene ran 3:44:49, improving her previous best time by 8½ minutes—even on a very warm and humid day. She not only didn't "die" at the end, but managed a final sprint the last 200 yards. She was inspired and elated, and wrote an article on her experience.

Running Slow in Order to Run Fast. Marlene's experience is typical for runners at all levels. Steady, relaxed running over several months is not only enjoyable, but cuts down on injuries and is the best base for competitive running. Not only can you run slow in order to run fast, but by carefully organizing slow running into a planned schedule, you can probably run faster than ever before.

Lydiard's Strategy Applied to Everyday Runners. Over the past 25 years I've worked with runners at clinics, in running camps, in our running stores and my training clubs and groups, and have developed a series of innovations and planning techniques that started with the concepts used by Lydiard, Bowerman, and Cooper.

I've come to visualize this program as a pyramid with a strong foundation of easy running, a transition zone of hill training, and finally a speed program that brings a runner to his or her peak for a race.

What's interesting is that these same principles used by world-class runners apply to runners of all levels. With these basic training concepts, not only do elite runners achieve world records, but beginners will get fit and have fun, joggers will be able to run their first races, and experienced runners will improve their personal records.

Starting Your Program. Your training program has already started. Your past exercise activity will be the basis upon which you'll build your long-range program. Adults who were active as children have a head start. So don't be surprised if a fellow sedentary office worker takes up running and improves faster than you. Start with what you're presently doing, so long as it's not already too much; then build in the specific workouts, rest and other adjustments described below.

Most of the runners I have counseled have initially *decreased* their mileage by adding strategic rest. This has allowed them to increase the quality of work on the hard days—and has invariably led to better performance. But even if you've been sedentary for many years, don't be discouraged; you can probably do things you never believed were possible, if you'll have patience and gradually build toward your goals.

Define Your Goals. First think about your goals. Why do you want to run? To lose weight, feel good, regain muscle tone, stay

fit year-round? All of these plus enter some races? Or become a competitive runner and race frequently? Think about what you want out of your running. What do you want to achieve in the next six and 12 months? Asking these questions will help you organize a plan and make your pursuit more effective.

Don't Use Anyone's Program But Your Own. The best training program for you is the one that meets your particular needs. This applies to beginners as well as to world-class runners. Don't adopt the successful program of a friend. Although he is succeeding, he may be improving on inborn talent "in spite" of his program. All of us have strengths, weaknesses and limitations which need to be considered in customizing a program. It's fine to try new training ideas, but experiment with only one at a time. Then blend the successful ones into your program to fit your own demands, rest needs, and current level of performance.

THE TRAINING PYRAMID

The training pyramid is normally a 4–6 month cycle with each stage building to the next. As I mentioned before, it is used by elite runners to improve endurance and speed, but in the following pages I'll show how *you* can use the pyramid concept to achieve your goals, whatever they may be. At the peak of the pyramid is the race the runner is aiming for. You can use the principles to achieve your race goal, or as a general guide to a balanced running program. Whether you race or not, these concepts will improve your running, make it more enjoyable, and develop your overall cardiovascular capacity and fitness.

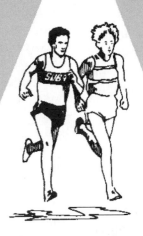

Speed: 35%

Continue long runs.
Cut total mileage 10%.
Replace hills with speedwork, once a week.
Gradually build number of reps.
Rest between long runs, speedwork, and races.
Do maximum eight weeks of speedwork
(except as noted on schedules).

Hill Training: 15%

Same as base period except for hill repeats
Once a week, run hills (3–7% grade), 50–200 yards.
Run uphill at 80–85% effort (about 5K race pace).
Walk downhill to recover.
Start with 4 hills; build up to 8–12.

Base Training: 50%

Daily runs, which are relaxed, easy, and comfortable
Long runs every other week
Pace: Run at comfortable speed; if in doubt, go slower.
Form work: 4–8 accelerations during daily run, twice a week
Races: At most, every other week and alternating with long run

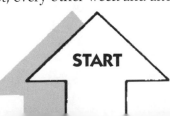

START

BASE TRAINING

Daily Runs. Your ultimate performance is governed by your base work—aerobic training. You can only improve a certain amount by speedwork. But it's the sustained period of long, steady running that is the foundation for running faster.

The base part of the pyramid consists of several months of steady aerobic running. Aerobic running develops a better circulatory system by strengthening the heart and increasing the amount of blood pumped through the circulatory system. This means nutrients and oxygen can get to the muscle cells more efficiently and wastes are more easily removed. Your muscles can do more work with less effort. You are building up your *vital transport system* in preparation for the speedwork phase which will ultimately help you run faster.

Long Runs. Long runs develop cardiovascular efficiency to its maximum. *They are the single most important element in your program.* The sustained pumping of the heart helps the heart, arteries and veins become more efficient in transporting the blood and allows the lungs to absorb oxygen more efficiently. When the muscles are pushed to their limits (as in a regularly scheduled, gradually increasingly long run) they will respond better and work longer because of this strengthening of the circulation system.

How long? If you're interested in running faster or racing—no matter how far down the line—here is what you do: Start with the distance of your longest run in the last three weeks and increase by one mile a week until you have reached 10 miles. At

that point, increase by two miles every two weeks. The intervening weeks will give your body a much-needed chance to recover and rebuild for the next long one. When you get up to 18 miles for a marathon or half-marathon, 15 for a 10K, or 10 miles for a 5K, go into a holding pattern. Don't go beyond these distances until your speed phase.

In the speed phase of your pyramid, you'll continue these long runs and for top performance, extend them to *beyond* the distance of the race you're aiming for. Ideally you should build up to a run of 10–12 miles for a 5K, 16–18 miles for the 10K, 17–19 miles for the half-marathon, and 28–30 for the marathon.

The other runs in your program will not change very much, if at all. *You will be increasing distance primarily through the long run, not through more miles each day.* You can run races during the base period, but don't need to. If you do, they should not be run at top speed, and should be run on weeks when there is no long run.

How fast? Long runs should be run very slowly—at least 2 minutes per mile slower than your goal pace for your target race. When in doubt, slow down and take more walk breaks, from the beginning. You can't run the long runs too slowly.

Note for Non-Competitive Runners. Long runs are used by competitive endurance runners of all levels. World-class racers have been using the principle for years now, and more and more weekend 10K or marathon runners are recognizing its value in improving overall speed and race performance. But the principle of the long run can be used by all runners, even those who run only 2–3 miles a day, three times a week. If you are not interested in racing or competing, just scale down the length of the long run as described above. The idea is to run longer one day every 2–3 weeks. If you run three miles a day during the week, start going four miles one day, then two weeks later, five miles. If five miles feels long enough, hold it at that, and have a five-mile run every two weeks. But if you want to, keep increasing a mile every two weeks—make that be a special day. It will give you more endurance, help burn more fat, get you in better condition —and make you feel better, even if you never intend to race.

Pace. On your slow runs during the week, go at least 1–1½ minutes per mile slower than your current goal pace. On long runs, run at least 2 minutes per mile slower than current goal pace. Even if you feel comfortable at a faster pace, slow down and learn to enjoy the slower running. This will help you recover faster so that you can do the other training later in the week. I run most of my daily runs and long runs 3 minutes per mile slower than I could run them and enjoy every one of them.

Form Work. Twice a week, on easy days, run 4–8 acceleration gliders *(see pp. 145–147)* during the run with complete recovery in between. For 100 yards, pick up the turnover of your feet and legs (RPMs) to a speed that is fast but not all-out, then coast for 20–50 yards. Keep the knees down, and don't bounce. You should feel like you're running close to your goal race pace, without straining the muscles or tendons in your legs. As you glide at the end, relax and gradually slow down. Keep it

under control. Think about your form then, but don't worry about it at other times while running.

Form is described in detail on pp. 138–149.

Races. Races can be run for practice, as stepping stones to the big race you are aiming for—but no more often than every other week. One per month is a better policy. Don't run them all-out, but use them as harder-than-normal runs (no faster than half the time difference between your mile pace for your race, and your relaxed training pace).

HILL TRAINING

Base period training gives you endurance and cardiovascular efficiency. Before jumping into speedwork, however, the body needs a period of transition to build strength. Hills prepare the muscles for faster running without going anaerobic.

After working with thousands of folks who've done hill training, I believe that this is the only strength and resistance training that helps distance runners, boosting their performance and strength on all types of terrain. Hills strengthen running muscles while they are running. This gives functional strength as opposed to the specific and limited strength of weight training.

Hills strengthen the main driving muscles—quadriceps, hamstrings and especially calf muscles. As the calf muscles get stronger, you can support your body weight farther forward on your feet and use the mechanical advantage of the ankle. This leads to more efficient running because the ankle is such an efficient mechanical lever.

As the base period develops the internal "plumbing," hill training develops *strength for running*. The legs get a taste of working hard without going into oxygen debt and without the hard impact or trauma of speedwork.

In the hill phase of the pyramid, the only real change from the base period is the hill workout one day a week. All other training remains the same. Most runners do hill work mid-week—on Tuesday or Wednesday.

Find a hill with an easy grade, about 3–7%. If it's too steep you can't develop a good, sustained drive and rhythm. Run at about 85% effort (slightly faster than 10K race pace) and walk down to recover. If you need more rest in between, take it. This is not supposed to be an anaerobic workout. Start with about 2–3 hills and increase by one a week until you can run 8–12 hills. Give yourself at least two days' rest between hill workouts and races or long runs.

Hill training usually lasts 4–6 weeks. Experienced, competitive runners can run two hill workouts a week, but be careful about this, because it's stressful and makes injury more likely.

Hill running form is described in detail on p. 129.

SPEED TRAINING

Your *base period* gives you endurance, and that, along with strengthening *hill training,* gets you ready for *speed.* As long as you continue the long runs, the speedwork will enable you to run faster for all distances. Each workout pushes the body farther than it went the week before. The working muscles thus gradually experience the

increased workload needed to accomplish your goal. The rest period that follows each speed session allows rebuilding for the next test. The final workouts in the speed phase will gradually build until they simulate race conditions.

In the early part of this century, speedwork consisted of running time trials and races. Athletes ran races without training in between. In between races the more ambitious ran time trials at their race distance. Training this way, they rarely increased their speed.

Interval training and *fartlek ("speed play," see pp. 71–72)* were introduced in Europe about 1920. These methods divided the race distance into several parts. Runners ran faster than race pace for a set distance, rested between segments and repeated the process numerous times. The number of repetitions increased each week until the endurance demands of the race were simulated. By breaking up the hard segments with rest periods, the overall stress of each workout was not as substantial as that required by a race. Whereas hard, sustained, effort tears the muscles down through gradual exhaustion, the rest intervals between speed accelerations keep the muscles from being overly fatigued.

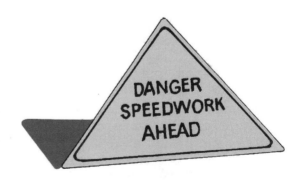

The 8-Week Rule: After about 8 weeks of speedwork, your performance will tend to peak. If you keep up intensive speedwork after this, you'll be risking injury, illness or fatigue. Note that in the half-marathon programs, the speed repetitions continue for a longer period of time.

Not for Beginners: Speedwork isn't for everyone. If you don't have a time goal, you don't need it. It puts a lot of stress on your body and increases the chances of injury. Speed training is a lot more damaging than long runs. On the positive side, however, it can train legs to go farther when tired, producing a faster time. Beginners should stay in the base period for the first one or two years. During this time, an occasional speed session would consist of merely accelerating faster than normal pace for portions of the run.

Speedwork is described in more detail on pp. 70–77.

AFTER THE PYRAMID

When you have finished the speed phase of a pyramid and have run your "big" race, it's time to recycle and begin the base part of a new pyramid. Going back to another base period is a relief after a hard period of speed and races. The wear and tear of your peaking period will be repaired, muscle fibers restored, and you'll have a greater cardiovascular capacity the next time around.

Like a sand pyramid on the beach, the wider the base, the higher the peak. Start with a solid base, get plenty of rest between hard workouts, and you'll improve your condition and performances. One pyramid can be the base for the next one, if you plan it that way. For example, a 5K or 10K pyramid in the spring will give you more leg speed which you'll need for use in your fall half-marathon pyramid (which gives you endurance for the next-spring 10K and etc . . .). A series of increasingly difficult workouts will lead you from one stage to the next and make possible the fulfillment of your goals.

> This has been an overall description of planning, goals, and the basic elements of this new approach to running. The chapters in the *Racing* section of the book *(starting on p. 89)* go into all the aspects of such a plan in greater detail.

6
YOUR RUNNING LOG

MUST YOU KEEP A LOG? Not necessarily. Some people apparently make great progress with little or no planning and lots of luck. You don't need a plan to run, or even to make progress with your running. Indeed, some of your greatest experiences will be the unplanned ones: the spontaneity of the daily run, a beautiful day in the woods, coming upon an unexpected wild animal, sunset, etc. But organization is what separates the runner from the jogger. Runners make more progress because they begin to schedule for their success, and schedule to avoid injuries, while joggers just get out there when they can.

Many runners will run for months, or years, without keeping a log. It seems like too much trouble, too fussy, or unnecessary. Yet eventually, perhaps through an injury, perhaps through the examples of friends, they'll start keeping a log, and then wonder how they ever ran without it.

The log is a motivator and an enforcer. The simple act of writing down your mileage is motivational. After several weeks you'll find yourself looking back through it to find reasons for "bad" days. You may *say* that you're only increasing mileage by 10% more per week, but your log will keep you honest. Only with the details written down can you go back and see what led you up to the present. Eventually you'll develop your own important items which, when totaled, will give you confidence or concern.

Finally, your log can be your daily and weekly "running planner." After scheduling your key races or challenges, you can fill in the long runs, group runs, speed sessions, or fun days that will keep you headed to your goal with fun built-in.

Plan for Your Goal. You need a plan to make maximum progress toward a goal. Since a common goal is to run "injury-free," you must plot your activity to keep from overdoing it. Time goals especially require a plan. A plan is a tool, a guide for inspiration. A beginner can lay out an easier path, avoid injury, and become addicted to running. A veteran can plan for variety, challenge, and improvement.

An effective plan will stage a series of small successes starting from your present training program. Each step feeds on the confidence developed from the last. Every plan must have the right combination of stress and rest for *you*.

A plan must also be flexible. Things change daily. At every step you should re-evaluate progress and adjust the log to reflect your current condition, ability, and other factors in your life. Successful plans are often changed en route to the goal.

A log helps speed up improvement and provides a sense of continuity over the long haul. Since a log is not only your plan for the future, but a record of your past improvement, it helps you pick things up when the doldrums set in. And a log may tell you the probable cause(s) of an injury so you can avoid the same mistakes next time.

There are many ways to log your runs. Some use a wall calendar, or an inexpensive school notebook. The logs that are designed for running make it easier to record data by asking you to fill in the blanks. There are several software and web log products, such as *PC Coach*, that allow you to sort through months or years to look for trends, causes of injuries, or reasons for success (admittedly more difficult to define).

Components of Your Log

- *Long runs.* Relaxed challenges. You may not be able to run faster each year, but you can run farther. This gives you a continuing feeling of progress and accomplishment. You get to know yourself well on the long ones.

- *Hard runs* help you improve your speed. Competitors will schedule a hard run about once a week during their speed phase. Most runners should schedule some transition work, usually hills, before jumping into speedwork.

- *Social runs* give you a chance to chat as you run, or take a quiet run with a good friend. Long and hard days should be balanced with easy ones; social runs can provide the leisurely "Sunday Bar-B-Q" atmosphere.

- *Form work.* Accelerations performed twice a week, year round, teach you to improve your running.

- *Scenic runs* are trips to beautiful running areas near home. If you cover the same course every day, scenic runs can get you out of the rut to enjoy some different terrain and scenery.

- *Races* are not just competitive experiences, they are ways to evaluate your running progress. Anticipating a race gives far more meaning to your daily runs and keeps you motivated. It's inspiring to see hundreds of people working toward a common goal and helping one another along the way.

- *Trips* provide variety and excitement. You can run in different parts of the country on business trips or vacations, or schedule specific running excursions to scenic areas. Running in unfamiliar areas often introduces you to instant friends. You may have more in common with runners you meet in another town than you do with your non-running next-door neighbors.

- *Rewards.* Positive reinforcement helps keep you on track. Too often runners progress gradually and don't realize the extent of the improvement. Rewards are as varied as the individuals who appreciate them: dinner out, clothes, shoes, etc. Small things for small improvements in your training program; bigger rewards for more significant time or distance goals.

- *Easy runs.* The other runs (and all of the above except for speedwork, races and form work) are run at an easy, comfortable pace.

- Be careful with Achilles tendon.
- Build long one to 18! (must slow down in beginning)
- Slow down in the beginning of each run!

sc= standard course	**in**= injury **sp**=speed **l**=long run **sn**= scenic **tr**=transcendental
gr= group run	**adj**= adjustments **fn**= fun **fb**= fat burning **nu**= nutrition
mn= mental training	**ag**= afterglow **so**=social

Monday

GOAL 35 min easy w/ 4-8 form accels
TIME 31 min
DISTANCE @ 3 mi
AM PULSE 52
WEATHER rainy-cold
TEMP 27°
TIME 5 (AM/**PM**)
TERRAIN rolling
WALK BREAK none

Jan 1
DATE

COMMENTS
1
2
③
4
5
6
7
8
9
10

Cloudy day — dreary. Had to force myself out!

* left Achilles felt tender — should have iced it but didn't.

This is the year to enjoy running!

Tuesday

GOAL 45 min easy (sn)
TIME 52 min
DISTANCE doesn't matter
AM PULSE 51
WEATHER sunny-dry
TEMP 48
TIME 6 (AM/**PM**)
TERRAIN mixed
WALK BREAK —

Jan 2
DATE

COMMENTS
1
2
3
4
5
6
7
8
⑨
10

very (↑)   Sunrise!
one of those rare days when the body didn't want to ... but the spirit craved for transcendental exertion. New trail — along river
    Very slow + very peaceful
(went slow in beginning — it worked!)

Wednesday

GOAL off — XT run in H₂0
TIME 33 min
DISTANCE —
AM PULSE 52
WEATHER —
TEMP —
TIME 6 (AM/**PM**)
TERRAIN
WALK BREAK

Jan 3
DATE

COMMENTS
1
2
3
4
5
6
7
8
9
10

(5 sets of 10) arm running weights

H₂0

3 sets of 2 minutes } new
then 15 min easy } flotation belt

walk for 15 min with Barb

Jeff's entries on a page out of Jeff Galloway's Training Journal *(above and right).*

Week of | Jan 1

Thursday — Jan 4

GOAL	35 min easy (SC)
TIME	45 min
DISTANCE	@ 6.5
AM PULSE	49
WEATHER	Cloudy
TEMP	40°
TIME	6 (PM)
TERRAIN	rolling
DATE	WALK BREAK —

COMMENTS

Great run with Barb, Wes + Sambo — who took out the pace too fast + died at the end. The rest of us caught up on the gossip. Achilles ached so I iced it for 15 minutes.

Friday — Jan 5

GOAL	45 min (sp) 5 × 800 meter
TIME	1:15
DISTANCE	7.5 mi
AM PULSE	53
WEATHER	45°
TEMP	sunny
TIME	5 (AM/PM)
TERRAIN	track
DATE	WALK BREAK 400m

COMMENTS

2:30
2:36
2:33
2:37
2:32
2:36

felt

Perform

My best workout in years!
- walked 400m between each
- struggled on last one

Achilles ached — iced 15 min

12 min warm up and warm down

Saturday — Jan 6

GOAL	Off
TIME	
DISTANCE	
AM PULSE	55
WEATHER	
TEMP	
TIME	(AM/PM)
TERRAIN	
DATE	WALK BREAK

COMMENTS

Kids soccer (Morn)

* Westin scores goal bouncing off his back
  1st goal of season!

Brennan's cross country (aft)
Invitational
* Brennan comes from 8th to 3rd in the last half mile. I'm so proud!

Sunday — Jan 7

GOAL	18 mi (I) easy!
TIME	2:53
DISTANCE	18 mi
AM PULSE	52
WEATHER	50°
TEMP	dry no wind
TIME	7 (AM/PM)
TERRAIN	flat
DATE	WALK BREAK 1 min/mi

COMMENTS

It was great to cover 18 miles — wish I had a group
longest run in 18 months!

but...
* went too fast in the first 5 miles
* Achilles hurt afterward — take 3 days off

Pulse is up — I'm not recovering — need more days off/week

Filling Out the Log. Here are the components of your running program. Once you know what you're going to do, you can pursue your plan with more enthusiasm.

Plan Your "Pyramid." Designate the time you would like to "peak," and count back. A 10K runner on a six-month program would allow eight weeks for speedwork. A half-marathoner should allow at least 12 weeks.

Pencil in the long runs, the hard runs and the races which will lead you to your goal. Look over the principles of daily and weekly mileage in the next chapter to help in your planning and see the charts on pp. 96–125. See how the whole picture looks and adjust where necessary.

Monitor Your Morning Pulse and Weight. A key entry for your daily log is your resting pulse rate, taken before you get out of bed each morning. Your body is less affected by external pressures like meals, work stress, etc., at this time. As soon as possible after waking, take your pulse and record it in the log. After two weeks, you should have a base line, an average. When your morning pulse rises more than 10% above base, it's a sign you've been working too hard and you need one or more days of reduced activity. By keeping tabs on yourself this way, you'll monitor patterns in your training and be able to add rest days before they are needed.

Also, be aware of daily weight loss. It takes about 35 miles of running to lose a pound of fat. If you lose a pound and didn't run that far the day before, it's dehydration: water loss. Right after rising, weigh yourself and record it in your log. When you drop more than two percent of body weight in a day, take a *very* easy day. When it drops three percent or more, take the day off. Should this happen, rehydrate yourself by drinking water and/or electrolyte fluids every hour or two, until your weight reaches the right level.

HEART RATE TRAINING

As the prices of heart rate monitors go down, more and more runners buy them and try to use them. I have mixed feelings about this. One of the greatest benefits of running is the development of intuitive monitoring of the many processes inside: pacing, possible over-exertion, when to push, when not to push. If we rely too much on technology to tell us what to do, we lose these instincts.

In fact, there's evidence that the use of intuition produces better progress and faster times. In a famous sports psychology study, the University of Wisconsin's Dr. Morgan showed that most world-class athletes associate with or monitor their stress signs, whereas a group of almost-world-class athletes disassociated or distracted themselves from the discomfort of a hard effort.

By training ourselves to use intuitive powers, which are extensive, we will become fine-tuned exercise machines, like world-class athletes. While our times won't be as fast, we can sense when to take an extra rest day, or walk break, when to push and when not to . . . before it's too late. Such monitoring will set us up for a program of maximum improvement, and/or continuous running enjoyment.

I don't believe in using the heart monitor as the first line of defense against overtraining, instead of intuition. But if you record the data and use it as a backup checking device, you have the best of both worlds. When in doubt, I rely on my gut instincts. If the heart monitor says, for example, that you could push harder in a speed or tempo workout, but you sense that this will require an extra day of recovery, don't push harder.

On most of your runs, your heart rate can tell you how hard you're working, relative to an all-out effort. It is particularly useful on speed workouts and races up to about 10K. After you have been tested to find your maximum heart rate, you will have some data to help you make decisions in workouts: how much rest, how fast, how far.

Be sure to get tested to determine your max heart rate. It's best to be tested under the supervision of a cardiologist or physiologist. Ask for a maximum heart rate test. Wear your heart monitor during the test if the doctor lets you. This will help you calibrate your instrument. Many of the heart monitors miss a beat or three every minute. It helps to know what your monitor registers, relative to the usually more reliable clinic equipment. In the unlikely event that you would have a medical problem under the stress of the test, you will have trained people there to deal with it.

At first the percentages seem complicated, but you'll become comfortable with these concepts with a few weeks of regular use. Your monitor can be a great tool to help you manage workload and fatigue. *Just don't let it tell you what to do.*

Benefits of a Heart Monitor

1. *Enforcing an easy day:* Most fitness/fun runners don't need a heart monitor. There are, however, a few "type A" runners who just can't hold back on their easy days, and become progressively more tired or injured. By keeping the rate below 65% of max on days that should be easy, these obsessive ones can keep their legs from becoming exhausted.

2. *Ensuring that you're doing accelerations, not sprints:* I mentioned in other chapters that some fast "gliding" on some of the mid-week runs can help you run more efficiently. You want these quicker-turnover glides of 50–100 yards or so to be at a faster pace than you would run normally, but without requiring a significant effort. Your heart rate will tell you whether you're doing this. If the rate on the gliders rises above 75% of max on an acceleration, shorten your stride, keep your feet lower to the ground, don't push off quite so hard, and glide. Keep adjusting until you get back down to 75%.

3. *Holding back at the end of long runs:* If you pace your long runs, from the beginning, 2 min./mi. slower than your goal pace (or slower) you should be registering 65% of max heart rate, or lower for most of the run—and no more than 70% of max at the end. If the rate rises above this during the first half, insert more walk breaks as necessary to keep the heart rate down. The only exception would be hot days (temperature above 70 degrees, particularly with high humidity). In this case, be as conservative as

you can, knowing that the weather itself will cause an elevation in heart rate. Walk most of the time if the rate reaches 88% or above.

4. *Establishing a resting heart rate:* As many days per week as you can, put on your monitor as soon as you arise for 10 minutes. Just lie down and listen to music. Most monitors will note your heart rate so that you can record it in your log or your computer. When the resting rate rises 5% above your baseline average, you should take an easy day. If it is above 10% higher, take the day off from running.

5. *Improving running form:* On a short mileage day during the week, warm up for 5–10 minutes, then go to a 400-meter track and do 4–6 accelerations (200–300 meters). Run for 100 meters, elevating heart rate to 80% of max. Continue at that effort level, timing yourself for 100 or 200 meters, staying at 80%. Walk for 2–3 minutes and do another one, trying to stay at 80%, while running a bit faster. If you do this regularly, your legs and feet will find a more efficient path, making you a smoother runner. You'll run easier and faster.

Using the Heart Monitor in a Speed Session

Warm Up: Do your usual warm-up, using the heart monitor if you wish — but it is not needed.

70% Rule: Once you know your max heart rate, and have calibrated your monitor, you are ready to go. Start each repetition, pushing the rate above 70%. Even on mile repeats, your heart rate for the speed rep should be at least 70%, and higher for 5K, 10K and half-marathon speed sessions.

Rest Until Heart Drops Below 65%: After running a speed repetition, you want to walk or jog very slowly to let the leg muscles recover. The heart rate is a great way to monitor this. Generally, I like to let the heart rate go below 65% of max before doing another speed repetition. *This may be the greatest benefit of heart monitors!*

Above 80%: During speedwork, you must push into the 80% zone to get faster, but too much running at this level will lead to over-training and stress injuries. On longer workouts (12×800 or 18×400) you often won't push above 80% for the first third of the workout. That's OK. Once you start getting into this zone, you want to keep from going higher, too soon. The repetitions in the second half of a hard speed workout will be generally over 80% — creeping up to 90%.

Above 90%: Some work in this zone is needed for top performance. The more you run above 90%, however, the longer you will have to recover from that workout. Try to limit the length of distance run at this level to the end of the workout, and only 25% of the distance of each repetition run above 90% (100 meters of a 400-meter repetition).

Tempo Runs: A common mid-week workout segment for time-goal athletes is "tempo" running, near goal race pace. The percentage allowed will increase in tempo work for short races, and decrease for longer ones. Lets assume that an 800-meter tempo segment is being run.

- *5K:* 70% for 200 meters, 75% for 200 meters, and no more than 80% for the final 400 meters.
- *10K:* 70% for 400 meters, 75% for 400 meters, and no more than 80% for the final 400 meters.

- *Half-Marathon:* 65% for 200 meters, 70% for 400 meters, and less than 80% for the final 200 meters.
- *Marathon:* 65% for 400 meters, below 75% for 400 meters, on most days. Below 85% in the last 2–3.

Easy Days Should Be Below 70%: Stay below 70% of max on all recovery days. It's OK to stay below 65%.

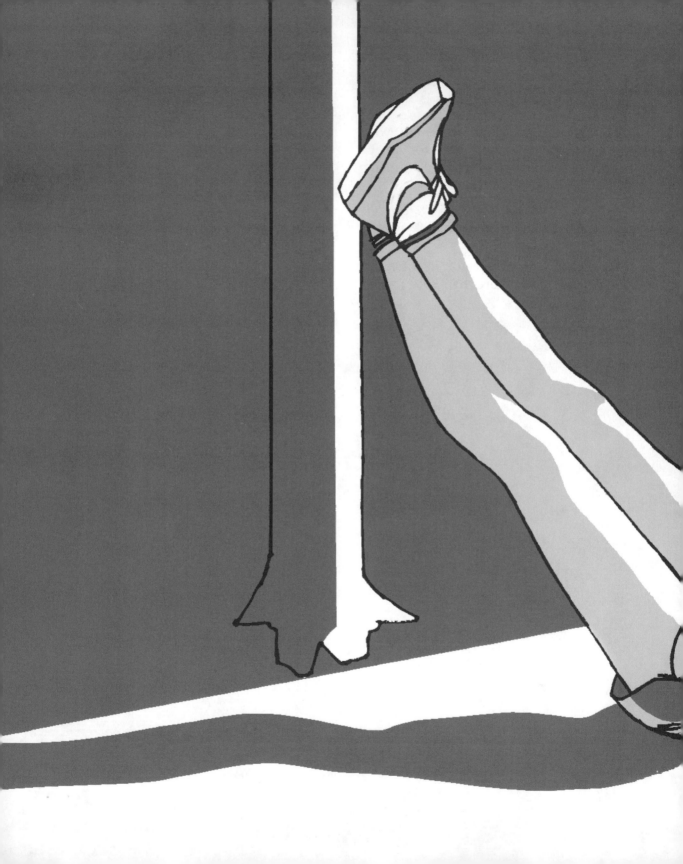

7
DAILY AND
WEEKLY MILEAGE
PROGRAMS

THE IMPORTANCE OF REST

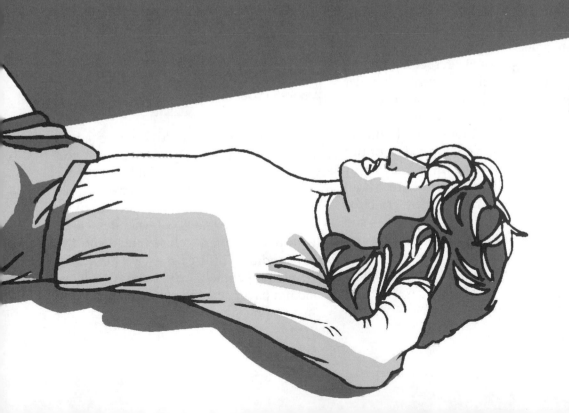

KENNY MOORE FINISHED FOURTH in the 1972 Olympic Marathon. He says he wouldn't have come nearly this far if he hadn't discovered the importance of rest. In his high school track days, Kenny didn't win a single race. After a year and a half of training, on the University of Oregon track team, he began to improve. He started to "beat" some of the better Oregon runners—at least in practice.

Excited by the prospect of becoming a winner, Kenny decided to train harder for a coming indoor track meet against Stanford and sneaked in some extra workouts to get ready. Confident at the starting line, he knew that none of his competitors had worked as hard as he had coming into this two-mile race. At the crack of the starting gun, he went with the leaders, but at the halfway point ran out of gas. He finished in one of his slowest times in years, 9:48.

While sitting in misery in the locker room he saw his coach, Bill Bowerman, heading toward him. "Good," he thought, "Bill's going to cheer me up with an inspiring talk." The internationally respected mentor, however, put a hand on Kenny's shoulder and read him the riot act. Bowerman had noticed Moore's extra workouts. He made his point quickly: Moore would run no more than three easy miles per day for two weeks or be kicked off the team. Kenny was insulted. He had worked harder than anyone else and was now being criticized for it. He knew he'd lose fitness—and races—under such a program. Determined to show that his coach was wrong, he followed the instructions to the letter. When he lined up against Washington State two weeks later, he was confident

he'd do poorly from lack of training and show up the "old man." This time he laid back at first, waiting for the out-of-shape "bear" to jump on his back. Instead, he found himself taking the lead at the mile and going on to win the race. His time: 8:48!

Although exalted by his fastest-ever time, he was humble as he thanked his coach. Bowerman knew Moore had pushed too hard without rest and that he'd come around if he took it easy. The sage of Eugene's Hayward Field track also knew that Kenny Moore was like most of us, and wouldn't rest unless confronted by the Wrath of God.

THE SECRET TO IMPROVEMENT

You cannot improve if you cannot run. *The single greatest cause of improvement is remaining injury-free.* If you're like most runners, you push it to the limit, and then Mother Nature steps in and forces you to rest. This slows your progress, for you must rebuild after each "down" period. But if you *build rest into your training program* you can avoid injuries and interruptions in your progress.

A common, overused running adage tells you to "listen to your body and you won't get injured." That would be great if it worked, but often either the signals are not strong enough or we're not listening attentively. A coveted goal will often cause us to push too far, to lose touch with the real condition of tired muscles. Or maybe we're preoccupied with other problems, and not paying careful enough attention to the warning signals.

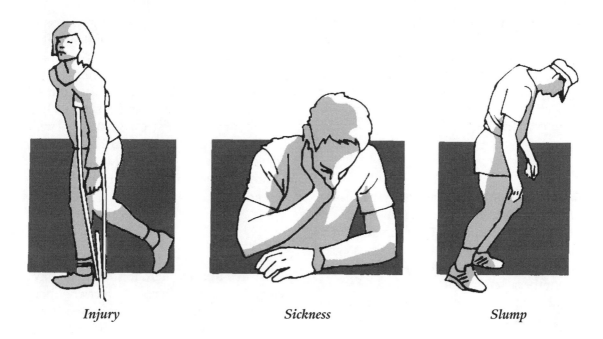

Injury *Sickness* *Slump*

Your body can also lie to you. When your muscles are overstressed, stress hormones mask tiredness. For a while the body slavishly responds to the mind's commands. When exhausted, the body draws upon its reserves; but reserves are limited, and once they've run out, you're at the crash point. This can have three results: *injury, sickness, or slump.*

- *Injury:* With reserves gone, muscles are so exhausted they cannot function normally. Weaker muscles try to take over the job and are usually overwhelmed. For example, the calf muscle is designed to provide much of your running power. When it gets tired it may shift some of the burden to the weak muscles on the inside of the lower leg. Shin splints and other shin problems often result by continuing to push, especially if you're a pronator (where the forefoot rolls excessively to the inside). In this way, pushing too far will quickly show you the weak links.

- *Sickness:* When the body is under prolonged stress, your resistance to disease is dramatically reduced. If a group of strong infectious germs wanders in, they're far more likely to find a comfortable home—at your expense and misery.

- *Slump:* If you are lucky enough to avoid injury or sickness, there's a "slump" waiting for you at the end of your exhaustion trip. Once you've hit rock bottom, there's no backing off. Your muscles won't respond even if you muster the will to drive them. You're going to feel tired, lacking in energy, and probably depressed until you build up your reserves again. This can last for weeks or months.

How can you avoid the above three undesirable conditions? *Rest* is the answer. Since "listening to your body" doesn't always work, you must build rest into your program—before it becomes the only choice and you're forced to take a long vacation from running.

STRESS + REST

Rx for Maximum Improvement. A basic and simple principle of getting stronger has been recognized in recent years. Coaches, sport physiologists, and top athletes agree that the most effective way to improve strength and endurance is to *stress*, and then *rest* the muscles. We've outlined the cellular aspects of stress/rest in the chapter on physiology *(see pp. 24–33)*. Now we're going to cover the application of this equation to your daily and weekly mileage programs.

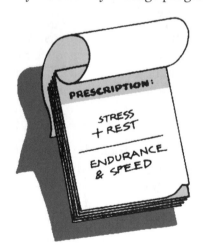

Rest is at least as important as stress in this formula. Muscles will rebuild stronger after being stressed, but *only* if they are given enough resting time. The trouble with most runners (especially the injured ones) is that they neglect the second half of the formula. You stress yourself—with speedwork, races, long runs, or weekly mileage increases. Then without adequate rest in between, you find yourself sidelined with an injury.

Individual muscle cells will do the work for which they have been prepared. When you push the muscles harder than you have before, they can become overwhelmed. They can no longer process oxygen and fuel efficiently and they build up large amounts of waste, primarily lactic acid. The mitochondria will try their best to process the energy needed, but are simply not able to do so. The circulation system becomes overloaded, the cell walls are physically "beaten up," swollen, and even broken in places. You have an injury, but it may not be extensive enough to cause serious problems.

After 48 hours of reduced activity most of these problems will be remedied. The walls of the cells, arteries and blood vessels will have been rebuilt stronger. The mitochondria are recharged and can process more energy. The capillaries will be working to remove wastes and deliver nutrients. Most runners need two easy days after every hard day for the rebuilding to take place.

Here is a chart of the specific effects of stress and rest:

Changes Inside the Muscle Cells		
	Results of Hard Run	**Results After Rest**
Mitochondria	Swollen, energy supplies depleted	Recharged
Cell Walls	Torn	Tears healed
Waste	Lactic acid buildup	Wastes removed, cells packed with nutrients

THE DAILY MILEAGE PROGRAM

Many runners know they should run easy after each hard day. Oregon's Bill Bowerman is credited with this concept. This seems obvious today, but it wasn't in my college days when I met Oregon steeplechaser Geoff Hollister. I was proud of my own progress under a system where I worked out hard each day. Back in the dark ages of my own running theories, it seemed that each day I slacked off, my competitors moved up a notch. I was amazed to learn from Geoff that the scores of national champions, recordholders and world-ranked runners from his alma mater thrived under a program that let them "loaf" every other day. We East Coast runners still believed we had to run harder each day to improve—and we were also injured much of the time.

The Easy-Day Rule. For most runners an easy day will mean no running. Elite athletes modify this by running fewer and slower miles on their easy days. Walking and other non-pounding cross-training activities will promote recovery better than hitting the couch by generating a gentle circulation of blood, oxygen and nutrients to speed the recovery (and strengthening) process. The late Dr. George Sheehan shifted to running every other day late in his running career. After several years of this, he ran his fastest marathon (3:01) at age 62. Jack Foster, the New Zealander who ran a 2:11

marathon at age 41, also shifted to this program, running three, or at most four days a week because otherwise he "inevitably came up with an injury after about 10 days." After about two years of this, he ran a 2:20 marathon at age 50. Jack also did some cycling on one non-running day per week.

Each runner will find his or her own pattern of daily rest periods. Kenny Moore found that when he was training for top performance, he needed two days of rest after hard days. He ran an easy 2–3 miles after a hard day, then an easy 8–10 miles the next day. Most runners would benefit more from a day of no running instead of the short run, but we have to find the combination that works best.

Each of us responds differently to hard work or long runs. Some will feel very tired that night, others the next day. Some may feel fine the day after and then wake up exhausted the second day. Likewise, a tiring workout will produce lingering effects for some and only minor aches, pains and fatigue for others. Even if you don't feel tired, it's best to take one or two easy days after a hard one.

How Many Days per Week? Research has shown that *you need at least three days of running per week for sustained improvement.* One or two days do comparatively little for you. At three days the improvement curve rises dramatically. Each day thereafter, improvement continues, but at a decreasing rate.

Those who run three days a week almost never get injured. When you consider the virtual certainty of injury from the six- or seven-day running week, even those with time goals should calculate the risks carefully before running more than five days. Your rest days should be spaced fairly evenly throughout the week. If you want to exercise on non-running days, you can improve endurance and strength through water running, cross-country ski machines, cycling, swimming, rowing, or other non-jarring activities. Only world-class runners can run seven days a week; but they, as well as other runners, can benefit physically as well as psychologically from a day or two of rest. *(See chart below.)*

Most runners can reach most of their goals by running 3–4 days a week. If you want more mileage, you can break up the mileage into two sessions on your running days.

How Much Rest After Races? Jack Foster believes you need one easy day for each mile of a race. The sustained drain of a race takes its toll. You shouldn't run another race or do speedwork until you have served your time according to "Foster's Rule." You could run a speed workout or race eight or more days after a 10K race, but no hard work should be attempted for 3–4 weeks after a marathon. No race should be run the weekend after a race longer than four miles. I've found that most runners should limit their race miles to 13 each month. This means you can run two 10K's, or two 5K's and a 10K, or a half-marathon each month—maximum.

How Much Rest After Speed? In speedwork—either intervals or fartlek *(see pp. 71–77)*—you're resting after each hard effort. This isn't like the uninterrupted strain of a race, so you don't need as much rest time. Most runners should only do one speed session a week; this will not normally overstress the system. If you're running a hard speed workout and a race in the same week, the race should be 5K or shorter. *(See Chapter 8, p. 68 for details on speedwork.)*

How Many Days a Week Should You Run?

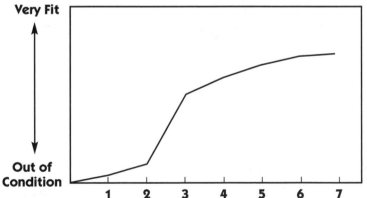

Note the dramatic increase in fitness from training three as opposed to two days a week. Over 95% of aerobic capacity is gained in training 4–5 days a week. Going beyond that point, the rate of orthopedic injuries rises drastically. (From *Computerized Running Training Programs,* James B. Gardner and J. Gerry Purdy)

THE WEEKLY MILEAGE PROGRAM

It's not enough to merely have easy days each week. A steady mileage program, at whatever level, leaves a residual tiredness that builds up, and eventually produces injury. You not only need the rest days after stress, but regularly scheduled rest weeks with reduced mileage, allowing the body to rebuild.

As you increase stress or even maintain the same load, tired muscle cells break down and must be replaced with fresh ones. When one group of cells becomes exhausted, the burden of carrying on is shifted to other, usually weaker muscle groups. Small tears and broken tissues are not healed completely by a few rest days within a steady mileage program. If you don't reduce overall mileage you will dig into reserves which eventually run out and leave you exhausted. Over time, the isolated small tears in the muscle fibers accumulate enough to cause an injury. If you're increasing mileage or speedwork, you are even more apt to face an injury.

The Easy-Week Rule. If you cut your mileage by 30% the second week and 50% the fourth week, you can avoid this mileage stress. This is a safety valve which allows your body to recover and shake off the accumulated stress and the physical abuse of running.

Some runners need more rest than others. Be conservative and find the pattern that works best for you. Don't be worried about losing conditioning. Studies have shown that athletes can cut their workouts by 50% for ten weeks and not lose significant fitness. In fact you may gain rather than lose by cutting back, because you return rested and less prone to injury.

Low-Mileage Ultras? Steve Boyer, a friend of mine from college, is a doctor and has had to regulate his running and racing addiction. He has run several marathons (a best time of 2:42) for which his weekly training miles varied between 20 and 45.

In preparing for the Mt. Hood (Oregon) 40-miler, he decided to test my low-mileage/long-run theory to its limits. A complicating factor was the altitude, and the rise and fall of the course (10,000 feet of gain and loss). Steve decided to spend his limited training time as specifically as possible for this difficult race.

He gradually built the long run to 30 miles with 2000 feet of vertical gain or did repeat hill repetitions with 7500 feet of vertical gain. Two weeks before the race he pre-ran the course very slowly. The day after each long run, he did not run, and gradually eased back into running (3–4 miles, 6–7 miles, etc.). The last week before the race he ran only 20 miles. Most weeks he ran less than 50 miles.

The results should be of interest to high-mileage advocates: In a strong field, including Bill Davis (third in one of the Western States 100's), Rae Clark (Tahoe 70-mile recordholder) and Frank Thomas (who holds the record for running across England), Steve finished second. He was six minutes behind the winner and later told me he thought he might have won had his ego not pushed him too fast (a 10-minute lead at 15 miles going up the first long hill).

Less Mileage for a Faster 10K — After Age 50. Lower mileage can also improve times for the middle distances. John Perkins found this out after three 2800-mile running years. He had reached plateaus with his marathon and 10K racing times despite his 50–70 miles per week, which included long runs and speedwork. After a disappointing finish in the New York City Marathon, he decided to give up racing and the hard training and run many fewer miles.

During an 18-month "vacation," John's competitive instincts didn't die. When he heard that a number of runners were improving performances with a program of reduced total mileage, a relaxed pace for the daily runs, and weekly speedwork, John decided to test the new theories.

For about nine months John reduced his weekly mileage from almost 60 to 39. He did a speed workout once a week with 8–10 440's at 82 seconds and gradually increased to 18 440's. Then he dropped to 10 440's, run at 74 seconds. This program helped him lower his 10K and 5K race times significantly.

John says he now feels strong from start to finish, whereas he used to feel lethargic, tired, and unresponsive. He's not afraid to challenge other runners, or to increase the pace slightly after the first mile. Before, he was tired throughout each race and was looking for the finish line after the first mile.

Following is a comparison of John's previous program—weekly mileage, pace, and races—and his new one.

Anthony Sandoval won the U.S. Olympic Marathon trials after several years of 100+ miles per week. The following year, during his M.D. residency he cut his mileage to about 40, running every other day, and ran 2:14 in the Boston Marathon.

RUNNING HOT AND COLD
In the Cold

Your lungs aren't going to freeze when you run outdoors in January. I've met many runners who've run in temperatures lower than −30° F and one Alaskan who ran in temperatures lower than −60° F with no damage to the breathing apparatus. After a visit to a good running or ski store you'll be ready to confront all the challenges that winter blows your way.

I've run in minus 30°. It was impossible for a guy from Atlanta to put on enough layers for that 5-miler. Even on a windless day, your running motion produces a significant wind-chill effect. All skin must be covered, with skin lubricant applied to the "holes": eyes, mouth, and neck area, underneath the edges. Breathing through a good ski mask will keep a warm-up zone in your mouth which should almost eliminate the chance of throat irritation due to breathing cold air. I needed a battery-operated sock warmer, for my toes took days to fully thaw out.

Previous Program	New Program
50–70 miles per week	30–50 miles per week
One hard 15+ mile run per week	One easy 12–15 mile run every other week
Pace for daily runs: 6:40–6:50	Pace for daily runs: 7:45–8:00
Raced most weeks	Races every other week
Best race times: 10K: 37:27 5K: 18:20	Best race times: 10K: 36:34 5K: 17:36

CLOTHING THERMOMETER

These are recommendations only; use the combination of layers that works best for you.

Degrees F	What to wear as it gets colder
60° +	Tank top or singlet and shorts
50–59	T-shirt and shorts
40–49	Long-sleeved T-shirt, shorts or tights or wind pants, mittens or gloves
30–39	Polypro long sleeve or long-sleeve T-shirt and another T-shirt, tights and shorts, socks, mittens or gloves, and a hat over your ears
20–29	Polypro top or thick long-sleeved T-shirt, another T-shirt layer, tights and shorts, socks, mittens or gloves, and a hat over your ears
10–19	Polypro top and thick long-sleeved T-shirt, tights and shorts, wind suit (top and pants), socks, thick mittens, and a thick hat over your ears
0–9	Two polypro tops, thick tights and shorts (and thick underwear or supporter for men), warm-up suit of Gore-Tex or a similar fabric, gloves and thick mittens, ski mask, a hat over your ears, and Vaseline covering any exposed skin
Minus 15	Two thick polypro tops, tights and thick polypro tights, thick underwear (and supporter for men), thick warm-up suit, gloves, thick (arctic) ski mask and a thick hat over your ears, Vaseline covering any exposed skin, thicker socks on your feet and other foot protection, as needed
Minus 20 and below	Add layers as needed

Stay in touch with the outdoor and ski shops for the warmest clothing that is still thin. Watch your feet. There are socks that may be heated up, not to mention other innovations.

Wear Layers—Not Heavy Coats

- Close to your skin, you'll want something warm. Polypropelene is one of several fibers that keep the warmth close to the skin, but allow extra heat and perspiration to escape. (Maxit makes an excellent selection of polypro clothing.)

- Add external layers, adjusting to the temperature and wind conditions.

- Cover up all extremities—hands, ears, toes—with extra layering.

- Men should wear an extra layer or two as underwear if necessary.

- In extreme cold (when the temperature or wind-chill factor is below 10°F [minus 11°C]), do not expose any skin, if possible. Even when there is minimal exposure, put Vaseline or other cold weather insulation and protection on any area that may incidentally be hit by the wind, such as your eyelids, etc.

- Be sure to coat your shoes or use socks that insulate your feet. Most running shoes are designed to let heat out and cold into your feet. This can cause frostbite on days colder than 32°F (or 0°C). Remember that running itself can generate a significant wind-chill effect on your feet.

- As you warm up while running, peel off each layer before you start sweating. Too much sweat accumulating will freeze and cause problems.

Warm-ups in Winter

In-and-out training will break up your winter exercise into segments, while keeping you from freezing. On very cold days, bundle up and exercise for a very few minutes indoors. You may walk, jog in place, use an indoor track, or exercise on the machines (cycle, rowing, stairs). Before you start sweating, go outdoors and you'll have a reservoir of warmth to get you down the road. Many runners in Canada's "snow belt" will do loops around their fitness club. The colder the day, the shorter the loop. If you plan to go back outdoors, do so before you start sweating.

Start your run or walk by going into the wind. This allows you to come back with the wind. If you start to get very warm, remove an outside layer of clothing or unzip your outer layer. A garment with long sleeves may be tied around your waist, or put it in your fanny pack—you may need it later. Survey any outdoor running route before running it, noting environments where you could seek refuge for at least a few minutes if you need to.

In the Heat

There's good and bad news about running in the heat. First, the bad news: When the temperature rises above 55°F (10°C), you're going to run more slowly and feel worse than you will at lower temperatures. But by gradually preparing yourself for increased temperatures and taking action from the beginning of hot-weather runs, you'll get a welcome dose of good news. You'll learn how to hydrate yourself, what to wear, and when and how much your body can take in hot weather, all of which will help you recover faster and run better than others of your ability on hot days. While even the most heat-adapted runners won't run as fast on hot days as they can on cold ones, they won't slow down as much nor will they feel as much discomfort as they did before becoming heat-acclimatized.

Note: Be sure to read the next section, Heat Disease Alert *(p. 63)*. Without knowing these concepts, you can get into serious trouble even on moderately warm days. Mark that section and revisit it several times during the warm season of the year. If you have any risk of heart disease, talk to a doctor trained in exercise before continuing.

Until the temperature rises to about 65° F, most runners don't notice much heat build-up, even though it is already putting extra burdens on the system. It takes most folks about 30 to 45 minutes of running (with or without walk breaks) to feel warm. But soon after that, if the temperature is above about 62° F, you're suddenly hot and sweating. On runs and especially races under those conditions, most runners have to force themselves to slow down. It's just too easy to start faster than you should when the temperature is between 60 and 69° F because it feels cool at first.

As the mercury rises above 65° F, your body can't get rid of the heat building up. This causes a rise in core body temperature and an early depletion of fluids through sweating. The internal temperature rise also triggers the rapid dispersion of blood into the capillaries of the skin, reducing the amount of that vital fluid that is available to the exercising muscles. Just when those workhorses are being pushed to capacity, they are receiving less oxygen and nutrients. What used to be a river becomes a creek and can't remove the waste products of exercise (such as lactic acid). As these accumulate, your muscles slow down.

Body Fat

The more body fat you have, the worse you'll feel as the temperature and humidity rise. I don't have any research on this, but my experience tells me that for every increase of 5 percent in body fat, the effects of heat and humidity are felt about 5 minutes sooner. For example, if a runner with 12 percent body fat feels severe heat discomfort after 45 minutes of running, then a runner with 22 percent body fat will feel it after 35 minutes, and a runner with 32 percent body fat after 25 minutes. Body fat acts like a blanket to hold heat in. It does too good a job during the summer.

Beat the sun, and you'll beat the heat.

The best time for hot weather running is before sunrise. The more you can run before sunrise, the cooler you will feel, compared with how you'll feel later in the day. The second-best time to run, by the way, is right after sunrise, unless the temperature cools off dramatically at sunset, which would make that time more favorable. In humid areas, however, it usually doesn't cool down much after sunset.

How to Stay Cool

Slow down early

Walk breaks, early and often, help you lower the exertion level, which conserves resources for the end and reduces heat build-up. The later you wait to slow down, the more dramatically you'll slow down at the end and the longer it will take to recover from the run.

Wear lighter garments

Loose-fitting clothes allow heat to escape. Don't wear cotton clothing. Sweat soaks into cotton, causing it to cling to your skin, increasing heat build-up. Several materials will wick the perspiration away from your skin: Coolmax, polypro, etc. As moisture leaves your skin, you receive the cooling effect that these types of materials are designed for.

No Hats! — Pour water over yourself

Up to 70 percent of the heat you can lose goes out through the top of your head. Hats keep the heat from being released through the best vent you have, the top of your head. Don't cover it up! It helps to regularly pour water over your hair (even if, like me, you are hair-challenged). Regularly pouring water on a light, polypro (or a similar material) singlet or tank top will keep you cooler.

Drink cold water

Not only does cold water leave the stomach of a runner quicker than any type of fluid, it produces a slight physiological cooling effect — and an even greater psychological cooling effect. But don't drink too much either. Most of us do well with between 6 and 10 ounces an hour during warm weather. Drink until you hear sloshing in your stomach, then stop. When the sloshing sound goes away, resume drinking.

Take a dip or a shower

On hot days, you can reduce heat build-up significantly if you spend 3 or 4 minutes in a pool or cold shower every mile or two. Do this several times and even the hottest day's run becomes manageable. The break in your run will not cause you to get out of shape. Over the span of a month, most runners get in more training this way because they don't overheat early.

Don't eat a big meal

Eating too much, particularly meals that are high in protein or fat, will put extra stress on your system when you exercise. Even worse is the probability that too much food loading will lead to unloading during the run. That can be embarrassing! Instead of big meals, eat light, easily digestible snacks, every hour or two. Many runners find it better not to eat anything within two hours or so of their hot weather run (although energy bars or PowerGel work well for most, when taken 1–2 hours before the run).

Training for hot weather

One day a week, you can train yourself to deal with the heat by inserting the hot segments below into your run, even if you are starting in the middle of winter. Of course, you need to run at least two other days per week, and you must do this heat training day every week. Before running each hot segment, read pp. 63–64 on symptoms of heat disease. At the first indication of symptoms, stop running before you get into trouble.

The process of heat training follows the same principles as conditioning for endurance and speed. By pushing yourself a little bit and then backing off, your body makes adaptations and can deal with the heat better the next time. On each run, warm up for at least 10 minutes of easy running (and walking), and ease off with at least 10 minutes of easy running (and walking) after the heat phase. If the outdoor temperature is cool, you may put on one or more layers of clothes, especially on the

Effects of Heat and Humidity

When it's	A 10-minute-per-mile pace becomes:	With humidity over 60 percent, the 10-minute-per-mile pace becomes:
55–60°	10:06	10:10
60–65	10:18	10:25
65–70	10:30	10:50
70–75	10:42	11:10
75–80	11:12	11:48
80–85	12:00	13:00
Above 85°	Forget it . . . take the day off or run for fun (with shower breaks).	

upper body, during the hot segment. You may also do these segments indoors. Take it very easy on these segments. You're only working on heat adaptation, not speed or intensity.

Schedule of Hot Segments

Week Number	Duration of Hot Segment
1	5–7 minutes
2	7–9 minutes
3	9–12 minutes
4	12–16 minutes
5	16–22 minutes
6	22–26 minutes

Adjusting for Heat

As the weather gets hotter, you must slow down your pace from the beginning. Also, in most places in North America, you'll need to make adjustments for the humidity. The higher the humidity, the sooner you'll feel the effect of the heat and the more difficult it will be to continue. Watch the weather reports and install a temperature and humidity gauge at your house. After a while, you'll learn the combination of the two that causes you discomfort and can avoid the times of the day when those conditions arise.

TALLAHASSEE SHOWERS

In Tallahassee, I discovered an outdoor shower beside the FSU track. Practically every afternoon during June, July, and August, I'd structure my runs so that I looped by the track at least every two miles. If my body heat built up more quickly, I'd cut the loop short and head for the shower. For those runs, I used special shoes that could be slipped on and off quickly without being unlaced. Without those regular dousings, I wouldn't have run half the distance I was able to cover.

Heat Disease Alert

Heat disease is a common health problem among endurance exercisers. This is a serious condition that has frequently resulted in death, even among highly trained, young athletes.

Symptoms

- Intense heat build-up in the head, significant headache, general overheating of the body
- General confusion and loss of concentration and muscular control

- Excessive sweating and then the cessation of sweating, a clammy skin, and excessively heavy breathing
- Extreme tiredness, upset stomach, muscle cramps, vomiting, and faintness

Risk factors

- Sleep deprivation
- Viral or bacterial infection
- Dehydration (avoid alcohol and caffeine)
- Severe sunburn and skin irritation
- Lack of acclimation to hot weather
- Overweight
- Lack of training for a specific training exercise
- Occurrence(s) of heat disease in the past
- Medications, especially cold medicines, diuretics, medicines for diarrhea, tranquilizers, antihistamines, atropine, and scopolamine
- Certain medical conditions including high cholesterol levels, high blood pressure, extreme stress, asthma, diabetes, epilepsy, drug use (including alcohol), cardiovascular disease, smoking, or a general lack of fitness

Prevention

- During hot weather, exercise at the coolest time (usually before sunrise).
- Pour water over the top of your head and clothes regularly.
- Drink water all day long, 4–8 oz. per hour when needed.
- Avoid caffeine, alcohol, and other drugs.
- Wear clothing that is light and loose.

- Eat small, lowfat snacks that you know will not cause you distress.
- Don't increase the duration or intensity of your exercise significantly.
- Slow down your pace even more to account for heat, humidity, and hills—especially in the beginning.
- Take walk breaks more often.
- See a physician who specializes in running and fitness before beginning the program if you have any questions about any of the conditions mentioned, or if you notice any significant change in body functions, immune response, and so on.

Take action!

Watch for heat disease in fellow runners when you run in a group or a race on a hot day, and take action if you think anyone is in trouble. Walk, cool off, and get help immediately.

Hyponatremia, or Water Intoxication

While extremely rare, this condition has caused death during or after long runs or marathons. Many runners become overly concerned about hyponatremia, and don't drink enough before, during and after a long run. The result is dehydration, which is much more likely to cause medical problems, and increase recovery time after long runs. As in all training components, use good common sense.

The underlying cause of hyponatremia is often severe dehydration, compounded by consuming only water in great quantities. Every marathoner should be aware of this condition, not only for self-protection.

If you see someone who seems to be going through the symptoms, a little attention can bring them around relatively quickly. If a member of your running group shows any of the symptoms below, stay in touch with that person for the next few hours to ensure that he or she is getting what is needed and is not alone. As always, when in doubt, get medical advice and care. A physician will have to determine whether an IV will help or not.

Causes

- Starting the run dehydrated, due to consuming alcohol the night before, not drinking enough fluid the day before, or eating a very salty meal the night before

  and/or

- Sweating excessively and continuously for more than 5 hours

  and/or

- Taking medication (within 48 hours of a long run) which messes up the fluid storage, and fluid balance systems

  and

- Drinking too much water, in a period of 1–2 hours, once the body is dehydrated

Signs that you may have it

- Hands and/or feet swell up twice normal size (or more)
- Nausea that leads to vomiting, continuous or several times
- Diarrhea which is continuous or repeated every 10 minutes or so
- Mental disorientation and confusion
- Severe cramping of the muscles for several miles

How to avoid it

1. Drink water in small doses during a long run—6–8 oz., no more often than every 25 minutes.

2. Don't drink if you hear a sloshing sound in your stomach.

3. After 2–3 hours of continuous, excessive sweating, eat salty pretzels, or mix a small packet of salt with your water, every 30 minutes or so.

4. Continue to eat or drink the salty food for an hour after a run of 5 hours or longer.

5. Drink a sip or so of water or electrolyte drink with every pretzel.

6. At the end of long runs, and for hours afterward, even if you are very thirsty, don't drink more than 8 oz. of water about every 30 minutes. It is OK to drink some electrolyte beverage which is not diluted.

7. The electrolyte beverages don't have enough sodium to get you back to balance, but the carbohydrate in them will slow down the absorption of the water.

CARS

- Remember: be prepared to give in quickly. Avoid confrontations. It doesn't matter if you were "right" if you get hit. Survival is the goal.

- *Run on the sidewalk* when you can. Try to find secluded residential areas, parks. Obviously, paths and trails are even better.

- *Run facing traffic* if you must run on the roads. Always be aware of the shoulder, curb, etc.—a place to leap if necessary. Be aware of traffic behind you. Many runners have been killed by drunks or passing cars coming from behind them as they ran "facing traffic."

- *Wear reflective gear at night.* Use strips of reflective tape, reflective shoelaces or reflective vests.

- *Understand the driver's mentality.* He may be in a hurry. He may be drunk. He may be overweight, and hate you for being trim and in good health. Don't assume that drivers will behave rationally.

DOGS

It's usually a matter of territory. Your problem is to figure out the dog's boundary lines. If you're in his zone, let him bark to get some of the aggressiveness out, then slow down and make your way cautiously out of his territory. If he keeps coming toward you, bend down and pick up a rock or stick; this in itself will usually scare him off.

Throw the rock or stick if he's particularly aggressive and bend down to get another. Carry a stick in dangerous dog areas and if you have to, hit him on the nose. You can also carry dog spray. Some postmen use a strong pepper solution which will drive a dog away without causing lasting discomfort.

RACING

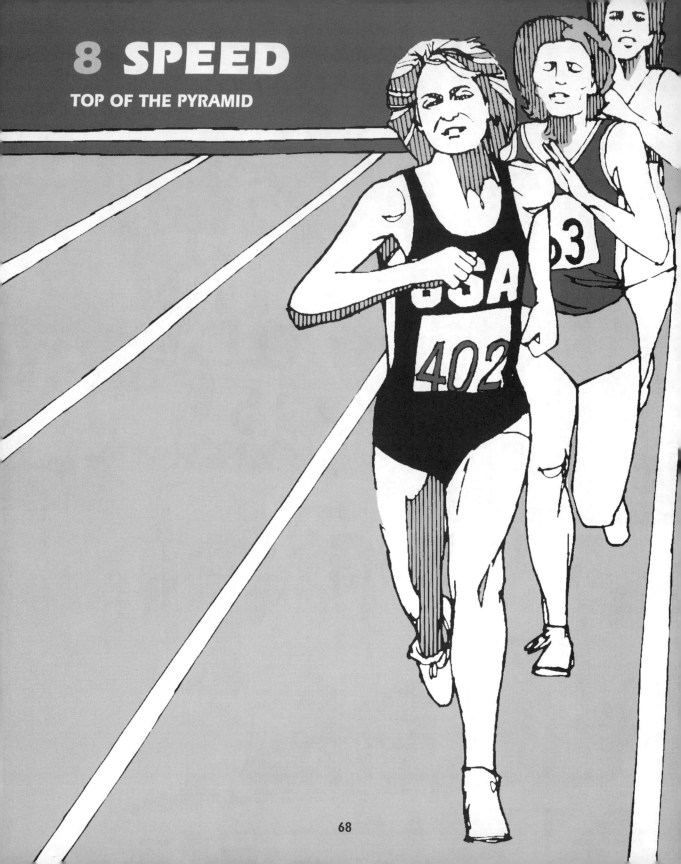

68

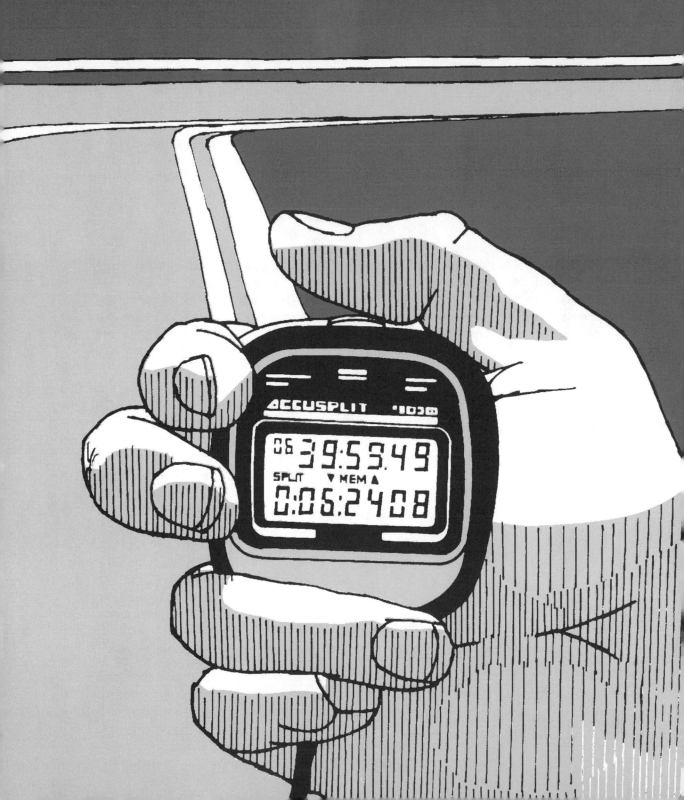

YOU CAN RUN FASTER! I've seen thousands of runners improve by making simple changes such as:

- Rearranging their schedules
- Adding rest
- Doing speedwork

The first rule is that your goals must be realistic. Setting a goal that is too ambitious will only lead to disappointment and frustration. But if you stage a series of goals that are within your reach, you'll build your running capacity *and* your confidence.

> **Note:** There's obviously a limit to how much you can improve. You'll reach plateaus at which your performance will level off, and sometimes even drop. A plateau may last a month or so, or even a year. As you get closer to your ultimate potential, the plateaus will tend to occur more often, and last longer.

Base Before Speed. Before attempting any speedwork, you must have built a good base, consisting of:

- One year of running
- At least two months (and preferably three) of aerobic running
- 4–6 weeks of hill training
- *See pp. 52–58 for details.*

YOU'RE AT THE TOP OF THE PYRAMID

During the base period you get your cardiovascular system ready to handle future speed demands. Whether you've run speedwork before or not, your base period will improve cardiovascular efficiency. Veterans find that base training also cleans out waste from a recent speed program.

Your hill training strengthens the key running muscles in your lower legs, allowing you to shift your weight a bit farther forward on your feet and to use your ankles for efficient mechanical advantage—gaining a stronger push-off. Now you're ready for the fast stuff!

The primary benefit of speedwork is to teach the body how to run anaerobically—to run fast when the muscles can't get enough oxygen. To run faster than you have ever run before, you must go beyond your capacity. Speed workouts take you *beyond* in a regular series of small extensions. By the end of a series of speed training sessions, you should have simulated the anaerobic demands of the race itself.

Each week you go beyond your efforts of the previous week. The lactic acid which pours into the muscles during the latter stages of a workout must be handled or the muscles will slow down. As the body restores the torn muscle cells and recharges the mitochondria *(see p. 25)*, it is able to go farther and faster before producing lactic acid.

How Much Can You Expect to Improve?	
Best Performance Last 6 Months	**Amount You Might Improve in 6-Month Pyramid**
50 min. 10K; 4:30 marathon	3–5 min. 10K; 30 min. marathon
42–50 min. 10K; 3:30–4:30 marathon	2–3 min. 10K; 15–20 min. marathon
38–42 min. 10K; 3:05–3:30 marathon	1–2 min. 10K; 8–15 min. marathon
35–38 min. 10K; 2:40–3:05 marathon	40 sec.–1 min. 10K; 5–10 min. marathon
32–35 min. 10K; 2:30–2:40 marathon	20–40 sec. 10K; 2–5 min. marathon

By dealing with this weekly dose of waste, the muscle cells learn how to cope with it. In some cases the muscles learn to process it out of the system more efficiently; in other cases they direct the waste into every available crevice. The mind learns that the body can go quite a bit farther even though it feels increasingly uncomfortable.

Speedwork brings you to a peak of performance and prepares you to race. When you have completed each of the small speed workouts in succession, you are at least physiologically ready to go. Of course you still have to take off at the crack of the gun and do it. Nevertheless you'll have the confidence of being prepared.

Endurance First. Before you can run a 10K fast, you must first be able to run a 10K. The first component of a speed program is a long run which increases each two weeks until it's longer than the race distance by at least 20%. Starting from the length of your longest run in the previous two weeks, add 1–2 miles once a week until you reach 11–12 miles. Then add 2–3 miles to each long one and run them every 14 days. You'll need this extra time between long runs. If your long runs exceed 17 miles, you should run them every third week.

Goal Race	Minimum Miles	For Top Performance
10K	8	15–17
Half-marathon	15	19–20
Marathon	26	28–30

You should include one-minute walk breaks, every 2–9 minutes from the beginning of all long runs, to make it easy for the body to adapt, and recover fast. These runs build endurance only and are not designed to improve speed. (Advanced runners will also benefit from walk breaks, at least one minute after 9 minutes of running). The pace of long runs should be at least two minutes per mile slower than you could race the distance that you're running on that day. When in doubt, slow down.

A Short History of Speedwork. Distance runners in the early 1900s believed that to run faster one must run repeated race simulations: full-speed races with rest in between. By the mid-1920s, athletes found they could improve more by breaking the race distance into many short segments and running each faster than race pace *with rest in between*. Two forms of speedwork thus emerged: *fartlek* and *interval training*.

FARTLEK

Fartlek is a Swedish word meaning *speed play*. It's a simple, natural form of speed training that can be worked into any daily run. During a run of a given distance, you accelerate — to the next telephone pole, to a tree, to any landmark. When you have pushed as long and as fast as you want (or can), you jog to recover. Then when you feel like it, you take off again.

Fartlek is speed training at your own pace. It is intuitive, free-form, without prescribed distances or speeds. You can run according to how you feel on that day, at that moment. Fartlek is speedwork, but it can be playful and creative.

Lasse Viren, the four-time Olympic gold medalist in 5K and 10K from Finland, did none of his speed training on the track during his 8 years of Olympic training. Fartlek can give you all the speed training you need, plus psychological strength benefits.

Fartlek Variations. Two popular fartlek variations are *hill fartlek* and *timed segments*. Hill fartlek begins with a normal non-stressful pace (about one minute slower per mile than 10K race pace). When you come to a hill, accelerate up and over the top—then jog to recover. When you recover, resume your original pace until the next hill.

In timed-segment fartlek, you run one minute, two minutes, three minutes, etc., slightly faster than race pace. After a gentle warmup of 10–20 minutes of easy running, then run 4–8 form accelerations *(see pp. 145–147)* before the first segment. Start each segment slightly slower than race pace, and insert 2–4 accelerations that are faster than race pace. Rest enough in between segments for recovery. The total number of segments is up to you. As in all speedwork, start with a few of them, and increase gradually on the once-a-week workout.

Not for Beginners. Fartlek does not give a beginner enough structure or feedback to learn a sense of pace. Many veterans who are already "pace-wise," however, can benefit from a fartlek session. While interval training gives the beginner exact feedback, it confines the veteran. Fartlek allows you to play with your limits of speed, tiredness, and endurance without stopping at the end of the lap. In this way you learn to cope with race-like discomfort and the anxiety of not knowing how long you can cope before slowing down. Beginners run a high risk of injury in fartlek training while veterans, more sensitive to stress, should know when to back off.

One week before the 1973 National Track Championships I tried to complete my first track workout of the year. The only hard work I had done that season was fartlek, and I needed timed feedback for confidence. After only a few ovals around the track, however, things weren't going right and I decided to quit. But it was a beautiful day, so instead of heading for the showers I found myself running down some of my favorite country roads.

Without realizing it, I increased the pace, accelerating for a while, letting off a little, then pouring it on again. I didn't feel particularly good that day, but my rhythm was smooth, so I just let it flow. Ironically, the workout was coming together although I felt bad and had to force myself to keep going.

I know now that this was one of the best workouts of my life and it led me to my best race. One week later, in the National AAU 6-mile at Bakersfield, California, I felt as I had when I started that earlier track workout: dumpy. For four miles I barely hung on in 12th place, and kept thinking about dropping out. Then my mind shifted into the same gear I had found on the roads. I moved up to fourth during the next mile and then took the lead. Although I was outkicked at the end, I ran my fastest time, 27:21.

When you have a good sense of pace, fartlek will prepare you best for rigorous races; it helps your mind shift gears. It can teach you to use your often-hidden powers of mental concentration to get beyond the barriers of discomfort and anxiety.

INTERVAL TRAINING

What Is It? Interval training breaks up the race distance into segments, called repetitions, or "reps." You run each rep slightly faster than goal race pace, then either jog or walk during the rest interval to recover. (Only advanced runners should jog; others should walk about half the distance of the repetition distance.) The number of reps is gradually increased over a series of weekly workouts. When preparing for the 10K race or less, the eventual total will be close to, or will equal, race distance. But the total distance of speedwork for a marathon will add up to only about one-half the race distance.

Repeating these segments may sometimes be boring, but the method gives you an invaluable lesson in judging pace. One of the most important skills of distance running is being able to intuitively feel whether you are running too fast or too slow. Interval training is exact and has several advantages over fartlek:

- With a measured distance, you get timed feedback on each lap.

- By controlling the pace of each rep, you'll learn how to run an even pace.

- When you first do speedwork, you are often lost when you try fartlek because you can only guess at distance, speed and total amount of work.

Basic Interval Training Principles

- *Choose the distance of your repetition: ¼ mile, ½ mile, or one mile.* It's typical to use 440 yards for a 5K or 10K, and half miles for the half-marathon.

- *Run each rep slightly faster (5–7 seconds × 440) than goal pace.* This makes race pace seem easier.

- *Hold back a little.* You need a tiring workout, but shouldn't "total" yourself. Finish the speed day feeling tired, yet capable of running more.

- *Walk between repetitions to recover.* For 5K and 10K speedwork, only advanced competitive runners should jog during recovery. When you start each speed program, start with a long rest period, walking at least half of the "rep" distance. If you recover easily, then decrease the rest interval. Walking is recommended for everyone during marathon speedwork.

- *Start with a few repetitions and increase the number in each weekly workout.* (See the charts on pp. 97–104 for a 5K, pp. 105–114 for a 10K, and pp. 115–125 for a half-marathon.) At the end of 10K speed training, you'll be doing 18–20 reps of a 400, with rest in between each one. At the end of half-marathon speed training you'll be doing about 10 reps of an 800, with rest in between.

- *Plenty of rest.* Take at least two days of rest after each speed day: at least one day off and at least one easy running day. If a given speed workout leaves you feeling tired, rest even more after the next one to avoid injury or lingering, dead-legged fatigue.

- *Length of speed program.* Speed programs for the 10K or shorter events are intense and should last no more than ten weeks.

Warm-up for Speedwork. Warming up properly is essential. Jumping into a speed session with cold muscles puts tremendous stress on any of your weak links and causes injury.

- Walk 5–10 minutes (longer if it's cold outside or you're stiff).
- Jog *slowly* for 10–20 minutes.
- Stretch *gently* if you usually stretch before running. Stretching before and after running doesn't help most runners, and may increase the chance of injury, so be very careful. An exception would be runners with iliotibial band injury.
- Run accelerations (5–8 × 100–200 yards.) Gradually increase speed to race pace or slightly faster, then decelerate. Take plenty of rest between each acceleration.
- Jog and walk slowly 3–5 minutes.
- Begin workout.

Warm-down After Speedwork. The warm-down is as important as the warm-up. If you stop abruptly, the lactic acid in the blood pools and you'll feel stiff the next day. No matter how tired you feel, keep moving.

- Jog slowly for 10 minutes after your last repetition. (Sometimes I barely move one foot in front of the other.)
- Ease into a walk for 5 minutes.
- Then into a slow walk for 10 minutes. You need to let the body down easy— don't drop it!
- *Note:* There are several incidents every year of runners who have heart attacks because they run from the track to the shower, or other standing activity, with no warm-down.

How Fast and How Long? The longer the reps, the slower the pace:

- *400 meter:* 5–7 seconds faster than goal pace.
- *800 meter:* 10 seconds faster than goal pace for 5K or 10K, 12–18 seconds faster than half-marathon goal pace.
- *1 mile:* 15–20 seconds faster than goal pace for 5K or 10K speedwork, 20–30 seconds faster for half-marathon/marathon speedwork.

There is obviously a trade-off here. The longer segments will more closely simulate race conditions, but make it harder to stay "on pace." The longer ones also take a longer recovery period. Walking between segments will speed recovery.

DEFINITIONS OF PACE

Goal pace: The speed which will lead you to your time goal.

Example: 5K goal of sub-25 minutes or a 10K goal of sub-50 minutes = 8 minutes/ mile or 2 minutes × 400 meter (one lap around a track) race pace.

Speed workout pace: Your pace for speed workouts.

Example: For a 5K or 10K, 400 reps are run 3–7 seconds faster than goal pace.

Where? Accurate distance is very important. A 400-meter track (¼-mile) is obviously a good choice for accuracy, but you can run roads, trails, athletic fields, anywhere, as long as the measurements are accurate. A car odometer and even highway markers are notoriously inaccurate. There are several running accelerometer devices (worn on the shoe) which are extremely accurate.

Fighting Boredom. As the number of segments grows, speed workouts become more difficult, and often boring. Running in a small group or with another runner helps. Some running clubs devote a day each week to group speedwork, offering a choice of several distances. A workout partner will make these difficult sessions easier and more interesting. Choose someone who will run on pace and who doesn't need to "win" each lap. When you work out with several runners, each should take the lead, alternating laps; after the rest period, another runner takes over the lead.

How Often? You should run one speed workout per week for the 5K-10K, and less frequently for the half-marathon (averaging about every other week).

SPEEDWORK ALTERNATIVES

Tempo Running. In this training mode, you're running race pace, or close to it for segments of about 2–5 minutes. I like to call this type of running "race rehearsal." It can be used as a replacement for another form of speed training, or as an extra speed session for very experienced runners.

Tempo running shouldn't build up an oxygen debt. You want to stay just below the level of exertion that would produce this. When in doubt, choose a pace that is slightly slower, especially at the beginning of a segment. When veterans use this as an extra speed session, they should never run a total workout distance that is more than about one-third of race distance. If this is a replacement for interval or fartlek training, the total distance could be the same as the distance of the replaced workout.

Race Rehearsal. It's very beneficial to have a few tempo sessions leading up to races, which are race rehearsals. On a measured course or track, run only a portion of the race distance (one-tenth to one-fourth of the distance), and run a few segments at race pace. If you plan to use walk breaks in the race itself, put them in as you plan. Time yourself and see if you're on pace.

Back to the Track. Joe Henderson, one of the original runner-writers, came into running from a competitive track background. He led thousands of runners into fun running in the '70s through his *Runner's World* editorials on long, slow runs. Track work practically dropped from his vocabulary. During the past few years, Joe has returned to the track—but not for the exhausting 15 × 440-yard sessions of his youth. He believes that running four 400's at or slightly faster than your current mile race pace builds speed without undue risk of injury. This workout is done once a week. You take as much rest as needed between repetitions.

Example:

- Current mile race pace: 8:00
- 400-yard pace: 2 minutes
- Workout: 4 × 400 with 400 or more walking or jog-walking in between
- Warm-up and warm-down: 10–20 minutes of slow jogging
- This is a low-stress speed workout which should improve your speed if you are not doing regular speedwork. Improvement under this program is limited, however, because the shorter speed sessions do not develop endurance. Increasing the long run every other week (to 12–16 miles for a 10K, for example) will allow these light speed sessions to produce better results.

Speeding on Sunday. For years, Monica Leerman tried to break 50 minutes in the 10K. She increased mileage, ran more races, and did regular speedwork, but nothing got her below the 50-minute threshold.

Then one winter, Monica changed tactics. Instead of running long on Sunday, she ran fast. Over a five-week period she ran a fast (7:15 pace average) three miles with some fartlek bursts. She shifted her weekly long run to mid-week, a 14–16 miler.

The new routine paid off. In a spring Avon 15K race, Monica ran the first 10K in 47:48, and held that pace to the end of the race. She could probably run even faster if she did some fine tuning with 4–8 form accelerations twice a week and 4–6 400 repetitions at about 7–10 seconds faster than race pace.

MOST FREQUENT CAUSES OF SPEED INJURIES

Speedwork is the second most frequent cause of running injuries. (Increasing total weekly mileage is the first.) *But I've discovered, over the years, that among those who do regular speedwork, it is the leading cause of injury.* By understanding how they happen, you can avoid most injuries.

These are the main reasons for speed injuries:

- *Inadequate warm-up or warm-down.* Be sure to follow a thorough warm-up procedure. By gradually getting the muscles active, you can avoid the trauma incurred when cold muscles go to maximum exertion. Likewise, it's cru-

cial to gradually ease off in a thorough warm-down.

- *Running too hard on easy days.* The speedwork and the long runs will take you to your goal. You must have easy running days in between these stress days to recover. If you run too fast on the easy days you'll gradually accumulate stress and tiredness which will lead to injury. A good easy-day pacing rule is to add 2 minutes per mile to what you feel you could race the distance you're running on the long run. When in doubt, slow down.

- *Sprinting.* Never run at top speed, not even in play, for there's great risk of injury. Even the form accelerations are designed to reach a maximum speed of only a hard one-mile pace. Never run the last portion of your workout sprinting.

- *Too many weeks of speed.* For races of 10K or less, speedwork should last no more than ten weeks. After this period, you run great injury risk by continuing. A half-marathon speed program should last no longer than 12 weeks.

- *Running faster on speed reps than you should.* If you're assigned a 2-minute 400-meter, you're more likely to get injured by running 1:55.

- *Too many hard days.* If you pack too many speed sessions, long runs and races into a short period of time, you're asking for trouble. Running slowly on the long runs and alternating weekends with races or easy runs will reduce stress. It's more important to complete the quality speed workouts and the long runs while minimizing races.

- *Inadequate transition.* Some runners try a "shortcut" up the pyramid by minimizing or eliminating hill work and/or the first few sessions. This forces the body to move too quickly from long slow running to intense speedwork. Jolting the muscles this way tears them down and makes the rebuilding long and difficult. Each hill and speed workout is part of a gradual program, a series of stepping stones in which you gradually apply stress and then recover.

- *On a bad day.* If you're not up to an interval work-out, quit. Try it the next day or the day after. If it still doesn't feel right, try a fartlek session or hill workout to simulate the intensity and duration of the interval work. If you suspect you're overly tired, take a low mileage week to recover and then try again.

GETTING OFF ON THE WRONG FOOT

An early burst of speed doesn't mean much unless you're competing in a 100-yard dash. A would-be shoe thief found this out in our Atlanta Phidippides store a few years ago. The young man came in, looked at several items, then grabbed a pair of shoes and sped out the door. He didn't realize he was in a true running store. The staff members—competitive runners to a man—drew straws to determine the lucky pursuer. While the thief gained ground in the first 200 yards, our salesman caught him at 600 yards and recovered the shoes from a quarry too tired to resist.

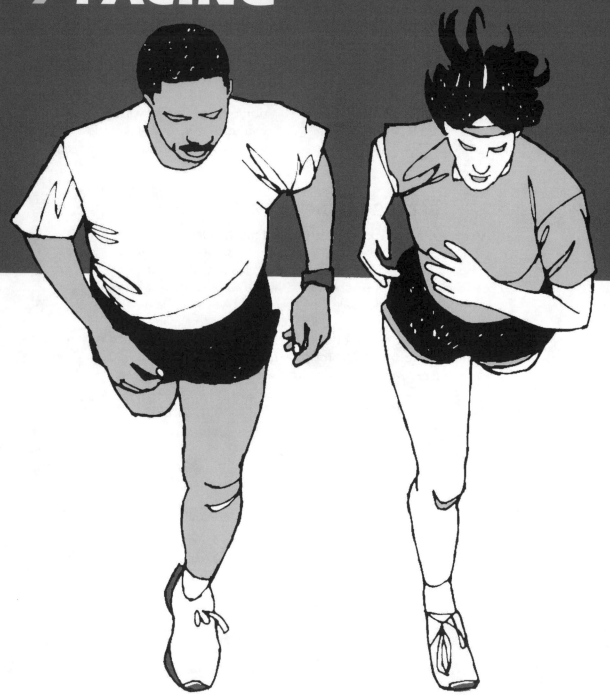

9 PACING

UNLESS YOU HAVE one of the new, high-tech accelerometer devices, it's always hard to tell how fast you are running. Slight physiological changes, tiredness, the weather, all affect your running speed. There are tests, however, which allow you to guess fairly accurately.

Speedwork as a Test. When you follow a speed program as indicated in the training charts, you're preparing yourself for a goal. It's also a gauge of fitness. If you were able to complete the workout about 10 days before the race in the assigned time, you're ready to run at your goal pace. If you finished the workout easily, or faster than expected (without realizing you were running faster), and recovered fast, you can expect to run faster than the goal pace. If you had trouble or couldn't complete the workout, you should readjust your goal to a slower time.

Test Races. If you schedule test races every other weekend leading up to the "big one," you'll get some valuable racing experience. After 2–3 such tests you should be able to estimate how fast your race goal should be. With a combination of speedwork and races as barometers, you can come up with an accurate estimate. Use the table *Predicting Your Race Performance (see pp. 266–269)* as a guide. While this has been a very reliable table over the span of a career, weather, hills, and turns on the course will slow down the race performance. I've run over 120 marathons, for example, and I've yet to see ideal conditions. Using the 5K distance as your test race, I'd recommend adding 30–60 seconds for a 10K and 5–10 minutes on a half-marathon.

Race Pace

In my senior year in high school, my training for the mile was going well. As I lined up against the South's best milers at the Florida Relays, I knew it was my day. Around the first turn I didn't have to strain to move ahead of all but one of the 60 competitors and registered a 59-second second lap (instead of my goal pace of 67 seconds). Running the fastest first lap of my life didn't faze me; I felt strong and was running smoothly. Coming off the last turn into the stretch, I accelerated and could almost touch the leader. Suddenly a gigantic 400-pound "bear" jumped on my back —or so it seemed. A tremendous surge of lactic acid turned my muscles into concrete. I stumbled along to the finish line in a daze, almost oblivious to the stream of runners going by me. Had I run even 2–3 seconds slower on the first lap, I probably could have run with strength to the finish.

Start Slow. Everyone knows you can get more out of a tank of gas by driving at an even speed. By stepping on the gas, then coasting, you ruin fuel economy. The same is true in racing. There's an old adage that for every second too fast per mile in the first half of the race, you'll run at least 2 seconds slower at the end. Moreover the problem increases if you run the first 2–3 miles too fast; *for every second too fast per mile in the first 2–3 miles of the race, you can be as much as 10 seconds slower at the end.*

Your body becomes more efficient as it warms up. The muscles, tendons, and joints work better after 10–20 minutes of activity. If you set up an inefficient situation at the beginning, it will be compounded throughout the rest of the race.

Recently I overheard one runner telling a friend he intended to run the first mile of the marathon in 8½ minutes. (His goal was a 7½-minute pace.) His more experienced friend just laughed. "You couldn't run the first mile that slow if you had three people hanging on your back!" Nevertheless, in spite of the adrenalin, excitement, and early-in-the-race speedsters, try to keep it down. You'll be glad later.

Run an Even-Paced Effort. If the course is perfectly flat with no wind, you can run an even pace throughout. But since most courses have hills and most days have wind, you must be realistic. Miles with hills should be run with the same effort as flat miles. Uphill segments will therefore be slower than "pace," and downhill segments faster. The same "even-effort" principle applies to running into the wind, but you cannot quite make up for time lost to a headwind, or to long or repeated hills.

Account for Heat. Most runners begin to slow down at 55° and start suffering at 65°. Of course, the body can adapt to heat

stress and push the threshold up a bit, but you'll never be able to run as fast on a 75° day as on a 45° one. High humidity is also a major problem. It's like a wet blanket—it doesn't allow much evaporation or perspiration and your body heat builds up.

If you try to run too hard in hot or humid conditions you'll hit "the wall" sooner than expected. Trying to maintain a goal pace in heat is like going out too fast early in the race. Temperatures generally increase hour by hour; therefore you must adjust your pace for the temperature expected at the end of the race.

Watch Out for Downhills. The Boston Marathon course goes sharply downhill for most of the first mile. On cool days, even experienced runners get caught up in the competition and fail to slow down when the course levels out. The results are often very fast times for the first ten miles and disappointing final results.

Be aware of your rhythm and pace after a hill. Time yourself carefully over the next mile or two and make sure you're not unconsciously going too fast.

Adjusting Race Pace for Heat

Estimated Temperature at Finish	Slower than Goal Pace	8-min./mile Pace Becomes
55–60°	1%	8:05
60–65°	3%	8:15
65–70°	5%	8:25
70–75°	7%	8:35
75–80°	12%	8:58
80–85°	20%	9:35
Above 85°	Forget it. Run for fun.	

Note: This chart is based upon my own experience in the heat and talking to other runners. It has no scientific verification, but I think you get the general idea.

Running "Bursts" in the Middle. Departing from an even pace can be disastrous at any point in the race. Competitive runners sometimes use "bursts" to gain a psychological edge. The idea is that these accelerations (usually 30–150 yards) put a runner ahead of an opponent or force him to spend energy to keep up. But the runner who does this is gambling that he's in better condition, or can demoralize the opposition and bluff into the lead. Bursts are an inefficient use of limited energy stores and I don't recommend them for the average runner.

What to Do When You Realize You've Run Too Fast? Don't slow down significantly below pace to compensate for going out too fast. If you already feel too tired or hot, slow down a small amount below goal pace (5–10 seconds a mile) for 2–3 miles. Never slow down dramatically below your goal pace, for this probably won't help you rest any more than cutting 5–10 seconds a mile. Don't assume you've blown it. You probably still have it in you to reach your goal. Just try to maintain your goal pace for the rest of the run.

WALK BREAKS

Our Running Heritage

As one who has proudly run for more than four decades, I find it hard sometimes to admit this, but here goes. Our bodies weren't designed to run continuously for long distances, especially distances as long as the marathon. Sure we can adapt, but there is a better way to increase endurance than by running continuously. By alternating walking and running, from the start, there's virtually no limit to the distance you can cover. Thousands of people in their forties and fifties with no exercise background have used the walk/run method to train for, and complete, a marathon after six months' training. Once we find the ideal ratio for a given distance, walk breaks allow us to feel strong to the end and recover fast, while building up the same levels of stamina and conditioning that we would have reached if we had run continuously.

Our ancient ancestors had to walk and run thousands of miles every year merely to survive. It is because they moved on to greener pastures and away from predators that we're here to philosophize about walk breaks. So it's a fact that each of us inherited an organism that was designed to move forward for long distances. As often happens with behaviors that promote survival, a series of complex and internally satisfying rewards has developed: the muscles relax, the creative and intuitive side of our brain is stimulated, and our spirits are energized. By getting out of the door and moving forward three or more times a week, even the most out-of-shape couch potato will discover this enhanced sense of self-worth and improved attitude.

Walking is our most efficient exercise pattern, but we can adapt to running and do well. Indeed, most walkers who add running to their exercise say they get a better boost in their after-exercise attitude. Running continuously, however, can quickly push us beyond the capacity of our leg muscles. When we alternate between walking and running, early and often, we are going back to the type of exertion that took our forebears across continents and over deserts and mountain ranges.

WALK BREAKS WILL...

- Allow those who can only run 2 miles to go 3 or 4 and feel fine
- Help beginners or heavy runners to increase their endurance to 5K, 10K or even the marathon in as little as six months
- Build up the endurance for runners of all abilities to go beyond "the wall"
- Allow runners over age 40 to not only do their first marathon but to improve times in most cases
- Help runners of all ages to improve times because legs are strong at the end
- Reduce the chance of injury and over-training to almost nothing

Walk Breaks Were Part of the Marathon—from the Beginning

Ancient Greek messengers such as the original marathoner Phidippides regularly covered distances of more than 100 kilometers a day by walking and running. The accounts of the original marathon race, in the 1896 Olympics, described significant periods of walking for all competitors, including the winner Spiros Louis.

Elite marathoners continue to use walk breaks. The great American marathoner, Bill Rodgers, has said many times that he had to walk at water stations during his marathon victories in Boston and New York City in order to get the water into his stomach (instead of wearing it on his shirt). To conserve his resources, Fabian Roncero took several walk breaks during his victory in the Rotterdam Marathon in 1998. He finished in 2 hours, 7 minutes, and 26 seconds, breaking the world record.

Running with Walk Breaks

Most runners will record significantly faster times when they take walk breaks because they don't slow down at the end of a long run. Thousands of veterans whose goal is to run faster have improved by 10, 20, 30 minutes and more in marathons by taking walk breaks early and often in the race. You can easily spot these folks: they're the ones who are picking up speed during the last 2–6 miles when everyone else is slowing down.

The title of marathoner has, from the beginning, been awarded to those who went the distance under their own power, whether they ran, walked, crawled, or tip-toed. When you cross that finish line, you've joined an elite group. About one-tenth of one percent of the population has done it. Don't let anyone take that great achievement away from you.

I've now done well over 100 marathons, about half of them without walk breaks. On every one of the walk-break marathons, I received the same sense of accomplishment, all of the internal rewards, and the indescribable exhilaration of finishing as on the non-walk-break marathons. But when I inserted walk breaks throughout, I was able to enjoy the accomplishment afterward.

Why Do Walk Breaks Work?

By varying the use of your muscles, your legs keep their bounce as they conserve resources. Walk breaks keep you from using up your resources early. By alternating the exertion level and the way you're using your running muscles, these prime movers have a chance to recover before they accumulate fatigue. On each successive walk, most or all of the fatigue is erased, giving you strength at the end. This dramatically reduces damage to the muscles, allowing you to carry on your life activities even after a marathon.

Walk breaks force you to slow down early in the run so that you don't start too fast. This conserves your energy, fluids, and muscle capacity. On each walk break, the running muscles make internal adaptations, which give you the option to finish under control, increase the pace, or go even further. When a muscle group, such as your calf, is used continuously step after step, it tires relatively soon. The weak areas get overused and force you to slow down later or scream at you in pain afterward. By shifting back and forth between walking and running muscles, you distribute the workload among a variety of muscles and increase your overall performance capacity. For veteran marathoners, this is often the difference between achieving a time goal or not.

Walk Breaks Can Eliminate Injury

Many runners who were injured during previous training programs (because they ran continuously) have stayed injury-free when they added walk breaks to long runs. If you don't walk from the beginning, your leg muscles fatigue more quickly and can't keep those lower extremities moving efficiently in their proper range of motion. The resulting wobble allows the leg to extend too far forward in an over-stride. This abuses the tendons and injures the small muscle groups that try to keep the body on its proper mechanical track but don't have the horsepower to control the body weight moving forward.

Walk breaks taken early in the run keep the muscles strong and resilient enough so that the legs can move with strength and efficiency throughout. This will significantly reduce or eliminate the excess stress around the knees, ankles, feet, etc. that produces injury. The little "back-up" muscle groups can stay in reserve and fine-tune the running motion after fatigue sets in.

When to Take Walk Breaks

The earlier you take the walk breaks, the more they help you! To receive maximum benefit, you must start the walk breaks in the first mile, before you feel any fatigue. If you wait until you feel the need for a walk break, you've already reduced your potential performance. Even waiting until the 2-mile mark to take the first break will reduce the resilience you could regain from walking in the first mile. To put it in shopping terms, would you like a discount? Walk breaks earn you a discount from the pounding on legs and feet. If you walk often enough, start early enough, and keep the pace slow enough, a 10-mile run leaves you no more tired than if you had run only 5 to 7 miles and a 20-miler makes you only as tired as a 12- to 15-mile run would.

Walk breaks can change a bad run into a regular one—and sometimes a into a great one. Sometimes we may not feel good as we start a run. Instead of quitting or suffering through (and then not wanting to run the next time), try a 1- to 2-minute walk break every 3 to 8 minutes. By breaking up your run early and often, you can still cover the distance you'd like to cover on that day, burn the calories you'd like to burn, and increase the chance that you'll enjoy the experience of running itself.

You don't need to take walk breaks on runs that are short enough and easy for you to run continuously. For example, if your current long run is 10 miles and you feel good as you start your Tuesday 5-miler, you don't need to put in walk breaks. If the walk breaks can make the experience better, however, take them!

When in Doubt, Walk

It's much better to take a 1-minute walk break every 5 minutes than to take a 5-minute walk every 25 minutes. By breaking up your run early—with even a short break—you allow for quicker and more effective recovery. If you're used to walking for 1 minute every 4 minutes but are not feeling good at the beginning of a run, walk for 2 minutes after running for 4, or for 1 minute after running for 2.

There's very little difference in benefit between these two intervals, but the more frequent break (a 1-minute walk after a 2-minute run) will keep the legs fresher. The longer you run continuously, the more fatigued the legs become. Remember that you lose only about 17 seconds when you walk for 1 minute. The short distance you lose on extra walking earlier will almost always be recovered at the end—because you kept your legs fresh. Those who put this concept to the test almost always find that taking more frequent walk breaks doesn't slow the overall time of long runs—when the long runs are done at the correct slow pace.

How Fast Should I Walk?

A slow walk is fine. When walking fast for 1 minute, most runners will lose about 15 seconds over running at their regular pace. But, even if you walk slowly, you'll lose only about 20 seconds. If you have a Type-A running personality and want to walk fast, make sure that you don't lengthen your walking stride too much. Monitor the tightness of your hamstrings and the tendons behind the knee. If you feel tension there, walk slowly with bent knees to keep that area relaxed. A slow walk is just as good as a fast one and may keep the leg muscles from getting tight.

Racewalking technique is also okay. As long as you receive qualified instruction and practice this regularly, racewalking will allow many runners to go faster during the walk breaks. Because a racewalk uses different muscle groups from those used in running, the prime running muscles are given time to recover and rebuild.

How Often Should I Walk?

As the long runs get longer, take the walk breaks more often. A runner who is comfortable running for 6 minutes and walking for 1 minute will, at 15 to 18 miles, take a break after every 5 minutes of running; at 20 miles, after every 4 minutes of running; and, at 23 miles, after every 3 minutes of running. But don't get too rigidly locked into a specific ratio of walk breaks.

Even if you run the same distance every day, you'll find that you'll need to vary the frequency of your walk breaks to account for speed, hills, heat, humidity, time off from training, etc. If you expect that your run will be more difficult or will require a longer recovery, take more frequent walk breaks (or longer walks); you may be surprised at how quickly you recover. On cold days, you may not need to take the walks as often (although it's not wise to reduce walk breaks in any run longer than 17 miles).

Can Walk Breaks Make Me Run Faster?

A survey of veteran marathoners showed an average improvement of 13 minutes when they put walk breaks into their marathon, rather than running continuously under the same conditions. By conserving the strength and efficiency of the running muscles through early walk breaks, you'll avoid the slowdown in the last 3 miles of a half-marathon, where most continuous runners lose their momentum. By making sure to walk before you get tired, you will be able to run with strength to the finish line, avoiding the 7- to 15-minute slowdown at the end. With proper speed training, pacing, and the right ratio of walking to running, you'll run faster during the last 6 to 8 miles because you walked early.

Do I Need to Take Walk Breaks on the Short Runs During the Week?

If you can now run continuously on shorter midweek runs, you don't have to take the walk breaks. If you want to take them, do so. Walk breaks on midweek runs will insure that you recover from the long runs as quickly as possible.

Do I Have to Take Walk Breaks at the End of My Runs If My Legs Are Tightening Up?

Take walk breaks as long as you can because they will speed your recovery. If your legs cramp up later during walk breaks then just shuffle through the breaks (by keeping your feet low to the ground and taking a short stride). At the end of a run, you want to stay as fluid as you can while still alternating the use of the muscle groups. Cramping at the end tells you to start more slowly in the next long run and to avoid dehydration the day before the run, the morning of the run, and during the run itself.

ARE WALK BREAKS FOR WIMPS?

A friend of mine in his late forties had been trying for years to run a 3:30 marathon, but 3:40 was as fast as he could run. According to the times of his 5K and 10K races, he should have been able to finish in about 3:25. He had done plenty of intense training in three different marathon campaigns, including high mileage, lots of speedwork, two runs a day, etc. Eventually, I told him that if he didn't run below 3:30 in his goal marathon, I'd return his check, and he sent in his entry form for my program. I never mentioned the walk breaks because I knew he would say something about "sissy stuff" and not sign up. I also knew that in the past he had probably over-trained for his goal and mainly needed to run with a group to slow down his pace on the long run.

After the very first session he came up to me, irate, and demanded his money back. "I can't do these walk breaks: they're wimpy!" I refused to return his check, reminding him that a deal was a deal. So he completed the program, complaining during just about every walk break. Secretly, he told friends in his pace group, he wasn't going to walk during the marathon itself.

On marathon morning, his group leader lined up with him and physically restrained him for 1 minute each mile, making him walk. Then, at 18 miles, the leader looked at my friend and said, "Well, you seem to have just enough life in your legs, so run along now!" And he did. His time was 3:25. He had run that marathon 15 minutes faster than ever before!

At first, he couldn't believe that he could improve that much while walking every mile. But when he analyzed his past marathons, he found that he had always slowed down in the last 6 to 8 miles. In this marathon, he kept picking up the pace after those first 18 miles and had knocked 5 minutes off his time in the last segment. He was forced to admit that the early and regular muscle shifts left his legs feeling strong and responsive all the way to the finish line.

EVEN A SHORT WALK BREAK WHEN TAKEN
EARLY AND REGULARLY WILL:

- Restore resiliency to the main running muscles before they fatigue—like getting a muscle strength booster shot each break

- Extend the capacity of the running muscles at the end of the run because you're shifting the workload between the walking and the running muscles

- Virtually erase fatigue with each early walk break by keeping your pace and effort level conservative in the early stages

- Allow those with some types of previous injuries to knees, ankles, hips, feet, etc. to train for marathons without further injury

- Leave you feeling good enough to carry on social and family activities

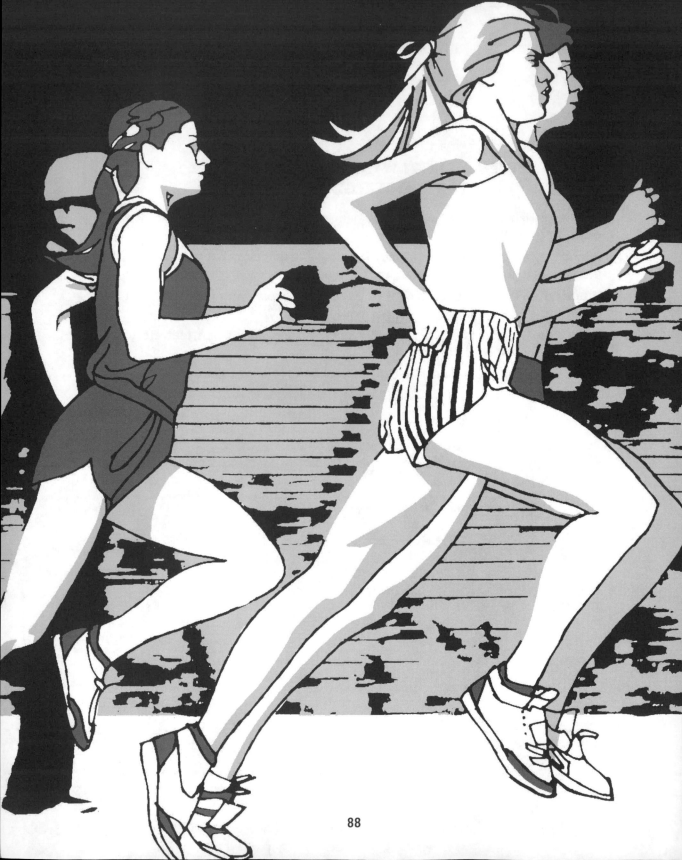

10
THE ART OF RACING
5K, 10K, HALF-MARATHON

Most of the information in this chapter refers to 5K–10K races.
Much of it can also be applied to half-marathons and races 30K (18.6 miles) or less.

JUST ABOUT ALL OF US have a competitive streak. Races can be an outlet for this tendency and give a special edge to running— whether you want to win, or just finish. On those days when motivation is low, the thought of an upcoming race can often get you out on the roads. You look forward to the excitement of a race—it's like deadline for a reporter, or a punctuation mark at the end of a sentence.

Races can actually be rewards for hard training. There's a positive atmosphere and contagious energy. Marking a race date on your calendar will give you a goal for structuring a running program.

Beware, however, for the excitement and stimulation of races can cause you to push your body too far and provoke injury. Races are intense. You may survive the race, but fail to rest afterward—and become injured. The thrill of participation and achievement often lures runners into the "twilight zone" that is part injury and part success. If all goes well and luck is with you, you may run your best time ever. But unfortunately, things are often not in balance, and by pushing too hard in a race, some parts of the body will be overstressed.

Race euphoria can give you illusions of strength and invincibility. The mind recovers quickly from a hard race, but it takes the body longer. The race is really the ego icing on the cake. Your time "under the lights" may give more meaning to your daily run, but it's second in importance to your overall fitness. Remember, the true benefits of running come from the peace and physical and psychological strength found in the daily run, not from a 20-second improvement in your race time.

I've come to believe that race times and age group awards are great for the ego. But you shouldn't let your ego determine your ultimate satisfaction from running. I've seen too many runners burn out because they start with a few races, then start measuring their progress only by time improvement. Finally they judge the quality of a run, or the status of another runner solely by the minutes and seconds in the race results, or PR (personal record), and quit running.

Setting Race Goals. Realism is the key to effective goal-setting. A 59-minute 10K runner cannot realistically project a 49-minute 10K by the end of the racing season. Even 54 minutes is too ambitious for that limited length of time.

Set goals you have a reasonable chance of achieving. We all have to deal with failure from time to time, but why push yourself into it? Set up a series of incremental goals, each leading to the other. Experiencing one small success after another builds confidence. Then if you surprise yourself and do better than anticipated, it's an unexpected thrill. *(See pp. 42–43.)*

Peaking

"Peaking" refers to a careful scheduling of key workouts at the end of the speed phase that can raise your performance potential to its highest level. Speedwork and long runs are scheduled to build the racing muscles to top efficiency.

The race training schedules *(see pp. 96–125)* bring you to a peak for each race. Peaking schedules are normally designed for 10K and shorter races. You must have enough quality work carefully planned to bring you up to—and keep you at—your peak.

Time your training peak to occur at the race of your choice about two weeks before the goal race. This gives you a "dry run" to evaluate your fitness, readjust if necessary and work out any last-minute bugs in the system.

The Day Before. I've always felt better running a few miles rather than none at all the day before a race less than half-marathon distance. This small amount doesn't tire me out, and keeps the muscles moving and the blood circulating. I enter the race feeling rested and fresh. But some runners feel better if they don't run at all. Most runners feel that walking a mile or two (as in strolling through the race expo, or mall) is better than no exercise at all, the day before a race.

Eating and Drinking Before the Race. A balanced diet is the best insurance against nutrition collapse. Don't change your diet right before a race, use the one that works best for you in daily life. As you get closer to the race, don't eat foods that are hard to digest, such as fried or fatty foods, milk, cheese, or other large amounts of protein. Avoid too much roughage.

Anything you eat 12–18 hours before the race won't be processed in time to help you. Instead, you'll be carrying it along. Since you don't want to "carbo-unload" during the race, avoid this excess baggage in the first place. Make lunch the day before the race your last solid-food meal. During the last 12–18 hours, cut solid foods and reduce total food intake. Fluids are crucial. Take 6–8 ounces of water or an electrolyte beverage every hour, especially the day before a race. This means 3–4 quarts a day—better safe than sorry.

Electrolytes are the minerals your body loses in exercising, particularly potassium and magnesium. Orange juice and the commercial sports drinks are good sources of these. Calcium is also important in maintaining heart rhythm, muscle contraction and healing. *(For more details on food and water before a race, see* Fuel, *p. 224.)*

Warming Up for the Race. Races bring you from a state of inactivity to top capacity rapidly. A warm-up should start slowly and gradually get the body moving. Slow running warms up the muscles, tendons and other mechanical apparatus simultaneously with the internal organs—and gets everything working as a unit.

Warming up for a race is psychological as well as physical. Work out a routine that becomes automatic. You'll start slowly, increase intensity to simulate race conditions, then rest and store up energy so you're ready to go. As you develop a set routine, you'll develop confidence, reducing pre-race anxiety.

Relaxing Is Part of the Warm-up. As I started my warmup for the 1972 Olympic trials 10K, I felt the usual surge of nervous anxiety; this was compounded by the fact that I was running with two formidable veterans, Frank Shorter and Jack Bacheler. As we ran along, warming up, I nervously tried to joke with my running partners, but I got only negative feedback. Finally I gave up and we ran a mile in silence until Frank's terse statement about the weather: "Sorta windy." Jack quickly replied, "Yeah, just like the Texas Relays."

A tense silence followed. I remembered that earlier in the year, on a windy track in Austin, Frank had suffered one of his few bad days of the year and Jack had won the 10K. The rivalry between the two was surfacing. I realized that each of them was as nervous and tense as I was — maybe more — and I suddenly relaxed.

I began looking forward to the race. Looking around at the other runners on the starting line — most of whom had defeated me in every race we'd run together — I saw scared faces and tunnel vision. I was ready to run!

The gun fired and we took off. I didn't expect to do well and settled into the back of the pack to watch the leaders battle it out. Besides, it was 95° — too hot for a fast time. So I chuckled to myself as teammate Frank Shorter led the pack through a suicidal first mile of 4:21.

Later, when I passed that one-mile mark, I moved past someone and out of last place. By two miles I'd passed two others who had been burned by the heat and Shorter's pace. By the halfway mark I was in the middle of the pack and gloating about doing better than expected.

Then something happened. As I passed another two runners, I realized almost everyone else in this race was falling apart, while I felt fine. At four miles, when I moved into fourth place, I began to worry about a mistake I'd later pay for dearly.

But no problems occurred. With slightly more than a mile to go, I moved into third place, then into second behind Shorter and qualified for the Munich Olympics. I don't remember touching the track during the last mile. I had learned a powerful secret.

Race Pacing. As the gun fires, go with the flow of energy and adrenalin. You can afford to go a little faster for the first 100–200 yards (to get a little better position in the crowd) without any bad effects, provided you slow down to race pace after that. An early burst will force those behind you to work harder to pass you, instead of the burden being upon you. Of course, big races like Bay to Breakers in San Francisco or Peachtree in Atlanta are so crowded you have no choice but to run them as fun runs.

Settle Down. Don't let the energy of the crowd pull you faster than your race pace for more than a few hundred yards. You'll have a sense of pace from your interval speedwork repetitions. In fact, run the first mile of your race about 10 seconds slower than race pace, to get thoroughly warmed up. Then get into your race pace and hold it; otherwise you'll miss your goal. Remember, for every second per mile you go too fast in the first half of the race, you'll run 5–10 seconds or more slower at the end.

I generally run my first mile of a marathon 15–20 seconds slower than goal pace. This warms me up and lets me relax. By the 3–5 mile points I've eased into my goal pace and I've never had trouble making up those few seconds during the last few miles.

Run Steady. Even-paced running is the most effective strategy, Whatever your fitness level, you'll have a faster time if you keep a steady, even pace. Energy and oxygen are used more effectively at a steady pace, and you keep heat build-up to a minimum. This means that uphill miles can be a bit slower, and the downhill ones a bit faster.

Beat the Heat. Another reason to start slowly and to run your own steady-effort pace race during the first half is to keep cool. Getting too hot slows you down severely, so watch it when it's 60° or more. The faster your body temperature rises, the more blood flows to the skin to reduce heat, and the more you sweat. Both reduce the amount of blood available to the muscles, which in turn determines oxygen supply and waste removal. When capillaries near the skin dilate to cool you off, they use a substantial amount of blood. Sweat loss ultimately reduces the blood supply.

Negative Split. If you maintain an even (and reasonable) pace in the first half, you'll actually speed up slightly during the second half: your body mechanics become more efficient as you run. By conserving your resources during the first half of the race, you'll have strength during the second half (a negative split in the second half).

Dehydration and Cooling. Drinking enough water is crucially important—especially in a race. Lately I've discovered that many of the undesirable aspects of racing—poor performance, muscle soreness, even injury—are partially or wholly attributable to dehydration. When you perspire, the water is drawn from the blood stream. If you haven't had enough water there'll be a shortage of this vital fluid for the cells and muscles. Glycogen won't be as efficiently converted to fuel, wastes won't be eliminated properly, and oxygen cannot be delivered quickly. With dehydration, all the stressful demands of racing are multiplied. To combat this:

- *Drink at least one full cup at each fluid station,* especially early in the race, even if you're not thirsty. (You become dehydrated before you realize you need water.) If you hear sloshing in your stomach, you have enough water and can by-pass that water stop.

- *Pour water on your head.* It cools your body, lowering your core temperature. I also believe, although I've seen no scientific verification, that in cooling your skin, you reduce the blood being diverted there. This makes more blood available for other vital body functions. Again, do this if the temperature is above 60 degrees F, even if you don't feel hot in the early stages of the race.

- *Stay on pace.* Take pride in being close to your projected pace for the various check points. When you do you'll be amazed at the number of runners you'll pass later on. When you're tired at the end, it's reinforcing and inspiring to pass a stream of runners.

Hurting. If you're going to race competitively (rather than "just for fun") you'll have to learn how to cope with exhausting discomfort. You'll also have to distinguish between the feeling that goes along with pushing yourself to a peak performance and the pain that means injury. Experienced athletes have learned to walk this tightrope very well. Of course you won't push things to the extent they do, but it's helpful for anyone interested in racing to know why all-out performance hurts, and to experience these feelings in smaller doses before the big race.

When you're working the muscles harder than you have before, they cannot get enough oxygen to perform smoothly. The glucose fuel that feeds them is in a sense fermented, and in powering the muscles, produces more wastes than your body can handle. What speedwork does—and you can see why it's important to go at it gradually—is to increase the ability of the muscle to use a limited supply of oxygen, and to continue performing when waste is present.

With each properly administered speed session you'll be pushing a little further and harder than before. The mitochondria will be slightly swollen, cell walls slightly torn and there'll be a buildup of lactic acid *(see p. 25)*. It will hurt. But with proper rest, everything will be repaired and strengthened. All of your performance systems respond to stress by becoming more efficient, so that you can respond to greater stress in the near future. The human organism is designed to get better after you've put it through the non-overwhelming stress of regular workouts, increasing your capacity to go farther and/or faster in your next one. It's called "the overload principle."

In training, you'll learn to live with this feeling. You'll take it in small doses in practice, so that the discomfort and temporary pain is not overwhelming in a race. You'll get better and better at accessing your tolerance. Although toward the end of the race you may feel that you'll never do this again, 30 minutes (or a few days) afterward, you'll be looking for the next one.

> **Note:** Certainly you should be careful. Heart patients must heed their physician's advice. Even seasoned athletes need to distinguish between discomfort on one hand, and true signs of spent muscles and actual endurance limits on the other.

Creative Distractions. Distraction is a strong ally. When you get into the tired zone, try to bluff your way through with positive thoughts. When these wear out, try distractions: passing the next runner, making it to the next telephone pole, or merely maintaining the same rhythm for the next five steps. At this point you may drift into a "cruising" state, into the creative and intuitive world of your right brain. Creative distractions will inspire more mental entertainment. *(For more information about motivation and mental strength, see* Mental Training, *p. 171.)*

Tapping the Source. If you can occasionally overcome the tiredness, and speed up when you'd normally slow down, you'll find a great source of strength and power.

Once you've tapped this source in running, you can do the same in other areas of your life when the going gets tough. You can discover this strength in a series of small excursions into the "twilight zone." At first you learn to tell when you've reached it. Next, you take small pushes into it. Next, bigger pushes. Some days you'll overestimate your capabilities and fall short. But if you're patient and keep at it, you can learn to utilize this strength on a regular basis.

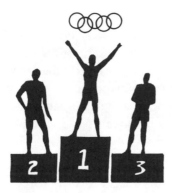

THE COUNTDOWN

The Week Before. Your work is over. Don't push too hard now or you'll be too tired to race well. Run short, easy workouts, no more than 1–3 miles the last three days. Let your racing muscles rest and rebuild. Eat a normal diet and drink 4–6 ounces of water per hour.

Two Nights Before. Get a good night's sleep.

The Night Before

- Pack your bag.
- Eat a very light meal or nothing. (I don't believe in carbo-loading the night before races, even marathons.)

- Drink 4–6 ounces of water every waking hour (unless you hear a sloshing sound in your stomach).
- Try to relax so you can sleep. But if you can't sleep, the race isn't lost. (I've run some of my best races after sleepless nights.)

Check List

- Shoes, socks, shirt, shorts, sweats or running suit
- Gloves, hat, turtleneck, etc., if cold
- Water (about a quart)
- Bandages and Vaseline
- $25–50 for registration, gas, food afterward, etc.
- Race number if sent to you in mail, 4 small safety pins
- Copy of *Race Morning* instructions *(see below)*

Race Morning

It's hard to remember all these things at the last minute. Photocopy these pages and put them in your bag the night before.

- After you wake, drink 4–6 ounces of water every half-hour.
- Drink your last water a half-hour before the race.
- Don't eat, it won't get processed in time to do you any good. (Those who need to boost their blood sugar level should eat the same food, in the same quantity that they have found works for them in other races or hard workouts.)
- 30–40 minutes before the race, start your warm-up.

Before You "Toe the Line"

- *Walk* 5 minutes to activate the running muscles gently and prepare the body for exertion, then jog for 1–2 minutes and walk for 1–2 minutes.

- *Jog* slowly 10–20 minutes. Start *very* slowly, then speed up gradually to a relaxed warm-up pace.

- *Stretch* gently if you need to stretch (ilio-tibial band injury, etc.). I've seen more problems when runners stretch before fast runs, than among those who don't stretch at all. If you have found stretching to be beneficial for you, then go ahead, but be very careful.

- *Walk* another 3–5 minutes to relax.

- About 10–15 minutes before the start, do some *accelerations* to get your body ready for race conditions. Do 5–10 × 50–100 yards. Start slowly, accelerate gradually to race pace, then ease back to a slow jog.

- *Walk* again, 3–5 minutes.

- About 5–10 minutes before the start, *relax*, sit down, walk around—whatever takes the edge off. Some runners put their legs above their heads, others meditate for 5 minutes.

- *Shift gears* as you line up. Tense muscles don't work smoothly. Joke, and enjoy the festive air, energy, and enthusiasm. This relaxes muscles throughout the body and gets them ready.

After the Gun

- Remember—go out slowly, settle into your pace, and hold it.

- If it's hot, pour water over your head and dampen clothes about 10 minutes before the race. Drink at every water stop.

- Relax during the race—enjoy the experience.

Right After the Race

- Keep walking. Try to walk a mile right afterward.

- Drink 6 ounces of a sports drink or some other dilute fluid every 20 minutes for three hours. If you have been sweating heavily for more than three hours, eat a salty food.

- Walk or walk-jog about 30–40 minutes later in the day. It will help you recover.

THE MORNING AFTER

- Walk/jog 30–40 minutes to get the stiffness out.

- Keep drinking 4–6 ounces of water (or electrolyte beverage) every waking hour.

- Wait at least a week before you (a) schedule your next race or (b) vow never to race again.

11
TRAINING CHARTS

On the following pages are training charts for 5K, 10K, and half-marathon races.

5K TRAINING PROGRAM: To Finish

Week #	Mon	Tue	Wed	Thu	Fri	Sat	Sun
1.	off or XT	10 min. run/walk	off or XT	10 min. run/walk	off or XT	off	1 mile run/walk
2.	off or XT	13 min. run/walk	off or XT	13 min. run/walk	off or XT	off	1.5 miles run/walk
3.	off or XT	15 min. run/walk	off or XT	15 min. run/walk	off or XT	off	2.0 miles run/walk
4.	off or XT	17 min. run/walk	off or XT	17 min. run/walk	off or XT	off	2.5 miles run/walk
5.	off or XT	19 min. run/walk	off or XT	19 min. run/walk	off or XT	off	3.0 miles run/walk
6.	off or XT	20 min. run/walk	off or XT	20 min. run/walk	off or XT	off	3.5 miles run/walk
7.	off or XT	20 min. run/walk	off or XT	20 min. run/walk	off or XT	off	**5K Race**
8.	off or XT	20 min. run/walk	off or XT	20 min. run/walk	off or XT	off	2–3 miles run/walk

This program assumes that you have not been running at all. If you are already doing more than is on this schedule, you can continue to maintain that schedule, as long as the legs are recovering quickly between runs.

1. You can do the long run on Saturday if you wish. In that case, take Friday off from exercise.

2. On your long runs, take more liberal walk breaks. If you are running 3 minutes and walking for 1 minute on your Tuesday runs, do 1–1 on the long runs. The pace of long runs should be at least two minutes per mile slower than a very conservative 5K race estimate.

3. On your Tuesday runs, take as many walk breaks as you need. Read the section on walk breaks and when in doubt, walk more.

4. XT means cross train. You can walk or do some form of non-pounding exercise, such as swimming, cycling, or exercise machines, for 10 minutes or so at an easy pace. If you are just starting to do any of these exercises (or are starting back after a layoff), start with only 5 minutes, and increase by 2–3 minutes each session. Water running is the best form of cross training.

5. In the 5K itself, most should take some walk breaks each mile, as you feel comfortable. Most runners should do the first 1–2 miles, taking the walk breaks as you have in the long runs. During the last mile you can cut out some or all of the walking, if you feel strong.

5K TRAINING PROGRAM: 45 min. goal

Week #	Mon	Tue	Wed	Thu	Fri	Sat	Sun
1.	off or XT	10 min. run/walk	off or XT	*(3 x 400) speed day	off or XT	off	1.5 miles run/walk
2.	off or XT	13 min. run/walk	off or XT	*(4 x 400) speed day	off or XT	off	2.0 miles run/walk
3.	off or XT	15 min. run/walk	off or XT	*(5 x 400) speed day	off or XT	off	2.5 miles run/walk
4.	off or XT	17 min. run/walk	off or XT	*(6 x 400) speed day	off or XT	off	3.0 miles run/walk
5.	off or XT	19 min. run/walk	off or XT	*(7 x 400) speed day	off or XT	off	3.5 miles run/walk
6.	off or XT	20 min. run/walk	off or XT	*(8 x 400) speed day	off or XT	off	4.0 miles run/walk
7.	off or XT	20 min. run/walk	off or XT	*(4 x 400) speed day	off or XT	off	**5K Race**
8.	off or XT	20 min. run/walk	off or XT	20 min. run/walk	off or XT	off	2–3 miles run/walk

This program assumes that you have been running at least at the level of running listed in the first week, for at least 2 months prior to the start of the program. If you are already doing more than this, you can continue to maintain that schedule, as long as the legs are recovering quickly between runs.

1. You can do the long run on Saturday if you wish. In that case, take Friday off from exercise.

2. On your long runs, take more liberal walk breaks. If you are running 3 minutes and walking for 1 minute on your Tuesday runs, do 2–1 on the long runs (or 2-minute walk and 2-minute run on bad days). The pace of long runs should be at least 1 minute per mile slower than your goal race pace (16+ min./mi.).

3. On your Tuesday runs, take as many walk breaks as you need. Read the section on walk breaks and when in doubt, walk more.

4. XT means cross train. You can walk or do some form of non-pounding exercise, such as swimming, cycling, or exercise machines, for 10 minutes or so at an easy pace. If you are just starting to do any of these exercises (or are starting back after a layoff), start with only 5 minutes, and increase by 2–3 minutes each session.

5. In the 5K itself, most should take some walk breaks each mile, as you feel comfortable. Most runners should do the first 1–2 miles, taking the walk breaks as you have in the long runs. During the last mile you can cut out some or all of the walking, if you feel strong. Be sure to move to the side of the road before taking walk breaks.

6.*Denotes speed day. Go to a local track. After a 4–5-minute warm-up, do the number of 400-meter laps assigned, running each in 3:28–3:30. Walk slowly for half a lap and repeat. Do a 4–5-minute warm-down afterward.

5K TRAINING PROGRAM: 38 min. goal

Week #	Mon	Tue	Wed	Thu	Fri	Sat	Sun
1.	off or XT	10 min. run/walk	off or XT	*(3 x 400) speed day	off or XT	off	2.0 miles run/walk
2.	off or XT	13 min. run/walk	off or XT	*(4 x 400) speed day	off or XT	off	2.5 miles run/walk
3.	off or XT	15 min. run/walk	off or XT	*(5 x 400) speed day	off or XT	off	3.0 miles run/walk
4.	off or XT	17 min. run/walk	off or XT	*(6 x 400) speed day	off or XT	off	3.5 miles run/walk
5.	off or XT	19 min. run/walk	off or XT	*(7 x 400) speed day	off or XT	off	4.0 miles run/walk
6.	off or XT	20 min. run/walk	off or XT	*(8 x 400) speed day	off or XT	off	4.5 miles run/walk
7.	off or XT	20 min. run/walk	off or XT	*(4 x 400) speed day	off or XT	off	**5K Race**
8.	off or XT	20 min. run/walk	off or XT	20 min. run/walk	off or XT	off	2–3 miles run/walk

This program assumes that you have been running at least at the level of running listed in the first week, for at least 2 months prior to the start of the program. If you are already doing more than this, you can continue to maintain that schedule, as long as the legs are recovering quickly between runs.

1. You can do the long run on Saturday if you wish. In that case, take Friday off from exercise.

2. On your long runs, take more liberal walk breaks. If you are running 3 minutes and walking for 1 minute on your Tuesday runs, do 2–1 on the long runs (or 2-minute walk and 2-minute run on bad days). The pace of long runs should be at least 1 minute per mile slower than your goal race pace (13:30+ min./mi.).

3. On your Tuesday runs, take as many walk breaks as you need. Read the section on walk breaks and when in doubt, walk more.

4. XT means cross train. You can walk or do some form of non-pounding exercise, such as swimming, cycling, or exercise machines, for 10 minutes or so at an easy pace. If you are just starting to do any of these exercises (or are starting back after a layoff), start with only 5 minutes, and increase by 2–3 minutes each session.

5. In the 5K itself, most should take some walk breaks each mile, as you feel comfortable. Most runners should do the first 1–2 miles, taking the walk breaks as you have in the long runs. During the second and third miles you can cut out some or all of the walking, if you feel strong. Be sure to move to the side of the road before taking walk breaks.

6.*Denotes speed day. Go to a local track. After a 4–5-minute warm-up, do the number of 400-meter laps assigned, running each in 2:52–2:55. Walk slowly for half a lap and repeat. Do a 4–5-minute warm-down afterward.

5K TRAINING PROGRAM: 30 min. goal

Week #	Mon	Tue	Wed	Thu	Fri	Sat	Sun
1.	off or XT	15 min. run/walk	off or XT	*(3×400) speed day	off or XT	off	2.0 miles run/walk
2.	off or XT	18 min. run/walk	off or XT	*(4×400) speed day	off or XT	off	2.5 miles run/walk
3.	off or XT	20 min. run/walk	off or XT	*(5×400) speed day	off or XT	off	3.0 miles run/walk
4.	off or XT	22 min. run/walk	off or XT	*(6×400) speed day	off or XT	off	3.5 miles run/walk
5.	off or XT	25 min. run/walk	off or XT	*(7×400) speed day	off or XT	off	4.0 miles run/walk
6.	off or XT	27 min. run/walk	off or XT	*(8×400) speed day	off or XT	off	4.5 miles run/walk
7.	off or XT	20 min. run/walk	off or XT	*(4×400) speed day	off or XT	off	**5K Race**
8.	off or XT	20 min. run/walk	off or XT	20 min. run/walk	off or XT	off	2–3 miles run/walk

This program assumes that you have been running at least at the level of running listed in the first week, for at least 2 months prior to the start of the program. If you are already doing more than this, you can continue to maintain that schedule, as long as the legs are recovering quickly between runs.

1. You can do the long run on Saturday if you wish. In that case, take Friday off from exercise.

2. On your long runs, take more liberal walk breaks. If you are running 4 minutes and walking for 1 minute on your Tuesday runs, do 3–1 on the long runs (or 2–1 on bad days). The pace of long runs should be at least 1 minute per mile slower than your goal race pace (11+ min./mi.).

3. On your Tuesday runs, take as many walk breaks as you need. Read the section on walk breaks and when in doubt, walk more.

4. XT means cross train. You can walk or do some form of non-pounding exercise, such as swimming, cycling, or exercise machines, for 10 minutes or so at an easy pace. If you are just starting to do any of these exercises (or are starting back after a layoff), start with only 5 minutes, and increase by 2–3 minutes each session.

5. In the 5K itself, most should take some walk breaks each mile, as you feel comfortable. Most runners should do the first 1–2 miles, taking the walk breaks as you have in the long runs. During the second and third miles you can cut out some or all of the walking, if you feel strong. Be sure to move to the side of the road before taking walk breaks.

6. *Denotes speed day. Go to a local track. After a 4–5-minute warm-up, do the number of 400-meter laps assigned, running each in 2:15–2:18. Walk slowly for half a lap and repeat. Do at least a 5-minute warm-down afterward.

5K TRAINING PROGRAM: 25 min. goal

Week #	Mon	Tue	Wed	Thu	Fri	Sat	Sun
1.	off or XT	18 min. run/walk	off or XT	*(5×400) speed day	off or XT	off	2.5 miles run/walk
2.	off or XT	20 min. run/walk	off or XT	*(6×400) speed day	off or XT	off	3.0 miles run/walk
3.	off or XT	22 min. run/walk	off or XT	*(7×400) speed day	off or XT	off	3.5 miles run/walk
4.	off or XT	25 min. run/walk	off or XT	*(8×400) speed day	off or XT	off	4.0 miles run/walk
5.	off or XT	27 min. run/walk	off or XT	*(9×400) speed day	off or XT	off	**5K Race**
6.	off or XT	30 min. run/walk	off or XT	*(10×400) speed day	off or XT	off	5.0 miles run/walk
7.	off or XT	20 min. run/walk	off or XT	*(4×400) speed day	off or XT	off	**5K Race**
8.	off or XT	20 min. run/walk	off or XT	20 min. run/walk	off or XT	off	2–4 miles run/walk

This program assumes that you have been running at least at the level of running listed in the first week, for at least 2 months prior to the start of the program. If you are already doing more than this, you can continue to maintain that schedule, as long as the legs are recovering quickly between runs.

1. You can do the long run on Saturday if you wish. In that case, take Friday off from exercise.

2. On your long runs, take more liberal walk breaks. If you are running 6 minutes and walking for 1 minute on your Tuesday runs, do 5–1 on the long runs (or 4–1 on bad days). The pace of long runs should be at least two minutes per mile slower than your goal race pace (10:00 min./mi.).

3. On your Tuesday runs, take as many walk breaks as you need. Read the section on walk breaks and when in doubt, walk more.

4. XT means cross train. You can walk or do some form of non-pounding exercise, such as swimming, cycling, or exercise machines, for 10 minutes or so at an easy pace. If you are just starting to do any of these exercises (or are starting back after a layoff), start with only 5 minutes, and increase by 2–3 minutes each session.

5. The 5K race in week 5 is a test race. Run the first mile 30 seconds slower than the goal pace. Try to run the goal pace during miles 2 and 3.

6. In the 5K race, pace yourself conservatively. The first mile should be about 5–10 seconds slower than goal pace. Then gradually increase the pace to the end of the race. The fastest mile should be mile #3.

7.* Denotes speed day. Go to a local track. After a warm-up of at least 5 minutes, do the number of 400-meter laps assigned, running each in 1:52–1:55. Walk slowly for half a lap and repeat. Do at least a 5-minute warm-down afterward.

5K TRAINING PROGRAM: 22 min. goal

Week #	Mon	Tue	Wed	Thu	Fri	Sat	Sun
1.	off or XT	20 min. run/walk	off or XT	*(6×400) speed day	off or XT	off	3.0 miles run/walk
2.	off or XT	22 min. run/walk	off or XT	*(7×400) speed day	off or XT	off	3.5 miles run/walk
3.	off or XT	25 min. run/walk	off or XT	*(8×400) speed day	off or XT	off	4.0 miles run/walk
4.	off or XT	28 min. run/walk	off or XT	*(9×400) speed day	off or XT	off	4.5 miles run/walk
5.	off or XT	30 min. run/walk	off or XT	*(10×400) speed day	off or XT	off	**5K Race**
6.	off or XT	30 min. run/walk	off or XT	*(12×400) speed day	off or XT	off	5.5 miles run/walk
7.	off or XT	25 min. run/walk	off or XT	*(5×400) speed day	off or XT	off	**5K Race**
8.	off or XT	30 min. run/walk	off or XT	30 min. run/walk	off or XT	off	3–5 miles run/walk

This program assumes that you have been running at least at the level of running listed in the first week, for at least 2 months prior to the start of the program. If you are already doing more than this, you can continue to maintain that schedule, as long as the legs are recovering quickly between runs.

1. You can do the long run on Saturday if you wish. In that case, take Friday off from exercise.

2. On your long runs, take more liberal walk breaks. If you are running 8 minutes and walking for 1 minute on your Tuesday runs, do 6–1 on the long runs (or 5–1 on bad days). The pace of long runs should be at least two minutes per mile slower than your goal race pace (9:00 min./mi.).

3. On your Tuesday runs, take as many walk breaks as you need—but you may not need to take them. Read the section on walk breaks and when in doubt, walk more.

4. XT means cross train. You can walk or do some form of non-pounding exercise, such as swimming, cycling, or exercise machines, for 10 minutes or so at an easy pace. If you are just starting to do any of these exercises (or are starting back after a layoff), start with only 5 minutes, and increase by 2–3 minutes each session. Water running is the best form of cross training.

5. The 5K race in week 5 is a test race. Run the first mile 30 seconds slower than the goal pace. Try to run the goal pace during miles 2 and 3.

6. In the 5K race, pace yourself conservatively. The first mile should be about 5–10 seconds slower than goal pace. Then gradually increase the pace to the end of the race. The fastest mile should be mile #3.

7.*Denotes speed day. Go to a local track. After a warm-up of at least 5 minutes, do the number of 400-meter laps assigned, running each in 1:35–1:40. Walk slowly for half a lap and repeat. Do at least a 5-minute warm-down afterward.

5K TRAINING PROGRAM: 19 min. goal

Week #	Mon	Tue	Wed	Thu	Fri	Sat	Sun
1.	off or XT	30 min. run/walk	off or XT	*(7 x 400) speed day	off or XT	off	4 miles run/walk
2.	off or XT	33 min. run/walk	off or XT	*(8 x 400) speed day	off or XT	off	5 miles run/walk
3.	off or XT	36 min. run/walk	off or XT	*(9 x 400) speed day	off or XT	off	6 miles run/walk
4.	off or XT	39 min. run/walk	off or XT	*(10 x 400) speed day	off or XT	off	7 miles run/walk
5.	off or XT	42 min. run/walk	off or XT	*(11 x 400) speed day	off or XT	off	**5K Race**
6.	off or XT	45 min. run/walk	off or XT	*(13 x 400) speed day	off or XT	off	9 miles run/walk
7.	off or XT	30 min. run/walk	off or XT	*(6 x 400) speed day	off or XT	off	**5K Race**
8.	off or XT	30 min. run/walk	off or XT	30 min. run/walk	off or XT	off	4–8 miles run/walk

This program assumes that you have been running at least at the level of running listed in the first week, for at least 2 months prior to the start of the program. If you are already doing more than this, you can continue to maintain that schedule, as long as the legs are recovering quickly between runs.

1. You can do the long run on Saturday if you wish. In that case, take Friday off from exercise.

2. On your long runs, take more liberal walk breaks. If you are running 9 minutes and walking for 1 minute on your Tuesday runs, do 7–1 on the long runs (or 6–1 on bad days). The pace of long runs should be at least two minutes per mile slower than your goal race pace (8:00 min./mi.).

3. On your Tuesday runs, take as many walk breaks as you need, but you may not need to walk. Read the section on walk breaks and when in doubt, walk more.

4. XT means cross train. You can walk or do some form of non-pounding exercise, such as swimming, cycling, or exercise machines, for 10 minutes or so at an easy pace. If you are just starting to do any of these exercises (or are starting back after a layoff), start with only 5 minutes, and increase by 2–3 minutes each session. Water running is the best form of cross training.

5. The 5K race in week 5 is a test race. Run the first mile 30 seconds slower than the goal pace. Try to run the goal pace during miles 2 and 3.

6. In the 5K race, pace yourself conservatively. The first mile should be about 5–10 seconds slower than goal pace. Then gradually increase the pace to the end of the race. The fastest mile should be mile #3.

7.*Denotes speed day. Go to a local track. After a warm-up of at least 5 minutes, do the number of 400-meter laps assigned, running each in 1:22–1:25. Walk slowly for half a lap and repeat. Do at least a 5-minute warm-down afterward.

5K TRAINING PROGRAM: 17 min. goal

Week #	Mon	Tue	Wed	Thu	Fri	Sat	Sun
1.	off or XT	30 min. run/walk	off or XT	*(7 × 400) speed day	off or XT	off	5 miles run/walk
2.	off or XT	33 min. run/walk	off or XT	*(8 × 400) speed day	off or XT	off	6 miles run/walk
3.	off or XT	36 min. run/walk	off or XT	*(9 × 400) speed day	off or XT	off	7 miles run/walk
4.	off or XT	39 min. run/walk	off or XT	*(10 × 400) speed day	off or XT	off	8 miles run/walk
5.	off or XT	42 min. run/walk	off or XT	*(12 × 400) speed day	off or XT	off	**5K Race**
6.	off or XT	45 min. run/walk	off or XT	*(14 × 400) speed day	off or XT	off	10 miles run/walk
7.	off or XT	30 min. run/walk	off or XT	*(6 × 400) speed day	off or XT	off	**5K Race**
8.	off or XT	30 min. run/walk	off or XT	30 min. run/walk	off or XT	off	4–8 miles run/walk

This program assumes that you have been running at least at the level of running listed in the first week, for at least 2 months prior to the start of the program. If you are already doing more than this, you can continue to maintain that schedule, as long as the legs are recovering quickly between runs.

1. You can do the long run on Saturday if you wish. In that case, take Friday off from exercise.

2. On your long runs, take more liberal walk breaks. If you are running 9 minutes and walking for 1 minute on your Tuesday runs, do 7–1 on the long runs (or 6–1 on bad days). The pace of long runs should be at least two minutes per mile slower than your goal race pace (7:30–8:00 min./mi.).

3. On your Tuesday runs, take as many walk breaks as you need, but you may not need to walk. Read the section on walk breaks and when in doubt, walk more.

4. XT means cross train. You can walk or do some form of non-pounding exercise, such as swimming, cycling, or exercise machines, for 10 minutes or so at an easy pace. If you are just starting to do any of these exercises (or are starting back after a layoff), start with only 5 minutes, and increase by 2–3 minutes each session. Water running is the best form of cross training.

5. The 5K race in week 5 is a test race. Run the first mile 30 seconds slower than the goal pace. Try to run the goal pace during miles 2 and 3.

6. In the 5K race, pace yourself conservatively. The first mile should be about 5–10 seconds slower than goal pace. Then gradually increase the pace to the end of the race. The fastest mile should be mile #3.

7. This is a minimal program. You may add an extra easy-running day on Friday or Monday.

8. *Denotes speed day. Go to a local track. After a warm-up of at least 5 minutes, do the number of 400-meter laps assigned, running each in 1:14–1:16. Walk slowly for half a lap and repeat. Do at least a 5-minute warm-down afterward.

10K TRAINING PROGRAM: To Finish

Week #	Mon	Tue	Wed	Thu	Fri	Sat	Sun
1.	off or XT	10 min. run/walk	off or XT	10 min. run/walk	off or XT	off	1 mile run/walk
2.	off or XT	13 min. run/walk	off or XT	13 min. run/walk	off or XT	off	1.5 miles run/walk
3.	off or XT	15 min. run/walk	off or XT	15 min. run/walk	off or XT	off	2.0 miles run/walk
4.	off or XT	17 min. run/walk	off or XT	17 min. run/walk	off or XT	off	2.5 miles run/walk
5.	off or XT	19 min. run/walk	off or XT	19 min. run/walk	off or XT	off	3.0 miles run/walk
6.	off or XT	20 min. run/walk	off or XT	20 min. run/walk	off or XT	off	3.5 miles run/walk
7.	off or XT	21 min. run/walk	off or XT	21 min. run/walk	off or XT	off	4.0 miles run/walk
8.	off or XT	22 min. run/walk	off or XT	22 min. run/walk	off or XT	off	4.5 miles run/walk
9.	off or XT	23 min. run/walk	off or XT	23 min. run/walk	off or XT	off	5.0 miles run/walk
10.	off or XT	24 min. run/walk	off or XT	24 min. run/walk	off or XT	off	5.5 miles run/walk
11.	off or XT	26 min. run/walk	off or XT	26 min. run/walk	off or XT	off	6.0 miles run/walk
12.	off or XT	20 min. run/walk	off or XT	20 min. run/walk	off or XT	off	**5K Race**
13.	off or XT	28 min. run/walk	off or XT	28 min. run/walk	off or XT	off	6.5 miles run/walk
14.	off or XT	20 min. run/walk	off or XT	20 min. run/walk	off or XT	off	**10K Race**
15.	off or XT	20 min. run/walk	off or XT	20 min. run/walk	off or XT	off	3–5 miles run/walk

This program assumes that you have not been running at all. If you are already doing more than is on this schedule, you can continue to maintain that schedule, as long as the legs are recovering quickly between runs.

1. You can do the long run on Saturday if you wish. In that case, take Friday off from exercise.

2. On your long runs, take more liberal walk breaks. If you are running 2 minutes and walking for 1 minute on your Tuesday and Thursday runs, do 2–2 on the long runs, or 1–1 (or 2-minute walk and 1-minute run on bad days). Many beginners will do mostly walking: for example, walk 4, run 1.

3. On your Tuesday and Thursday runs, take as many walk breaks as you need. Read the section on walk breaks and when in doubt, walk more.

4. XT means cross train. You can walk or do some form of non-pounding exercise, such as swimming, cycling, or exercise machines, for 10 minutes or so at an easy pace. If you are just starting to do any of these exercises (or are starting back after a layoff), start with only 5 minutes, and increase by 2–3 minutes each session.

5. The 5K race, two weeks before the goal 10K race will give you a "dress rehearsal" for the big day. Be sure to line up in the back of the crowd, and take walk breaks as you have been doing in your shorter runs during the week. If you are feeling strong during the last mile, you may reduce some of the walk breaks. Do not sprint, especially at the end.

6. In the 10K itself, most should take some walk breaks each mile, as you feel comfortable. Most runners should do the first 1–2 miles, taking the walk breaks as you have in the long runs. During the last mile you can cut out some or all of the walking, if you feel strong. Be sure to move to the side of the road before taking walk breaks.

10K TRAINING PROGRAM: 90 min. goal

Week #	Mon	Tue	Wed	Thu	Fri	Sat	Sun
1.	off or XT	10 min. run/walk	off or XT	*(4 x 400) speed day	off or XT	off	2.5 miles run/walk
2.	off or XT	13 min. run/walk	off or XT	*(5 x 400) speed day	off or XT	off	3.0 miles run/walk
3.	off or XT	15 min. run/walk	off or XT	*(6 x 400) speed day	off or XT	off	3.5 miles run/walk
4.	off or XT	17 min. run/walk	off or XT	*(7 x 400) speed day	off or XT	off	4.0 miles run/walk
5.	off or XT	19 min. run/walk	off or XT	*(8 x 400) speed day	off or XT	off	4.5 miles run/walk
6.	off or XT	21 min. run/walk	off or XT	*(9 x 400) speed day	off or XT	off	5.0 miles run/walk
7.	off or XT	23 min. run/walk	off or XT	*(10 x 400) speed day	off or XT	off	5.5 miles run/walk
8.	off or XT	25 min. run/walk	off or XT	*(11 x 400) speed day	off or XT	off	6.0 miles run/walk
9.	off or XT	27 min. run/walk	off or XT	*(12 x 400) speed day	off or XT	off	6.5 miles run/walk
10.	off or XT	29 min. run/walk	off or XT	*(13 x 400) speed day	off or XT	off	**5K Race**
11.	off or XT	30 min. run/walk	off or XT	*(14 x 400) speed day	off or XT	off	7.0 miles run/walk
12.	off or XT	20 min. run/walk	off or XT	*(5 x 400) speed day	off or XT	off	**10K Race**
13.	off or XT	20 min. run/walk	off or XT	20 min. run/walk	off or XT	off	3–5 miles run/walk
14.	off or XT	25 min. run/walk	off or XT	25 min. run/walk	off or XT	off	4–6 miles run/walk

This program assumes that you have been running at least at the level of running listed in the first week, for at least 2 months prior to the start of the program. If you are already doing more than this, you can continue to maintain that schedule, as long as the legs are recovering quickly between runs.

1. You can do the long run on Saturday if you wish. In that case, take Friday off from exercise.

2. On your long runs, take more liberal walk breaks. If you are running 3 minutes and walking for 1 minute on your Tuesday runs, do 2–1 on the long runs (or 2-minute walk and 2-minute run on bad days). The pace of long runs should be at least 1 minute per mile slower than your goal race pace (16+ min./mi.).

3. On your Tuesday runs, take as many walk breaks as you need. Read the section on walk breaks and when in doubt, walk more.

4. XT means cross train. You can walk or do some form of non-pounding exercise, such as swimming, cycling, or exercise machines, for 10 minutes or so at an easy pace. If you are just starting to do any of these exercises (or are starting back after a layoff), start with only 5 minutes, and increase by 2–3 minutes each session.

5. The 5K race, two weeks before the goal 10K race will give you a "dress rehearsal" for the big day. Be sure to line up in the crowd where you should be, according to the projected pace. Most races have pace signs; if not, ask several people and move forward or back, as needed. Take walk breaks as you have been doing in your shorter runs during the week. If you are feeling strong during the last mile, you may reduce some of the walk breaks. Do not sprint, especially at the end. Be sure to move to the side of the road before taking walk breaks.

6. In the 10K itself, be sure to line up in the crowd where you should be, according to the projected pace. Most races have pace signs; if not, ask several people and move forward or back, as needed. Take walk breaks as you feel you need to. If you are feeling strong during the last mile or two, you may reduce some of the walk breaks. Do not sprint, especially at the end. Be sure to move to the side of the road before taking walk breaks.

7.* Denotes speed day. Go to a local track. After a 4–5-minute warm-up, do the number of 400-meter laps assigned, running each in 3:28–3:30. Walk slowly for half a lap and repeat. Do a 4–5-minute warm-down afterward.

8. Before your goal race, write another goal on your calendar, 2–4 weeks after the 10K. It doesn't have to be another race: a scenic run, a social run with friends, etc. This will keep you motivated to maintain your great training program.

10K TRAINING PROGRAM: 70 min. goal

Week #	Mon	Tue	Wed	Thu	Fri	Sat	Sun
1.	off or XT	15 min. run/walk	off or XT	*(5×400) speed day	off or XT	off	3.0 miles run/walk
2.	off or XT	17 min. run/walk	off or XT	*(6×400) speed day	off or XT	off	3.5 miles run/walk
3.	off or XT	19 min. run/walk	off or XT	*(7×400) speed day	off or XT	off	4.0 miles run/walk
4.	off or XT	20 min. run/walk	off or XT	*(8×400) speed day	off or XT	off	4.5 miles run/walk
5.	off or XT	21 min. run/walk	off or XT	*(9×400) speed day	off or XT	off	5.0 miles run/walk
6.	off or XT	23 min. run/walk	off or XT	*(10×400) speed day	off or XT	off	5.5 miles run/walk
7.	off or XT	25 min. run/walk	off or XT	*(11×400) speed day	off or XT	off	6.0 miles run/walk
8.	off or XT	27 min. run/walk	off or XT	*(12×400) speed day	off or XT	off	6.5 miles run/walk
9.	off or XT	29 min. run/walk	off or XT	*(13×400) speed day	off or XT	off	7.0 miles run/walk
10.	off or XT	31 min. run/walk	off or XT	*(14×400) speed day	off or XT	off	**5K Race**
11.	off or XT	32 min. run/walk	off or XT	*(15×400) speed day	off or XT	off	7.5 miles run/walk
12.	off or XT	20 min. run/walk	off or XT	*(6×400) speed day	off or XT	off	**10K Race**
13.	off or XT	20 min. run/walk	off or XT	20 min. run/walk	off or XT	off	3–5 miles run/walk
14.	off or XT	25 min. run/walk	off or XT	25 min. run/walk	off or XT	off	4–6 miles run/walk

This program assumes that you have been running at least at the level of running listed in the first week, for at least 2 months prior to the start of the program. If you are already doing more than this, you can continue to maintain that schedule, as long as the legs are recovering quickly between runs.

1. You can do the long run on Saturday if you wish. In that case, take Friday off from exercise.

2. On your long runs, take more liberal walk breaks. If you are running 4 minutes and walking for 1 minute on your Tuesday runs, do 3–1 on the long runs (or 3-minute walk and 2-minute run on bad days). The pace of long runs should be at least 1 minute per mile slower than your goal race pace (12:00+ min./mi.).

3. On your Tuesday runs, take as many walk breaks as you need. Read the section on walk breaks and when in doubt, walk more.

4. XT means cross train. You can walk or do some form of non-pounding exercise, such as swimming, cycling, or exercise machines, for 10 minutes or so at an easy pace. If you are just starting to do any of these exercises (or are starting back after a layoff), start with only 5 minutes, and increase by 2–3 minutes each session.

5. The 5K race, two weeks before the goal 10K race will give you a "dress rehearsal" for the big day. Be sure to line up in the crowd where you should be, according to the projected pace. Most races have pace signs; if not, ask several people and move forward or back, as needed. Take walk breaks as you have been doing in your shorter runs during the week. If you are feeling strong during the last mile, you may reduce some of the walk breaks. Do not sprint, especially at the end. Be sure to move to the side of the road before taking walk breaks.

6. In the 10K itself, be sure to line up in the crowd where you should be, according to the projected pace. Most races have pace signs; if not, ask several people and move forward or back, as needed. Take walk breaks as you feel you need to. If you are feeling strong during the last mile or two, you may reduce some of the walk breaks. Do not sprint, especially at the end. Be sure to move to the side of the road before taking walk breaks.

7.* Denotes speed day. Go to a local track. After a 4–5-minute warm-up, do the number of 400-meter laps assigned, running each in 2:50–2:52. Walk slowly for half a lap and repeat. Do a 4–5-minute warm-down afterward.

8. Before your goal race, write another goal on your calendar, 2–4 weeks after the 10K. It doesn't have to be another race: a scenic run, a social run with friends, etc. This will keep you motivated to maintain your great training program.

10K TRAINING PROGRAM: 59 min. goal

Week #	Mon	Tue	Wed	Thu	Fri	Sat	Sun
1.	off or XT	18 min. run/walk	off or XT	*(6×400) speed day	off or XT	off	3.5 miles run/walk
2.	off or XT	20 min. run/walk	off or XT	*(7×400) speed day	off or XT	off	4.0 miles run/walk
3.	off or XT	22 min. run/walk	off or XT	*(8×400) speed day	off or XT	off	4.5 miles run/walk
4.	off or XT	24 min. run/walk	off or XT	*(9×400) speed day	off or XT	off	5.0 miles run/walk
5.	off or XT	26 min. run/walk	off or XT	*(10×400) speed day	off or XT	off	5.5 miles run/walk
6.	off or XT	28 min. run/walk	off or XT	*(11×400) speed day	off or XT	off	6.0 miles run/walk
7.	off or XT	30 min. run/walk	off or XT	*(12×400) speed day	off or XT	off	6.5 miles run/walk
8.	off or XT	30 min. run/walk	off or XT	*(13×400) speed day	off or XT	off	7.0 miles run/walk
9.	off or XT	30 min. run/walk	off or XT	*(14×400) speed day	off or XT	off	7.5 miles run/walk
10.	off or XT	32 min. run/walk	off or XT	*(15×400) speed day	off or XT	off	**5K Race**
11.	off or XT	30 min. run/walk	off or XT	*(16×400) speed day	off or XT	off	8.0 miles run/walk
12.	off or XT	20 min. run/walk	off or XT	*(7×400) speed day	off or XT	off	**10K Race**
13.	off or XT	20 min. run/walk	off or XT	20 min. run/walk	off or XT	off	3–5 miles run/walk
14.	off or XT	25 min. run/walk	off or XT	25 min. run/walk	off or XT	off	4–6 miles run/walk

This program assumes that you have been running at least at the level of running listed in the first week, for at least 2 months prior to the start of the program. If you are already doing more than this, you can continue to maintain that schedule, as long as the legs are recovering quickly between runs.

1. You can do the long run on Saturday if you wish. In that case, take Friday off from exercise.

2. On your long runs, take more liberal walk breaks. If you are running 5 minutes and walking for 1 minute on your Tuesday runs, do 4–1 on the long runs (or 3-minute walk and 1-minute run on bad days). The pace of long runs should be at least 1 minute per mile slower than your goal race pace (11:00+ min./mi.).

3. On your Tuesday runs, take as many walk breaks as you need. Read the section on walk breaks and when in doubt, walk more.

4. XT means cross train. You can walk or do some form of non-pounding exercise, such as swimming, cycling, or exercise machines, for 10 minutes or so at an easy pace. If you are just starting to do any of these exercises (or are starting back after a layoff), start with only 5 minutes, and increase by 2–3 minutes each session.

5. The 5K race, two weeks before the goal 10K race will give you a "dress rehearsal" for the big day. Take walk breaks as you have been doing in your shorter runs during the week, if needed.

6. In the 10K itself, be sure to line up in the crowd where you should be, according to the projected pace. Take walk breaks as you feel you need to.

7.* Denotes speed day. Go to a local track. After a 4–5-minute warm-up, do the number of 400-meter laps assigned, running each in 2:14–2:17. Walk slowly for half a lap and repeat. Do a 4–5-minute warm-down afterward.

10K TRAINING PROGRAM: 49 min. goal

Week #	Mon	Tue	Wed	Thu	Fri	Sat	Sun
1.	off or XT	20 min. run/walk	off or XT	*(6×400) speed day	off or XT	off	4.0 miles run/walk
2.	off or XT	22 min. run/walk	off or XT	*(7×400) speed day	off or XT	off	4.5 miles run/walk
3.	off or XT	24 min. run/walk	off or XT	*(9×400) speed day	off or XT	off	5.0 miles run/walk
4.	off or XT	26 min. run/walk	off or XT	*(10×400) speed day	off or XT	off	5.5 miles run/walk
5.	off or XT	28 min. run/walk	off or XT	*(11×400) speed day	off or XT	off	6.0 miles run/walk
6.	off or XT	30 min. run/walk	off or XT	*(12×400) speed day	off or XT	off	6.5 miles run/walk
7.	off or XT	30–32 min. run/walk	off or XT	*(14×400) speed day	off or XT	off	7.0 miles run/walk
8.	off or XT	30–34 min. run/walk	off or XT	*(15×400) speed day	off or XT	off	7.5 miles run/walk
9.	off or XT	30–36 min. run/walk	off or XT	*(16×400) speed day	off or XT	off	8.0 miles run/walk
10.	off or XT	30–34 min. run/walk	off or XT	*(12×400) speed day	off or XT	off	**5K Race**
11.	off or XT	30–32 min. run/walk	off or XT	*(18×400) speed day	off or XT	off	8.5 miles run/walk
12.	off or XT	20 min. run/walk	off or XT	*(8×400) speed day	off or XT	off	**10K Race**
13.	off or XT	20 min. run/walk	off or XT	20 min. run/walk	off or XT	off	3–5 miles run/walk
14.	off or XT	25 min. run/walk	off or XT	25 min. run/walk	off or XT	off	4–6 miles run/walk

This program assumes that you have been running at least at the level of running listed in the first week, for at least 2 months prior to the start of the program. If you are already doing more than this, you can continue to maintain that schedule, as long as the legs are recovering quickly between runs.

1. You can do the long run on Saturday if you wish. In that case, take Friday off from exercise.

2. On your long runs, take more liberal walk breaks. If you are running 6 minutes and walking for 1 minute on your Tuesday runs, do 5–1 on the long runs (or 4-minute walk and 1-minute run on bad days). The pace of long runs should be at least 1 minute per mile slower than your goal race pace.

3. On your Tuesday runs, take as many walk breaks as you need. Read the section on walk breaks and when in doubt, walk more.

4. XT means cross train. You can walk or do some form of non-pounding exercise, such as swimming, cycling, or exercise machines, for 10 minutes or so at an easy pace. If you are just starting to do any of these exercises (or are starting back after a layoff), start with only 5 minutes, and increase by 2–3 minutes each session.

5. The 5K race, two weeks before the goal 10K race will give you a "dress rehearsal" for the big day. Take walk breaks as you have been doing in your shorter runs during the week.

6. In the 10K itself, be sure to line up in the crowd where you should be, according to the projected pace. Take walk breaks as you feel you need to.

7.*Denotes speed day. Go to a local track. After a 4–5-minute warm-up, do the number of 400-meter laps assigned, running each in 1:52–1:55. Walk slowly for half a lap and repeat. Do a 4–5-minute warm-down afterward.

10K TRAINING PROGRAM: 44 min. goal

Week #	Mon	Tue	Wed	Thu	Fri	Sat	Sun
1.	off or XT	25 min. run/walk	off or XT	*(6 × 400) speed day	off or XT	off	4.0 miles run/walk
2.	off or XT	27 min. run/walk	off or XT	*(8 × 400) speed day	off or XT	off	4.5 miles run/walk
3.	off or XT	29 min. run/walk	off or XT	*(9 × 400) speed day	off or XT	off	5.5 miles run/walk
4.	off or XT	31 min. run/walk	off or XT	*(10 × 400) speed day	off or XT	off	6.0 miles run/walk
5.	off or XT	30–33 min. run/walk	off or XT	*(11 × 400) speed day	off or XT	off	6.5 miles run/walk
6.	off or XT	30–35 min. run/walk	off or XT	*(12 × 400) speed day	off or XT	off	7.5 miles run/walk
7.	off or XT	30–36 min. run/walk	off or XT	*(13 × 400) speed day	off or XT	off	8.0 miles run/walk
8.	off or XT	30–36 min. run/walk	off or XT	*(14 × 400) speed day	off or XT	off	8.5 miles run/walk
9.	off or XT	30–38 min. run/walk	off or XT	*(16 × 400) speed day	off or XT	off	9.0 miles run/walk
10.	off or XT	30–38 min. run/walk	off or XT	*(17 × 400) speed day	off or XT	off	**5K Race**
11.	off or XT	30–40 min. run/walk	off or XT	*(18 × 400) speed day	off or XT	off	10 mile run
12.	off or XT	20 min. run/walk	off or XT	*(8 × 400) speed day	off or XT	off	**10K Race**
13.	off or XT	30 min. run/walk	off or XT	30 min. run/walk	off or XT	off	3–6 miles run/walk
14.	off or XT	30–39 min. run/walk	off or XT	30 min. run/walk	off or XT	off	5–8 miles run/walk

This program assumes that you have been running at least at the level of running listed in the first week, for at least 2 months prior to the start of the program. If you are already doing more than this, you can continue to maintain that schedule, as long as the legs are recovering quickly between runs. You may add an additional day of training, if you have already been running 4 days a week. This would be on Friday, and would be a very easy 2–3 mile run.

1. You can do the long run on Saturday if you wish. In that case, take Friday off from exercise.

2. On your long runs, take more liberal walk breaks. If you are running 8 minutes and walking for 1 minute on your Tuesday runs, do 6–1 on the long runs (or 5–1 on bad days). The pace of long runs should be at least two minutes per mile slower than your goal race pace.

3. On your Tuesday runs, take as many walk breaks as you need—but you may not need to take them. Read the section on walk breaks and when in doubt, walk more.

4. XT means cross train. You can walk or do some form of non-pounding exercise, such as swimming, water running, cycling or exercise machines, for 10 minutes or so at an easy pace. If you are just starting to do any of these exercises (or are starting back after a layoff), start with only 5 minutes, and increase by 2–3 minutes each session. Water running is the best form of cross training.

5. In the 5K and the 10K races, pace yourself conservatively. The first mile should be about 5–10 seconds slower than goal pace. Then gradually increase the pace to the end of the race. The fastest mile should be the last mile, but do not sprint!

6. *Denotes speed day. Go to a local track. After a 4–5-minute warm-up, do the number of 400-meter laps assigned, running each in 1:39–1:42. Walk slowly for half a lap and repeat. Do a 4–5-minute warm-down afterward.

10K TRAINING PROGRAM: 39 min. goal

Week #	Mon	Tue	Wed	Thu	Fri	Sat	Sun
1.	off or XT	25 min. run/walk	off or XT	*(7×400) speed day	off or XT	off	5.0 miles run/walk
2.	off or XT	27 min. run/walk	off or XT	*(8×400) speed day	off or XT	off	6.0 miles run/walk
3.	off or XT	29 min. run/walk	off or XT	*(9×400) speed day	off or XT	off	7.0 miles run/walk
4.	off or XT	31 min. run/walk	off or XT	*(10×400) speed day	off or XT	off	8.0 miles run/walk
5.	off or XT	30–33 min. run/walk	off or XT	*(11×400) speed day	off or XT	off	9.0 miles run/walk
6.	off or XT	30–35 min. run/walk	off or XT	*(12×400) speed day	off or XT	off	10.0 miles run/walk
7.	off or XT	30–36 min. run/walk	off or XT	*(13×400) speed day	off or XT	off	**5K Race**
8.	off or XT	30–36 min. run/walk	off or XT	*(14×400) speed day	off or XT	off	12.0 miles run/walk
9.	off or XT	30–38 min. run/walk	off or XT	*(16×400) speed day	off or XT	off	**5K Race**
10.	off or XT	30–38 min. run/walk	off or XT	*(18×400) speed day	off or XT	off	13–14 miles run/walk
11.	off or XT	30–40 min. run/walk	off or XT	*(20×400) speed day	off or XT	off	**5K Race**
12.	off or XT	20 min. run/walk	off or XT	*(8×400) speed day	off or XT	off	**10K Race**
13.	off or XT	30 min. run/walk	off or XT	30 min. run/walk	off or XT	off	3–6 miles run/walk
14.	off or XT	30–39 min. run/walk	off or XT	30 min. run/walk	off or XT	off	5–8 miles run/walk

This program assumes that you have been running at least at the level of running listed in the first week, for at least 2 months prior to the start of the program. If you are already doing more than this, you can continue to maintain that schedule, as long as the legs are recovering quickly between runs. You may add an additional day of training, if you have already been running 4 days a week. This would be on Friday, and would be a very easy 4–5 mile run.

1. You can do the long run on Saturday if you wish. In that case, take Friday off from exercise.

2. On your long runs, take more liberal walk breaks. If you are running 8 minutes and walking for 1 minute on your Tuesday runs, do 6–1 on the long runs (or 5–1 on bad days). The pace of long runs should be at least two minutes per mile slower than your goal race pace (8:30 min./mi.).

3. On your Tuesday runs, take as many walk breaks as you need—but you may not need to take them. Read the section on walk breaks and when in doubt, walk more.

4. XT means cross train. You can walk or do some form of non-pounding exercise, such as swimming, water running, cycling or exercise machines, for 10 minutes or so at an easy pace. If you are just starting to do any of these exercises (or are starting back after a layoff), start with only 5 minutes, and increase by 2–3 minutes each session. Water running is the best form of cross training.

5. In the 5K and the 10K races, pace yourself conservatively. The first mile should be about 5–10 seconds slower than goal pace. Then gradually increase the pace to the end of the race. The fastest mile should be the last mile, but do not sprint!

6.*Denotes speed day. Go to a local track. After a 4–5-minute warm-up, do the number of 400-meter laps assigned, running each in 1:28–1:31. Walk slowly for half a lap and repeat. Do a 4–5-minute warm-down afterward.

10K TRAINING PROGRAM: 34 min. goal

Week #	Mon	Tue	Wed	Thu	Fri	Sat	Sun
1.	off or XT	30–45 min. run/walk	off or XT	*(7×400) speed day	XT	off	6.0 miles run/walk
2.	off or XT	30–45 min. run/walk	off or XT	*(8×400) speed day	XT	off	7.0 miles run/walk
3.	off or XT	30–45 min. run/walk	off or XT	*(9×400) speed day	XT	off	8.0 miles run/walk
4.	off or XT	35–45 min. run/walk	off or XT	*(10×400) speed day	XT	off	9.0 miles run/walk
5.	off or XT	35–45 min. run/walk	off or XT	*(11×400) speed day	XT	off	10.0 miles run/walk
6.	off or XT	35–45 min. run/walk	off or XT	*(12×400) speed day	XT	off	11.0 miles run/walk
7.	off or XT	40–45 min. run/walk	off or XT	*(13×400) speed day	XT	off	**5K Race**
8.	off or XT	40–50 min. run/walk	off or XT	*(14×400) speed day	XT	off	13.0 miles run/walk
9.	off or XT	40–50 min. run/walk	off or XT	*(16×400) speed day	XT	off	**5K Race**
10.	off or XT	40–50 min. run/walk	off or XT	*(18×400) speed day	XT	off	15 miles run/walk
11.	off or XT	40–50 min. run/walk	off or XT	*(20×400) speed day	XT	off	**5K Race**
12.	off or XT	20 min. run/walk	off or XT	*(8×400) speed day	XT	off	**10K Race**
13.	off or XT	30 min. run/walk	off or XT	30 min. run/walk	XT	off	3–6 miles run/walk
14.	off or XT	30–45 min. run/walk	off or XT	30 min. run/walk	XT	off	8–15 miles run/walk

This program assumes that you have been running at least at the level of running listed in the first week, for at least 2 months prior to the start of the program. If you are already doing more than this, you can continue to maintain that schedule, as long as the legs are recovering quickly between runs. You may add an additional day of training, if you have already been running 4 days a week. This would be on Monday, and would be a very easy 3–6 mile run. During the Tuesday run, I recommend that you insert 4–8 acceleration gliders. (See pp. 145–147.)

1. You can do the long run on Saturday if you wish. In that case, take Friday off from exercise.

2. On your long runs, take more liberal walk breaks. At the very least, when the long run reaches 10 miles, take a 1-minute walk break, after running for 8–9 minutes. When in doubt, take the walk breaks more frequently. The pace of long runs should be at least two minutes per mile slower than your goal race pace (about 8:00 min./mi.).

3. XT means cross train. You can walk or do segments of non-pounding exercise, such as swimming, water running, cycling or exercise machines, for 10–20 minutes or so at an easy pace. If you are just starting to do any of these exercises (or are starting back after a layoff), start with only 5 minutes, and increase by 2–3 minutes each session. Water running is the best form of cross training.

4. In the 5K and the 10K races, pace yourself conservatively. The first mile should be about 5–10 seconds slower than goal pace. Then gradually increase the pace to the end of the race. The fastest mile should be the last mile, but do not sprint!

5.*Denotes speed day. Go to a local track. After a 4–5-minute warm-up, do the number of 400-meter laps assigned, running each in 1:14–1:16. Walk slowly for half a lap and repeat. Do a 4–5-minute warm-down afterward.

Week #	Mon	Tue	Wed	Thu	Fri	Sat	Sun
HALF-MARATHON TRAINING PROGRAM: To Finish							
1.	off or XT	10 min. run/walk	off or XT	10 min. run/walk	off or XT	off	1 mile run/walk
2.	off or XT	13 min. run/walk	off or XT	13 min. run/walk	off or XT	off	2 miles run/walk
3.	off or XT	15 min. run/walk	off or XT	15 min. run/walk	off or XT	off	3 miles run/walk
4.	off or XT	17 min. run/walk	off or XT	17 min. run/walk	off or XT	off	4 miles run/walk
5.	off or XT	20 min. run/walk	off or XT	20 min. run/walk	off or XT	off	5 miles run/walk
6.	off or XT	23 min. run/walk	off or XT	23 min. run/walk	off or XT	off	6 miles run/walk
7.	off or XT	25 min. run/walk	off or XT	25 min. run/walk	off or XT	off	7 miles run/walk
8.	off or XT	27 min. run/walk	off or XT	27 min. run/walk	off or XT	off	8 miles run/walk
9.	off or XT	30 min. run/walk	off or XT	30 min. run/walk	off or XT	off	10 miles run/walk
10.	off or XT	30 min. run/walk	off or XT	30 min. run/walk	off or XT	off	5 miles run/walk
11.	off or XT	30 min. run/walk	off or XT	30 min. run/walk	off or XT	off	12 miles run/walk
12.	off or XT	30 min. run/walk	off or XT	30 min. run/walk	off or XT	off	6 miles run/walk
13.	off or XT	30 min. run/walk	off or XT	30 min. run/walk	off or XT	off	14 miles run/walk
14.	off or XT	30 min. run/walk	off or XT	30 min. run/walk	off or XT	off	6 miles run/walk
15.	off or XT	30 min. run/walk	off or XT	30 min. run/walk	off or XT	off	**Half-Marathon**
Continuation Schedule							
	off or XT	30 min. run/walk	off or XT	30 min. run/walk	off or XT	off	5–6 miles run/walk

This program assumes that you have not been running at all. If you are already doing more than is on this schedule, you can continue to maintain that schedule, as long as the legs are recovering quickly between runs. If your long run is already longer than 1 mile, you may begin on the week which has a long run as long as you're currently running.

1. You can do the long run on Saturday if you wish. In that case, take Friday off from exercise.

2. On your long runs, take more liberal walk breaks. If you are running 2 minutes and walking for 1 minute on your Tuesday and Thursday runs, do 2–2 on the long runs, or 1–1 (or 2-minute walk and 1-minute run on bad days). Many beginners will do mostly walking: for example, walk 3, run 1.

3. On your Tuesday and Thursday runs, take as many walk breaks as you need. Read the section on walk breaks and when in doubt, walk more.

4. XT means cross train. You can walk or do some form of non-pounding exercise, such as swimming, cycling, or exercise machines, for 10 minutes or so at an easy pace. If you are just starting to do any of these exercises (or are starting back after a layoff), start with only 5 minutes, and increase by 2–3 minutes each session.

In the half-marathon race, most should take some walk breaks each mile, as you feel comfortable. Most runners should do the first 11 miles, taking the walk breaks as you have in the long runs. During the last 2 miles you can cut out some or all of the walking, if you feel strong.

HALF-MARATHON TRAINING PROGRAM: 2:45 goal

Week #	Mon	Tue	Wed	Thu	Fri	Sat	Sun
1.	off or XT	15 min. run/walk	off or XT	15 min. run/walk	off or XT	off	3 miles run/walk
2.	off or XT	17 min. run/walk	off or XT	17 min. run/walk	off or XT	off	4 miles run/walk
3.	off or XT	20 min. run/walk	off or XT	20 min. run/walk	off or XT	off	5 miles run/walk
4.	off or XT	23 min. run/walk	off or XT	23 min. run/walk	off or XT	off	6 miles run/walk
5.	off or XT	25 min. run/walk	off or XT	25 min. run/walk	off or XT	off	7 miles run/walk
6.	off or XT	27 min. run/walk	off or XT	27 min. run/walk	off or XT	off	8 miles run/walk
7.	off or XT	30 min. run/walk	off or XT	30 min. run/walk	off or XT	off	10 miles run/walk
8.	off or XT	30 min. run/walk	off or XT	30 min. run/walk	off or XT	off	3×800m
9.	off or XT	30 min. run/walk	off or XT	30 min. run/walk	off or XT	off	12 miles run/walk
10.	off or XT	30 min. run/walk	off or XT	30 min. run/walk	off or XT	off	**5K Race**
11.	off or XT	30 min. run/walk	off or XT	4–5×800m	off or XT	off	14 miles run/walk
12.	off or XT	30 min. run/walk	off or XT	30 min. run/walk	off or XT	off	5–6×800m
13.	off or XT	30 min. run/walk	off or XT	30 min. run/walk	off or XT	off	15 miles run/walk
14.	off or XT	30 min. run/walk	off or XT	6–7×800m	off or XT	off	6 miles run/walk
15.	off or XT	30 min. run/walk	off or XT	30 min. run/walk	off or XT	off	**Half-Marathon**
Continuation Schedule							
	off or XT	30 min. run/walk	off or XT	30 min. run/walk	off or XT	off	5–6 miles run/walk

This program assumes that you have been running the amount listed in week #1. If you are not doing that, spend a week or two on the beginning schedule. If you are already doing more than is on this schedule, you can continue to maintain at the higher amount, as long as the legs are recovering quickly between runs. If your long run is already longer than 3 miles, you may begin on the week which has a long run as long as you're currently running.

1. You can do the long run on Saturday if you wish. In that case, take Friday off from exercise.

2. On your long runs, take more liberal walk breaks. If you are running 3 minutes and walking for 1 minute on your Tuesday and Thursday runs, do 2–1 on the long runs, or 1–1 on bad days. Make sure that you're doing your long runs at least 2 minutes per mile slower than your goal pace. It's OK to go slower than that.

3. On your Tuesday and Thursday runs, take as many walk breaks as you need. Read the section on walk breaks and when in doubt, walk more.

4. XT means cross train. You can walk or do some form of non-pounding exercise, such as swimming, cycling, or exercise machines, for 10 minutes or so at an easy pace. If you are just starting to do any of these exercises (or are starting back after a layoff), start with only 5 minutes, and increase by 2–3 minutes each session.

5. The 800-meter repeats, on weeks 8, 11, 12, and 14 will help you build the speed you need for a time goal of your choice. Do these on a 400-meter track. After a 5-minute warm-up, run each 800m in 6 minutes and 10 seconds. Walk for a full 400-meter lap and repeat. Warm down with a slow 5 minutes of running and 5 minutes of walking.

6. Remember that it doesn't benefit you to run faster than the pace assigned for the workout. If you're struggling to run the time assigned for your 800-meter reps, your time goal is too ambitious and should be adjusted.

7. Running the 5K race, on week #10, will give you a "reality check" on your time goal. For a 2:45 goal, you'll want to run a time of 33:30 or faster in the 5K race. In this race, you can reduce the number of walk breaks in order to run a fast time, for you, on that day. If you run slower than this, you should adjust to a slower time goal using the prediction table in this book.

In the half-marathon race, most should take some walk breaks each mile, as you feel comfortable. (Be sure to move to the side of the road before walking.) Most runners should take a one-minute walk break as you have in the long runs, for at least the first 10 miles. During the last few miles you can cut out some or all of the walking, if you feel strong.

HALF-MARATHON TRAINING PROGRAM: 2:20 goal

Week #	Mon	Tue	Wed	Thu	Fri	Sat	Sun
1.	off or XT	15 min. run/walk	off or XT	15 min. run/walk	off or XT	off	3 miles run/walk
2.	off or XT	17 min. run/walk	off or XT	17 min. run/walk	off or XT	off	4 miles run/walk
3.	off or XT	20 min. run/walk	off or XT	20 min. run/walk	off or XT	off	5 miles run/walk
4.	off or XT	23 min. run/walk	off or XT	23 min. run/walk	off or XT	off	6 miles run/walk
5.	off or XT	25 min. run/walk	off or XT	25 min. run/walk	off or XT	off	7 miles run/walk
6.	off or XT	27 min. run/walk	off or XT	27 min. run/walk	off or XT	off	8 miles run/walk
7.	off or XT	30 min. run/walk	off or XT	30 min. run/walk	off or XT	off	10 miles run/walk
8.	off or XT	30 min. run/walk	off or XT	30 min. run/walk	off or XT	off	3×800m
9.	off or XT	30 min. run/walk	off or XT	30 min. run/walk	off or XT	off	12 miles run/walk
10.	off or XT	30 min. run/walk	off or XT	30 min. run/walk	off or XT	off	**5K Race**
11.	off or XT	30 min. run/walk	off or XT	4–5×800m	off or XT	off	14 miles run/walk
12.	off or XT	30 min. run/walk	off or XT	30 min. run/walk	off or XT	off	5–6×800m
13.	off or XT	30 min. run/walk	off or XT	30 min. run/walk	off or XT	off	15 miles run/walk
14.	off or XT	30 min. run/walk	off or XT	6–7×800m	off or XT	off	6 miles run/walk
15.	off or XT	30 min. run/walk	off or XT	30 min. run/walk	off or XT	off	**Half-Marathon**
Continuation Schedule							
	off or XT	30 min. run/walk	off or XT	30 min. run/walk	off or XT	off	5–6 miles run/walk

This program assumes that you have been running the amount listed in week #1. If you are not doing that, spend a week or two on the beginning schedule. If you are already doing more than is on this schedule, you can continue to maintain at the higher amount, as long as the legs are recovering quickly between runs. If your long run is already longer than 3 miles, you may begin on the week which has a long run as long as you're currently running.

1. You can do the long run on Saturday if you wish. In that case, take Friday off from exercise.

2. On your long runs, take more liberal walk breaks. If you are running 4 minutes and walking for 1 minute on your Tuesday and Thursday runs, do 3–1 on the long runs, or 2–1 on bad days. Make sure that you're doing your long runs at least 2 minutes per mile slower than your goal pace. It's OK to go slower than that.

3. On your Tuesday and Thursday runs, take as many walk breaks as you need. Read the section on walk breaks and when in doubt, walk more.

4. XT means cross train. You can walk or do some form of non-pounding exercise, such as swimming, cycling, or exercise machines, for 10 minutes or so at an easy pace. If you are just starting to do any of these exercises (or are starting back after a layoff), start with only 5 minutes, and increase by 2–3 minutes each session.

5. The 800-meter repeats, on weeks 8, 11, 12, and 14 will help you build the speed you need for a time goal of your choice. Do these on a 400-meter track. After a 5-minute warm-up, run each 800m in 5:10 seconds. Walk for a full 400-meter lap and repeat. Warm down with a slow 5 minutes of running and 5 minutes of walking. Remember that it doesn't benefit you to run faster than the pace assigned for the workout. If you're struggling to run the time assigned for your 800-meter reps, your time goal is too ambitious and should be adjusted.

6. Running the 5K race, on week #10, will give you a "reality check" on your time goal. For a 2:20 goal, you'll want to run a time of 29 minutes or faster in the 5K race. In this race, you can reduce the number of walk breaks in order to run a fast time, for you, on that day. If you run slower than this, you should adjust to a slower time goal using the prediction table in this book.

In the half-marathon race, most should take some walk breaks each mile, as you feel comfortable. (Be sure to move to the side of the road.) Most runners should do the first 11 miles, taking the walk breaks as you have in the long runs. During the last few miles you can cut out some or all of the walking, if you feel strong.

HALF-MARATHON TRAINING PROGRAM: 1:59 goal

Week #	Mon	Tue	Wed	Thu	Fri	Sat	Sun
1.	off or XT	30–40 min. run/walk	off or XT	30–40 min. run/walk	off or XT	off	6 miles run/walk
2.	off or XT	30–40 min. run/walk	off or XT	30–40 min. run/walk	off or XT	off	7 miles run/walk
3.	off or XT	35–40 min. run/walk	off or XT	35–40 min. run/walk	off or XT	off	8 miles run/walk
4.	off or XT	35–40 min. run/walk	off or XT	5×800m	off or XT	off	9 miles run/walk
5.	off or XT	40 min. run/walk	off or XT	40 min. run/walk	off or XT	off	10 miles run/walk
6.	off or XT	40 min. run/walk	off or XT	40 min. run/walk	off or XT	off	**5K Race**
7.	off or XT	40 min. run/walk	off or XT	40 min. run/walk	off or XT	off	12 miles run/walk
8.	off or XT	40 min. run/walk	off or XT	40 min. run/walk	off or XT	off	6×800m
9.	off or XT	40 min. run/walk	off or XT	40 min. run/walk	off or XT	off	14 miles run/walk
10.	off or XT	40 min. run/walk	off or XT	7×800m	off or XT	off	**5K Race**
11.	off or XT	40 min. run/walk	off or XT	8×800m	off or XT	off	16 miles run/walk
12.	off or XT	40 min. run/walk	off or XT	40 min. run/walk	off or XT	off	10×800m
13.	off or XT	40 min. run/walk	off or XT	40 min. run/walk	off or XT	off	17 miles run/walk
14.	off or XT	40 min. run/walk	off or XT	40 min. run/walk	off or XT	off	6–7×800m
15.	off or XT	30 min. run/walk	off or XT	30 min. run/walk	off or XT	off	**Half-Marathon**
Continuation Schedule							
	off or XT	30 min. run/walk	off or XT	30 min. run/walk	off or XT	off	5–6 miles run/walk

This program assumes that you have been running the amount listed in week #1. If you are not doing that, spend the weeks necessary to gradually build to that level. If you are already doing more than is on this schedule, you can continue to maintain at the higher amount, as long as the legs are recovering quickly between runs. If your long run is already longer than 6 miles, you may begin on the week which has a long run as long as you're currently running.

1. You can do the long run on Saturday if you wish. In that case, take Friday off from exercise.

2. On your long runs, take more liberal walk breaks. If you are running 5 minutes and walking for 1 minute on your Tuesday and Thursday runs, do 4–1 on the long runs, or 3–1 on bad days. Make sure that you're doing your long runs at least 2 minutes per mile slower than your goal pace. It's OK to go slower than that.

3. On your Tuesday and Thursday runs, if your legs are feeling fresh enough, run at projected race pace for a mile, take a short walk break and repeat. You can do as many as 2 of these with at least 4 minutes of walking and slow jogging between each set of 2 miles (4 miles total). This "rehearses" your body for race pace. If your legs haven't been recovering well, run the Tuesday and Thursday runs very slowly, with walk breaks.

4. XT means cross train. You can walk or do some form of non-pounding exercise, such as swimming, cycling, or exercise machines, for 10 minutes or so at an easy pace. If you are just starting to do any of these exercises (or are starting back after a layoff), start with only 5 minutes, and increase by 2–3 minutes each session.

5. The 800-meter repeats (6 x 800m, for example) will help you build the speed you need for a time goal of your choice. Do these on a 400-meter track. After an easy 5-minute warm-up, run each 800m in 4:28–4:30. Walk for a full 400-meter lap and repeat. Warm down with a slow 5 minutes of running and 5 minutes of walking. Remember that it doesn't benefit you to run faster than the pace assigned for the workout. If you're struggling to run the time assigned for your 800-meter reps, your time goal is too ambitious and should be adjusted.

6. Running the 5K races, on weeks #6 and #10, will give you a "reality check" on your time goal. For a 1:59 goal, you'll want to run a time of 25:00 or faster in the 5K race. In this race, you can run as fast as you wish, realizing that most 5K PR's are done by running the second half faster than the first. If you run slower than this, you should adjust to a slower time goal using the prediction table in this book.

In the half-marathon race, most should take some walk breaks each mile (30–60 seconds each), as you feel comfortable. (Be sure to move to the side of the road.) Most runners, during the first 10 miles, should take a 60-second walk break every mile. During the last few miles you can cut out some or all of the walking, if you feel strong.

HALF-MARATHON TRAINING PROGRAM: 1:45 goal

Week #	Mon	Tue	Wed	Thu	Fri	Sat	Sun
1.	off or XT	35–40 min. run/walk	off or XT	35–40 min. run/walk	off or XT	off	6 miles run/walk
2.	off or XT	35–40 min. run/walk	off or XT	35–40 min. run/walk	off or XT	off	7 miles run/walk
3.	off or XT	35–40 min. run/walk	off or XT	35–40 min. run/walk	off or XT	off	8 miles run/walk
4.	off or XT	35–40 min. run/walk	off or XT	35–40 min. run/walk	off or XT	off	9 miles run/walk
5.	off or XT	40 min. run/walk	off or XT	40 min. run/walk	off or XT	off	10 miles run/walk
6.	off or XT	40 min. run/walk	off or XT	40 min. run/walk	off or XT	off	**5K Race**
7.	off or XT	40 min. run/walk	off or XT	40 min. run/walk	off or XT	off	12 miles run/walk
8.	off or XT	40 min. run/walk	off or XT	40 min. run/walk	off or XT	off	5×800m
9.	off or XT	40 min. run/walk	off or XT	40 min. run/walk	off or XT	off	14 miles run/walk
10.	off or XT	40 min. run/walk	off or XT	6×800m	off or XT	off	**5K Race**
11.	off or XT	40 min. run/walk	off or XT	7×800m	off or XT	off	16 miles run/walk
12.	off or XT	40 min. run/walk	off or XT	40 min. run/walk	off or XT	off	10×800m
13.	off or XT	40 min. run/walk	off or XT	40 min. run/walk	off or XT	off	17–18 miles run/walk
14.	off or XT	40 min. run/walk	off or XT	40 min. run/walk	off or XT	off	6–7×800m
15.	off or XT	30 min. run/walk	off or XT	30 min. run/walk	off or XT	off	**Half-Marathon**
Continuation Schedule							
	off or XT	30 min. run/walk	off or XT	30 min. run/walk	off or XT	off	5–6 miles run/walk

This program assumes that you have been running the amount listed in week #1. If you are not doing that, spend the weeks necessary to gradually build to that level. If you are already doing more than is on this schedule, you can continue to maintain at the higher amount, as long as the legs are recovering quickly between runs. If your long run is already longer than 6 miles, you may begin on the week which has a long run as long as you're currently running.

1. You can do the long run on Saturday if you wish. In that case, take Friday off from exercise.

2. On your long runs, take more liberal walk breaks. If you are running 6 minutes and walking for 1 minute on your Tuesday and Thursday runs, do 5–1 on the long runs, or 4–1 on bad days. Make sure that you're doing your long runs at least 2 minutes per mile slower than your goal pace. It's OK to go slower than that.

3. On your Tuesday and Thursday runs, if your legs are feeling fresh enough, run at projected race pace for a mile, take a short walk break and repeat. You can do as many as 3 of these with at least 4 minutes of walking and slow jogging between each set of 2 miles. This "rehearses" your body for the race. If your legs haven't been recovering well, run the Tuesday and Thursday runs very slowly, with walk breaks.

4. XT means cross train. You can walk or do some form of non-pounding exercise, such as swimming, cycling, or exercise machines, for 10 minutes or so at an easy pace. If you are just starting to do any of these exercises (or are starting back after a layoff), start with only 5 minutes, and increase by 2–3 minutes each session.

5. The 800-meter repeats (6 x 800m, for example) will help you build the speed you need for a time goal of your choice. Do these on a 400-meter track. After an easy 5-minute warm-up, run each 800m in 3:50. Walk for a full 400-meter lap and repeat. Warm down with a slow 5 minutes of running and 5 minutes of walking. Remember that it doesn't benefit you to run faster than the pace assigned for the workout. If you're struggling to run the time assigned for your 800-meter reps, your time goal is too ambitious and should be adjusted.

6. Running the 5K races, on weeks #6 and #10, will give you a "reality check" on your time goal. For a 1:45 goal, you'll want to run a time of 22:13 or faster in the 5K race. In this race, you can run as fast as you wish, realizing that most 5K PR's are done by running the second half faster than the first. If you run slower than this, you should adjust to a slower time goal using the prediction table in this book.

In the half-marathon race, most should take some walk breaks each mile (30–45 seconds), as you feel comfortable. (Be sure to move to the side of the road.) Most runners, during the first 8 miles, should take a 40–60-second walk break every mile. During the last few miles you can cut out some or all of the walking, if you feel strong.

HALF-MARATHON TRAINING PROGRAM: 1:29 goal

Week #	Mon	Tue	Wed	Thu	Fri	Sat	Sun
1.	off or XT	40 min. run/walk	off or XT	40 min. run/walk	off or XT	off	6 miles run/walk
2.	off or XT	40 min. run/walk	off or XT	40 min. run/walk	off or XT	off	7 miles run/walk
3.	off or XT	40 min. run/walk	off or XT	40 min. run/walk	off or XT	off	8 miles run/walk
4.	off or XT	40 min. run/walk	off or XT	5×800m	off or XT	off	9 miles run/walk
5.	off or XT	40 min. run/walk	off or XT	6×800m	off or XT	off	10 miles run/walk
6.	off or XT	7×800m	off or XT	40 min. run/walk	off or XT	off	**5K Race**
7.	off or XT	40 min. run/walk	off or XT	9×800m	off or XT	off	12 miles run/walk
8.	off or XT	40 min. run/walk	off or XT	40 min. run/walk	off or XT	off	11×800m
9.	off or XT	40 min. run/walk	off or XT	40 min. run/walk	off or XT	off	14 miles run/walk
10.	off or XT	40 min. run/walk	off or XT	13×800m	off or XT	off	**5K Race**
11.	off or XT	40 min. run/walk	off or XT	15×800m	off or XT	off	16 miles run/walk
12.	off or XT	40 min. run/walk	off or XT	40 min. run/walk	off or XT	off	16×800m
13.	off or XT	40 min. run/walk	off or XT	40 min. run/walk	off or XT	off	18 miles run/walk
14.	off or XT	40 min. run/walk	off or XT	40 min. run/walk	off or XT	off	6–7×800m
15.	off or XT	30 min. run/walk	off or XT	30 min. run/walk	off or XT	off	**Half-Marathon**
Continuation Schedule							
	off or XT	30 min. run/walk	off or XT	30 min. run/walk	off or XT	off	5–6 miles run/walk

This program assumes that you have been running the amount listed in week #1. If you are not doing that, spend the weeks necessary to gradually build to that level. If you are already doing more than is on this schedule, you can continue to maintain at the higher amount, as long as the legs are recovering quickly between runs. If your long run is already longer than 6 miles, you may begin on the week which has a long run as long as you're currently running.

1. You can do the long run on Saturday if you wish. In that case, take Friday off from exercise.

2. On your long runs, take more liberal walk breaks. If you are running 8 minutes and walking for 1 minute on your Tuesday and Thursday runs, do 6–1 on the long runs, or 5–1 on bad days. Make sure that you're doing your long runs at least 2 minutes per mile slower than your goal pace. It's OK to go slower than that.

3. On your Tuesday and Thursday runs, if your legs are feeling fresh enough, run at projected race pace for a mile, take a short walk break and repeat. You can do as many as 3 of these with at least 4 minutes of walking and slow jogging between each set of 2 miles (max total is 6 miles). This "rehearses" your body for the race. If your legs haven't been recovering well, run the Tuesday and Thursday runs very slowly, with walk breaks.

4. XT means cross train. You can walk or do some form of non-pounding exercise, such as swimming, cycling, or exercise machines, for 10 minutes or so at an easy pace. If you are just starting to do any of these exercises (or are starting back after a layoff), start with only 5 minutes, and increase by 2–3 minutes each session.

5. The 800-meter repeats (6 x 800m, for example) will help you build the speed you need for a time goal of your choice. Do these on a 400-meter track. After an easy 5-minute warm-up, run each 800m in 3:50. Walk for a full 400-meter lap and repeat. Warm down with a slow 5 minutes of running and 5 minutes of walking. Remember that it doesn't benefit you to run faster than the pace assigned for the workout. If you're struggling to run the time assigned for your 800-meter reps, your time goal is too ambitious and should be adjusted.

6. Running the 5K races, on weeks #6 and #10, will give you a "reality check" on your time goal. For a 1:29 goal, you'll want to run below 19 minutes in the 5K race. In this race, you can run as fast as you wish, realizing that most 5K PR's are done by running the second half faster than the first. If you run slower than this, you should adjust to a slower time goal using the prediction table in this book.

In the half-marathon race, most should take some walk breaks each mile (15–30 seconds), as you feel comfortable. (Be sure to move to the side of the road.) Most runners should take a 20–30-second walk break each mile for the first 6 miles. After that, you can cut out some or all of the walking, if you feel strong.

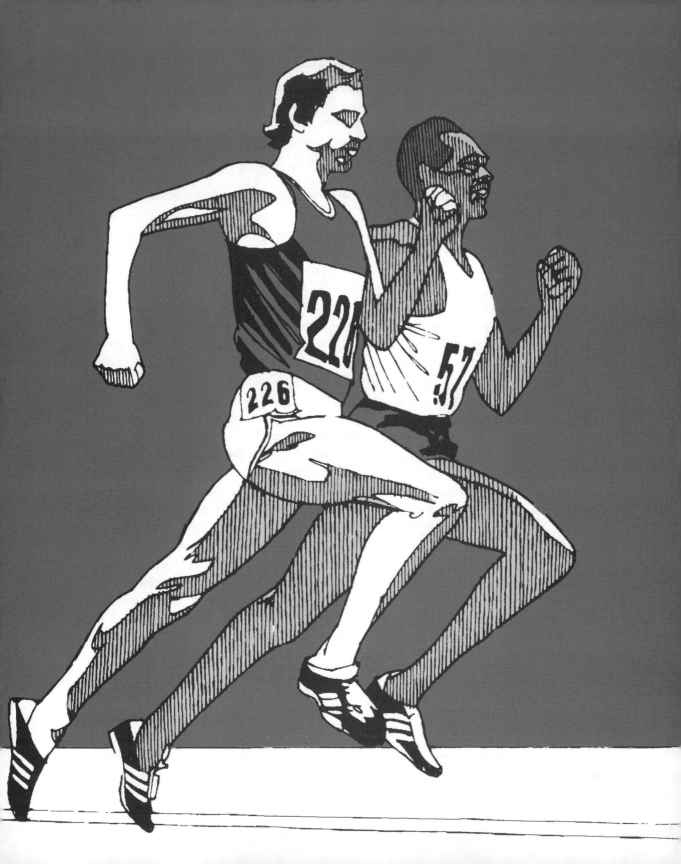

12
THE ADVANCED COMPETITIVE RUNNER

WORKOUTS FOR THE ADVANCED COMPETITIVE RUNNER

RUNNERS WITH AT LEAST four years of speed-work have often found the need for an extra "push" to top performance. These experienced runners usually have muscles and tendons that can handle more abuse, and their years of experience should (but don't always) keep them from overtraining. The principles here are the same; the workouts differ in degree, not kind.

If you try these workouts, follow all the guidelines in Chapter 7, pp. 50–66, especially the easy-week concept. An easy week is especially important after these workouts, since you'll be pushing your body harder than other runners.

Don't be a slave to weekly mileage. The workouts that lead to your goal are the long runs, the speed days, and form work. Weekly mileage during the speed phase is unimportant. It's better to slack off before you need to, than to overtrain and suffer the consequences. Taking extra days off each week can reduce your injury risk significantly (i.e., it is better to cover 25 miles in a 3- or 4-day running week, than to run 5–6 days a week).

> **Note:** Runners must often make sacrifices in order to excel. Performance work demands extra time, which may be taken away from work, family or friends. It can also make you high-strung or difficult to be around. I don't have a solution to this problem—it's really a matter of priorities. If you're an advanced competitor, being aware of the trade-off can make you think about balancing your running with other important elements in your life. Or if you have a friend who is training hard, perhaps this chapter will help you understand the demands of competitive running. (See Five Stages of the Runner, pp. 12–19.)

Greater Injury Risk. Advanced runners often feel invincible, immune to normal running problems. In fact, in spite of their greater experience and stronger running muscles, they are injured more often than the average runner for one simple reason: they run harder and longer. *Speed training is the leading cause of injury among those who do speedwork.*

Those who have been close to the fire know the meaning of warmth and have probably been burned. Usually, runners who have experienced injury-producing workouts become sensitive to early signs of overstress and hopefully will know when to stop. They have learned the necessity of strategic rest.

Greater Need for Rest. Greater stress means greater need for rest. Advanced runners must take their two easy weeks a month and two rest days after a hard or long day. Even when you feel recovered, you must take these breaks. When there is a hint of lingering tiredness, you must have patience and realize that an extra rest day will do more for your ultimate performance than another hard day in a tired state. Rest cannot be compromised without disaster —sooner or later.

Pulse Rate and Weight Maintenance. It's very important for a veteran competitive runner to check pulse rate and body weight daily. As soon as you wake up—before getting out of bed—check your pulse. Then step on the scales. *See p. 46 for details.*

Heart Rate Monitors (that monitor pulse). Those who are doing regular speed training can benefit from a pulse monitor more than other runners. *See pp. 46–49 for more details on how these can help.*

Common Mistakes

- *Pacing.* Advanced runners often run too fast on days that should be slow and easy. Long runs build endurance, hills build strength, and speedwork develops speed. The runs between should be slow, recovery experiences, about 2 minutes per mile slower than 10K race pace. *When in doubt, go slower.*

- *High-powered weekends.* Don't run a race and a long run the same weekend. This stresses the system. Long-run weekends can be alternated with race weekends.
- *Too much speed.* Speedwork should not continue beyond the periods listed in the charts or you will encounter fatigue, sickness, or injury.

One Day Off Per Week. Yes, you too! Advanced runners tend to be compulsive. Force yourself to take at least one day off per week, usually before the long-run day. This must be scheduled and adhered to. Competitors who are over 40 should take 2 days per week off, and those over 50 will usually improve if they put all their training into 4 days per week (instead of 5–7 days).

Goals. Like other runners, advanced competitors often have a general performance goal but are not specific about when they want to achieve that goal. They end up bouncing from one race to the next. They lose the edge gained by top European distance runners who plan for a specific performance peak and reach that goal by scheduling for it.

To make optimal progress, goals need to be scheduled at least six months in advance with a training pyramid *(see pp. 36–37)*. Races, long runs, and speed workouts can be carefully interwoven and strategically staged for maximum results.

Goals should not be too ambitious. By moving gently from one goal to the next, you build a foundation of success which leads to other successes. The most successful goal setters I have known plan to be at top performance during a 4–6 week period. That allows them to make the constant adjustments necessary along the way, instead of being a slave to a daily schedule made up months in advance.

THE ADVANCED TRAINING PROGRAM

Endurance. A long, slow run should be taken every other week. Gradually increase to beyond the race distance. The maximum long run for a 10K is 15–17 miles, and for the half-marathon, 18–21 miles. The extra distance builds extra endurance and almost assures better performance. When you have gone farther than the race distance, you can maintain a faster pace in the race. The extra long runs give you a better cardiovascular base, which will help you get more out of your speedwork.

Hills. Advanced runners can run a hill workout once a week during the base period. By running 4–8 hills, you can develop lower leg strength, which allows you to shift the body weight forward and push off strongly on your forefoot. This increases speed.

During the hill period of the pyramid, advanced runners can do two hill workouts per week. One could build to 4–8 hills of yards, 300–600 meters long at a 10K pace. The second workout should be shorter and faster: 6–10 × 80–150 meters, at 5K pace. These must be coordinated with races; they're usually done on Tuesdays and Thursdays, with long runs or races on weekends. Be sure to warm up thoroughly before these workouts. No sprinting!

Speed. During the speed phase, hill workouts are replaced by intervals or fartlek. Advanced runners will find the speed workouts excellent preparation for their goals. Because of your speedwork experience, you should be able to jog (rather than walk) between repetitions and take less rest between repetitions (half the repetition distance or less). The reduced rest gives the body a higher level of anaerobic conditioning. If more rest (or walking) is needed to complete the number of reps in the time assigned, take it.

A second, faster speed session (usually Thursday) can be done each week to increase leg turnovers and mechanics. Here you lower the 400 pace of the main workout by about five seconds. This is a shorter workout and you take the complete rest in between reps. Don't sprint. Run with a relaxed form, at a pace that is at or slightly faster than race pace, picking up the rhythm. *Examples:* 3–5 × 400, or 6–8 × 200, or 2 × 300; 1 × 400, 2 × 220.

The second, shorter hill workout could be alternated with this second speed workout, if you feel the need for strength or more hill training. The longer hill workout is abandoned during the speed phase.

An alternative to the long speed sessions is training for a shorter race. Half-marathoners could do speedwork designed for the 10K; 10K specialists would train for the 5K, etc. Endurance is maintained through long runs and racing endurance is fine-tuned through hard, continuous runs (tempo runs).

Half-marathon runners would run the repeat 400s of a 10K speed program (*see pp. 105–114*) on Thursday or Friday after a long run and again on Tuesday or Wednesday before the next long one. The repetitions would be run 5–7 seconds faster than the current 10K goal pace and would gradually build in number to 20.

10K runners would shift to a maximum of 12 × 400, but would run each about 3–5 seconds faster than a 5K goal pace.

Advanced Fartlek Principles

This trains your mind as it conditions your body. There is no end of the track to shoot for, so you quickly learn your limits. You want to push yourself to near the limit and stay there. As you make progress in your fartlek training, you learn your potential as never before. Because this workout more closely resembles a race, it takes more recovery time. For every easy day after an interval workout, take two easy days after these fartlek sessions. One of these every two weeks is plenty. In a race, you never know when the pace will pick up. Fartlek, with its intermittent accelerations—and no complete rest in between—gets you ready for this situation.

- Set distance at race distance (a maximum of 12 miles).
- Warm up by running an easy ½–1½ miles.
- Run a fairly *hard base* pace, about 5–10% *slower* than race pace.
- Run *accelerations* starting at race pace.
- Vary length of accelerations: 50–350 yards; 400–600 yards; 800–1000 meters. Occasionally throw in a fast 50. You can use the shorter ones to recover when you really need it.
- Return to base pace—not a jog—immediately after each acceleration. (This is the tough part.)
- Run segments of 1–5 minutes.
- Warm down the final 1–2 miles. Jog and relax after the hard running.
- Fartlek is free-form. You can be creative and tailor it to suit your exact speed needs. If you find yourself getting left in the dust at the end of a race, work hard on your accelerations at the end of a workout. If you find others pulling away from you in the middle, work on your mid-workout accelerations.

Advanced Interval Training

Interval workouts can also be creative. First, cover the basics by building the total number of reps to approximately race distance and keep the speed slightly below race pace. Then you can tailor your workouts to help you where you need it most.

Veterans should be able to take less rest between repetitions, You can jog between reps at a faster pace and still recover. Sometimes this also means you must take rest days, so listen to your body.

Longer repetition distances also help simulate race conditions. Instead of 20×400, a 10K runner could run 10×800—or even 5×1 mile. There's no need to keep the same distance throughout. Run a 600, then a mile, then a 400. The guidelines are the same as for other runners: start with the equivalent of $6–8 \times 400$, gradually build up through the weeks to 20×400. Don't run more than eight weeks of this intense speedwork. After that, you must return to your aerobic base period.

Here's a fartlek/interval innovation that's worked well for me: mile repeats are my base. My goal race pace is my "base pace" for each mile. Within the four laps I run several accelerations, one about 500 yards, and 2–3 others 50–100 meters. After each acceleration, I try to come back to the base pace.

Advanced runners may choose between fartlek or interval training or may mix them. In any case, these two stressful workouts need to be carefully mixed with races and long runs so there is adequate rest between each. *If you run more than one race or long run per week, you will run great risk of injury.*

The following workouts are listed only as guidelines that can be inserted into a 10K or half-marathon program. Remember,

you are running these for form and speed. You don't have to complete them as listed. Your goal is to stay bouncy and strong throughout the workout. If you start feeling tired, or begin dragging, cut the distance of the reps in half. If this doesn't help, abandon the workout.

Sample Two-Week Schedule							
Week	Mon	Tue	Wed	Thu	Fri	Sat	Sun
1	Easy	Intervals	Easy	Acceleration glider	Easy	Off	Long (15–18)
2	Easy	Fartlek	Easy	Acceleration glider	Easy	Off	Long (8–15 or race)

Acceleration Gliders

When done every 3 days or so, these little "pick-ups" will warm up your legs while they improve your running form. These are not sprints, and are not hard to do. Your mission is to play with your momentum, while running with less effort. The acceleration part is easy to do on a short stretch of downhill. Simply pick up the turnover of your feet (not your stride length) on the downhill, propelled by gravity, touching lightly with your feet. As you "coast" onto flat ground, maintain that increase without any significant effort. Then let the momentum gradually decrease, back to your easy running pace for that day. Your goal is to glide very smoothly, even with a quicker turnover. *(See "Acceleration Gliders in Six Easy Steps" on pp. 145–147.)*

Barefoot Running

If you like, and have the proper surface, barefooted running can help. This develops a quicker response from your foot, reducing shock and improving leg turnover. Shoes block some of the crucial rhythmic

feedback from your feet. Best is a smooth, well-groomed grass course, with no rocks or glass. Ease into barefoot running, at first doing only one or two 50-yard bursts (no sprinting). Two or three days later, run 2–3, etc. (Remember: You don't have the cushion of running shoes, so there's more impact. By jumping into this too soon and too fast, you can injure vital muscles and tendons.)

Only veteran barefoot runners should try loose sand. There are many potential hazards. Sand running is resistance work, not rhythmic running, and can be substituted for a hill workout with proper care. It helps to develop extra strength, but there is correspondingly extra stress. With the "aqua socks" type of foot covering (used by windsurfers, etc.) you can get about the same foot response and have some protection.

Peaking

The veteran should be more "fine-tuned" than other runners and can therefore benefit most from a careful peaking strategy.

Beyond the Plateau

Often veteran runners will tell me they just can't seem to get beyond that 3:05 marathon, or 38-minute 10K, etc., try as they might. I've heard similar complaints over the years, have thought about it and come up with a few suggestions. If you've reached a plateau (it can be either slower or faster times than the above examples), here's what you might do to break through to a new performance level:

- Try a temporary reduction in job-related stress. Take your annual vacation 2–3 weeks before the marathon. Get away from the computer and phone.

- Train at a higher altitude than where you'll be racing. (This helps mentally, too.)

- Switch to a lighter racing shoe. This will improve your efficiency and performance provided you're still getting enough cushion. Half-marathoners should not choose the lightest racing flat, but a lightweight training shoe.

- Reduce your body fat (provided you have fat and weight to spare). Reduce fat and sugar intake and increase your mileage slowly and gradually. *(See* Fat-Burning, *p. 233.)*

IN THE LONG RUN

Most runners don't realize how long it takes to fully develop their endurance-running potential. Often after running two, three or four years, they reach a plateau and consider their best time unsurpassable. The truth is, and it will probably surprise you, *it takes about ten years to build your strength, speed and endurance* to its full potential in running—no matter what the starting age.

RACING STRATEGY FOR THE ADVANCED COMPETITIVE RUNNER

In the media, too much credit is given to the racing strategies of victorious athletes. From what I've seen, many runners win in spite of their strategies, or fail because they do not tailor their strategies to their abilities. An example of this was Steve Prefontaine, America's top 5K runner in the early 1970s. Pre was unbeatable in the U.S., but because of poor strategy couldn't win in Europe, where he raced each summer. In practically every race, less-talented runners would leave him behind with a finishing kick. After one of these summers, he told me that he merely needed more and faster speedwork—which he proceeded to do. The next summer, after finishing second, third and fourth in Europe, he discovered that determination and hard speedwork cannot install fast-twitch muscle fibers that Mother Nature left out.

Leading up to the 1972 Olympics, Pre again changed his racing strategy. He decided to run hard for the last mile of the 5K race to put his competitors into oxygen debt and "burn the kick outta them." As planned, he took the lead with four laps to go and increased the pace. Unfortunately, he burned no one out but himself. Lasse Viren, the Finnish superstar, accelerated dramatically with two laps to go and held that hard pace until the end—hitting the tape far in front of everyone else. Had Pre waited until the last two laps, he probably would have given Viren a good race.

Front Runners. Occasionally front runners will win a race but usually they just set up a fast race for the eventual winner. Front runners try to build up a lead and demoralize the competition. Usually they become victims of "the wall." They go out at a much faster pace than they can maintain, slow down dramatically during the last third of the race, and are passed by the eventual winner who is running at a more even pace.

The front runner feeds on the confidence of being the leader. This mental energy and optimism propels the front runner to a hard, fast race. Although experienced front runners don't often win, they consistently finish high in their peer group, and often run faster times when they lead from the start.

By pushing the pace throughout the race, front runners get an excellent workout. If they don't overtrain between races, they improve their condition race by race and are able to hold their fast pace for a longer distance in successive races.

Wait and Kick: The Lazy Method for Speedsters. If you're blessed with natural speed and find it's still there at the end of the race, you can afford to be lazy: wait and kick. Big kickers let others do the pacing. As members of the lead pack jostle for position, they drop back and save their energy.

The biggest problem for the kicker is staying with the leaders until the finish line is in sight. If you drop too far behind the pack, it takes great mental energy to catch up. Lead pack runners get increased energy from the exhilaration (and paranoia). They often try to "waste" the kickers by forcing a hard pace early on or by running a series of speed bursts.

As distance racing becomes more competitive at all levels, more races will be decided by the kick. Every runner, regardless of ability, can benefit from a regular program of accelerations that will develop speed. Runners with a kick who do regular quality speedwork and regular long runs are difficult to beat.

Kickers need to have some fartlek training sessions that train them to relax as the pace gradually picks up. The bottom line is that you must train to be ready for any race tactic used by your opponents.

Stronger Arms for a More Powerful Kick. If everything else is equal between two runners, the runner with stronger arms and shoulders may run slightly faster in the sprint to the finish. For a short period, moving your arms faster makes you run faster. Jim Ryun lifted weights throughout his career. Frank Shorter, Olympic marathon champion, has said that weight training helps him run as much as three seconds faster for the last lap of a 10K, but added that he thinks only highly competitive endurance runners in the top of their age groups will benefit significantly from weight training.

How to Develop a Kick

- Continue two acceleration sessions per week year-round. Work on rhythm and driving quickly off each foot. Never run these at top speed; run at your current mile race pace, occasionally running at 800 race pace.

- During the speedwork phase, do an extra session of accelerations after speedwork: 1×300, 1×200, 2×150 meters, etc. The 150's are run to the end of the track straightaway from the middle of the curve. Take lots of rest between each acceleration.

- Work on driving with strength and lightness. Don't let your hands get in the way: keep the palms down and let your wrists relax.

- Remember that you'll be tired at the end of these speed sessions. It's easy to injure yourself by pushing too hard. Monitor yourself carefully and back off if there's any feeling of strain.

- Warm down with at least one easy mile of *slow* jogging.

Bursting: A Strategy That Often Backfires. Some runners who have been frustrated by being out-sprinted at the end of races will try to "burn" the kick out of kickers by bursting (accelerating) in the middle or late stages of the race. The theory is the same as that of the front runner: by going with the burster, the kicker will use up his fast-twitch energy stores and reduce the power of the kick; but if he doesn't accelerate, the kicker lets the burster get so far ahead that the final kick can't carry him to victory.

The theory seldom works in a race. The burster usually gets worn out by the inefficiency of accelerating in a long race. Generally the kicker and others will let the burster go and then gradually and efficiently speed up and reel him in. Rarely does a kicker fall prey to the trick and match strides with the burster.

When it's common knowledge that a runner is the best in a given race, he can use bursting to separate himself from the rest of the pack. Otherwise, improving runners can hang on to a better runner and then run over their head in the final sprint. The "star" can sometimes discourage his competitors by a burst or two in the middle.

Pick It Up in the Final Mile. The smart runner maintains an even pace until the final stage of the race and then applies the strategy best suited to his or her capabilities. If you don't have much of a kick, your best strategy, in my opinion, is that of a sustained final mile or two.

Experiment to define *your* final stage of the race. For a 10K it might range from $\frac{1}{2}$–2 miles. In a half-marathon, it might be the last mile or the last three. Most runners find they can concentrate best if the distance is around 1–1 $\frac{1}{2}$ miles or less.

Until that point, an even pace is best. If you keep track of your peer group and maintain mental contact, you'll find yourself moving up on them as the miles pass. Then you'll have the added energy and enthusiasm of passing people in the last part of the race; it's also demoralizing to your competitors.

To run the kick (and determination) out of a speedster, you must run hard for a sustained distance. Gradually accelerate and put the pressure on. Don't go so fast at first that you can't hold it to the end; but try to make it hurt a little. Then when you reach the halfway mark of your final push, go a bit harder. This long drive is hard on you, but it's harder on your opponents who haven't trained for it. They also don't know how long you can hold your acceleration. In many cases it wears the kicker's sprint muscles out so they cannot accelerate at the end. The best way to train for this is to run the last few repetitions of your hillwork or speedwork sessions harder than the earlier segments.

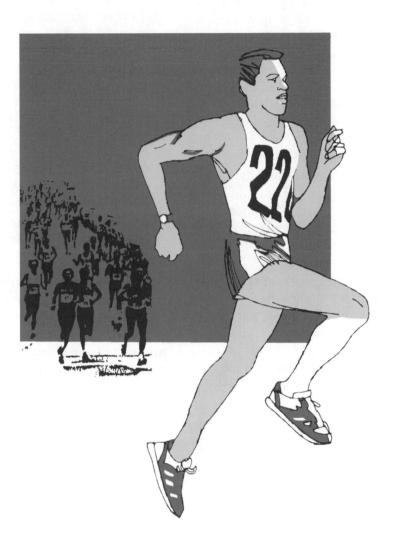

TOO MUCH OF A GOOD THING

As I've mentioned, running is an addictive activity. Once you've run long enough to experience the stimulating effects of endurance exercise, it's hard to turn back. You feel so *good*, you never want to let it slide. Your body is used to its daily fix of oxygen, a better attitude, increased circulation, and calming endorphins.

Yet running, like many other pursuits, can be carried too far—from habit to obsession. A highly motivated, hard-driving person may ride the pendulum swing from an overweight, sedentary lifestyle to an almost constant preoccupation with running, racing, and weight. The solution soon becomes the problem.

Physical symptoms are obvious early warning signs of burnout. When activity is increased dramatically or too many races are run, injury is probably just down the road. There are also mental signs of going too far. You may not feel like running, you may be depressed, or you may experience radical behavior changes.

Early Warning Signs. Your body has hormones that keep you going under periods of stress. Sometimes you may feel even better than normal when overstressed. Try to be aware of the early signs of stress so you can back off when they occur and avoid injury or breakdown. These early signs are:

- *Restlessness at night*
- *Higher pulse rate in the morning.* If it's 10% higher, cut back 50% on distance, and run each mile one minute slower. If it's 20% higher, stop running for 1–3 days.

- *Soreness in the feet.* If your feet remain sore for a week, stop running for 2–3 days.
- *Pain in your "weak links."* If in doubt, take a day or two off to get the healing process started.
- *Change in appetite.* If you suddenly feel like eating more, or less, it may be due to overstress.
- *Lack of desire.* Usually your desire to run will be rekindled during the run, even if things were dragging at first. But if you have three or more days when the flame is not rekindled, take a 3-day rest.
- *Feeling dead at the beginning and end of a run.* Again, take a 1–3-day lay-off.

When running is no longer a joy and a release from the pressures of the world, but a manic pursuit, then family, friends and job are likely to suffer. Some runners —you probably know a few like this— jump into it so strongly they let everything *else* go. Ironically, they begin to lose the motivation even to run—although they keep pounding away, day after day. They're miserable, but don't know it.

I've seen many, many burnouts in my running career, with varying shades of disaster: divorce, separation, friendships ended, social contacts severed, careers interrupted, etc. The best advice I can give you to avoid this sad state of affairs is to first, be aware of the early warning signals— recurring injuries, depression, loss of motivation, irritability, fixation—and make necessary course corrections. Secondly, try to keep things balanced and in harmony, and *let running enhance, not rule, your life.*

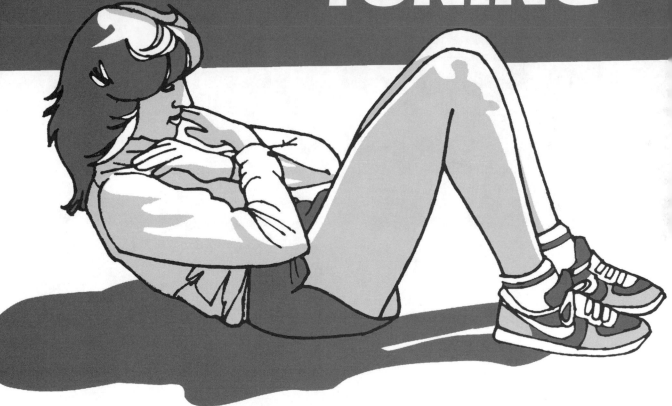
TUNING

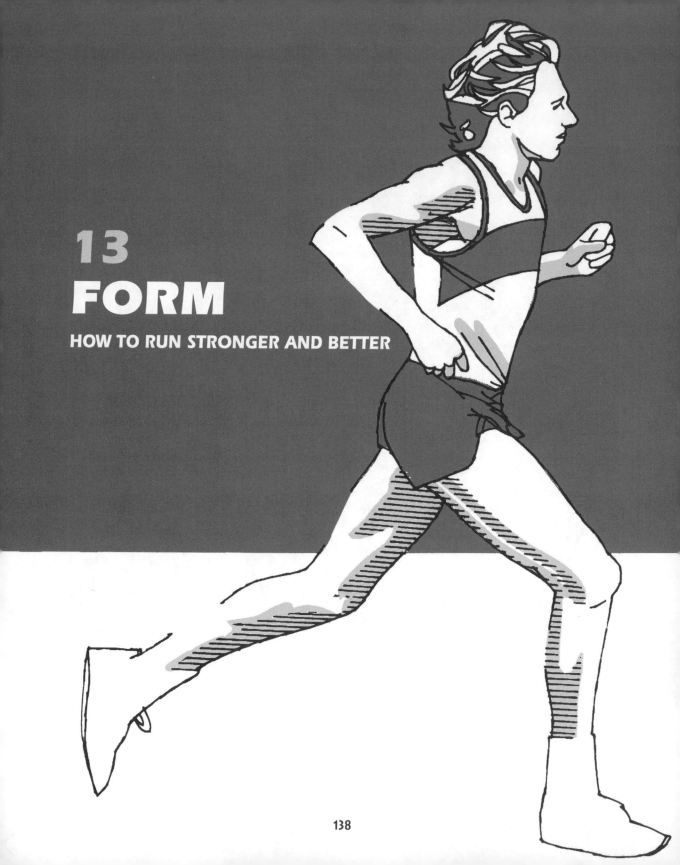

13
FORM
HOW TO RUN STRONGER AND BETTER

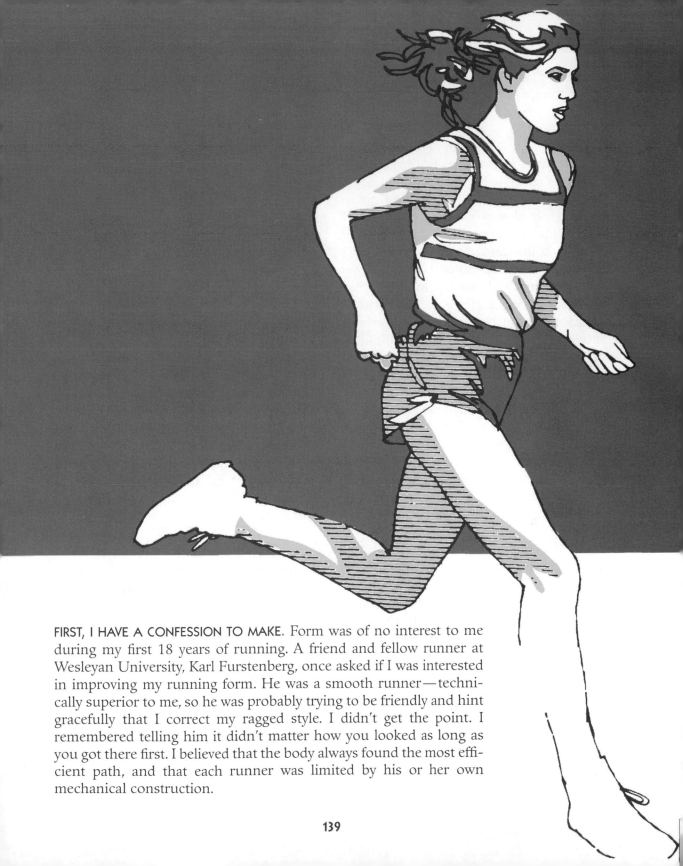

FIRST, I HAVE A CONFESSION TO MAKE. Form was of no interest to me during my first 18 years of running. A friend and fellow runner at Wesleyan University, Karl Furstenberg, once asked if I was interested in improving my running form. He was a smooth runner—technically superior to me, so he was probably trying to be friendly and hint gracefully that I correct my ragged style. I didn't get the point. I remembered telling him it didn't matter how you looked as long as you got there first. I believed that the body always found the most efficient path, and that each runner was limited by his or her own mechanical construction.

More than ten years later, however, my "lazy" form was getting me into trouble. In my earlier days, I had instinctively sprung off the forefoot—using the flick of each ankle for propulsion. Later I found I could rest the lower leg muscles by "cruising"— leaning slightly back and shuffling along. This more relaxed pattern allowed me to run slightly slower with less effort. As I slipped into this "cruise" mode for most of my workouts and races, I was losing power—and races. Since I wasn't using the springing and driving muscles, they were not strong and ready. The "cruise" muscles are not designed for power and acceleration—and they often were pulled or strained when I used them for that purpose. My running form was drifting.

Then I met Arthur Lydiard. The coach of New Zealand Olympic champions believed that form work helped good runners become great. I tried his suggestions and later developed some form principles of my own that have helped runners of all abilities run better and faster with the same effort.

One problem with learning form from a book (as opposed to a coach) is that you can read all the particulars, but then when you're out running it's impossible to remember everything. What I'll do here is list the general principles of good form. Some of them will ring a bell with you; you'll also recognize things in your own running style that need improvement.

Over the past three decades, I've videotaped thousands of runners at my Lake Tahoe running camp, giving improvement suggestions to almost every one. Fitness runners usually need to eliminate extraneous motion and shuffle more. Competitive folks focus on using their mechanical efficiency and strength. All benefit from making little adaptations to run smoother and stronger.

But don't go out and practice all these tips at once. It'll only confuse you. The *Points on Form* section that follows is an overall review of good form and something which you can refer back to whenever you want to fine-tune things. The section after that, *Three Tips on Form*, lists three basic principles that are fairly easy to remember and that you can work on right away.

POINTS ON FORM

There is no single prescription for efficient running, for we are all put together differently. These points on form are general principles of body mechanics that can be applied to all runners. Be sensitive to your own structure and abilities and never force a particular running style on yourself that doesn't feel right.

> **One other thing:** Good form is something all runners—regardless of ability or experience—can work on. Racers are naturally interested in improving form, for it will help them run faster. But beginners and non-competitive runners will also benefit from understanding some of these principles, for good form will make anyone's running smoother and more enjoyable.

Erect Posture. Your running will be most efficient if your posture is erect, perpendicular to the ground (and the force of gravity).

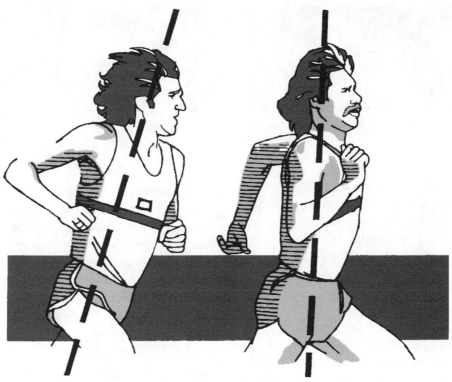

The most efficient way to run is to have your head, neck, and shoulders erect, as at right. When you're leaning forward, as at left, you're always fighting gravity.

Check your form as you run by storefronts in a shopping center. If your body parts are lined up properly, you'll feel like you're moving forward as one unit—head, torso, hips, knees, and ankles all together. The storefront windows will tell you if your head or shoulders, etc., are leaning too far ahead or behind.

Feet Low to the Ground. It is the "revolutions per minute" of your feet and legs that reduce pounding and improve speed and efficiency. Every runner will benefit when the feet lightly touch and barely leave the ground. This allows you to improve turnover or "RPM's" of the feet and legs, which improves speed for most runners.

Relaxed Body. If your body is relaxed and balanced by being erect, you won't have to spend energy keeping your head, neck, shoulders, etc., aligned. The muscles of your jaw and face should be so relaxed that they bounce and shake as you run. Relax your upper body; it's just going along for the ride and you don't want to divert energy into this area.

Moving Forward. All motion should be directed straight ahead. Hips, shoulders, arms and legs should be pointing forward —not side-to-side and certainly not leaning back. This may sound obvious, but just look at the next runner you see for wobbles, sways, and backward lean. I'll be charitable and not ask you to look at yourself—yet.

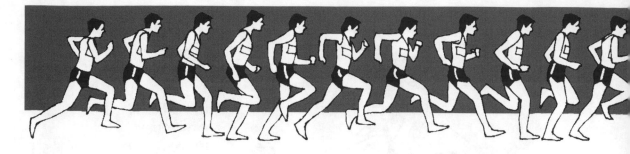

Arms. The main function of the arms is coordination with the legs. At the completion of each arm swing, a nerve signal tells the legs to work again. When held in a relaxed swing fairly low and close to the body, very little effort is required to keep your arms in place and you'll tend to get a quicker response from your feet. But if you hold your arms out from your body, your arms and shoulders will tire quickly. In general, the less arm swing, the better. The arm motion won't help you run faster or farther, but too much arm motion can slow you down through upper body fatigue. Less is more!

Let gravity do your arm work. Keep the top of your hands up, not to the side, and wrists relaxed and floppy. Let your legs lead and your arms follow your leg motion. Your hand can rise as high as the middle of your chest and back as far as the seam on your pants. *Most of your arm movement should be in the lower arms; the upper arms should not move very much.* Practice in front of a mirror. Don't try to run with your arms, just let them relax and follow the rhythm of your feet.

Arm-swing Tip: Keep your fingers slightly cupped and relaxed, palms down; let your hands slightly knick the outside of your shorts with each swing. If you find your hands and arms getting tight, shake them loosely and then put your thumb and forefinger together. This should keep the tension in a small arc between the two fingers.

Hips. Hips should simply be in alignment, directly underneath head and shoulders. Some of us slouch as we stand, walk or run and let the hips shift back and tilt one way or the other. This puts a major mechanical link out of position, and can cause hip and knee discomfort and injury.

Legs. Sprinters lift their knees high. Endurance runners do not. Sprinters must achieve maximum stride length, leg speed and power. You can't run very long like that. You should also avoid a high back kick. Increasing speed in long runs comes from a quicker turnover of legs due to ankle action; high knee lift and back kick will slow this down and divert power up or behind you instead of pushing you down the road.

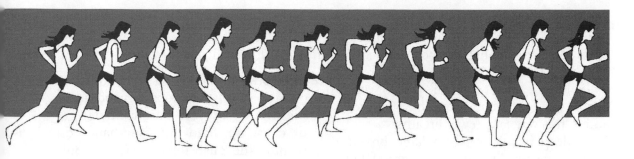

Ankle Efficiency. The ankle is a highly efficient lever. As you strengthen your lower leg muscles, you'll be able to naturally move your ankle into position for an efficient release. This saves energy because the mechanics of the ankle do most of the work instead of the leg muscles. Your calf muscles will conserve energy, and the hamstring muscles are only needed for fine-tuning when you use your ankles. In other words, this is a "lift off" instead of a "push off." See drawing below on how to take advantage of ankle power.

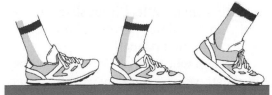

Heel landing: For cushion and to respond to your body alignment (left).

Ankle angle: Quickly shift forward so ankle is in position to push strongly (center.)

Foot push: When put in position, the ankle will automatically spring forward (right).

Stride Length. Believe it or not, a longer stride will not lead to faster running. *Experienced competitive runners find that their stride length shortens as they run faster.* A key to faster running is stride frequency. If you increase the speed of your footfall and get a good strong pushoff, you'll improve. Most runners I've worked with who have stride problems, have too long a stride (often by only an inch or two, however).

Quick and Light. You should touch lightly with each step. As your form improves, the sound of your feet decreases—as the direct force of each ankle-push increases. Top runners prance along, because they use the flick of the ankle and save energy that would otherwise be demanded by hamstrings and other major muscles.

Once you have overcome inertia by starting your run, you want to refine your form and use it to your advantage. You are trying to minimize the effect of gravity rather than overcome it; you do this by touching lightly, with quick turnover, flowing with the momentum you've produced. If you feel like your running easier, lighter and quieter, you're doing it the right way.

Deep Breathing. When you are inactive you need only a small part of your lung capacity. When you run, you need to use much more. Deep breathing or "belly breathing" makes running easier. If your posture is erect you can utilize more of your lung capacity. With your chest forward you're better aligned for deep breathing.

To feel what it's like to get your chest forward, take a deep breath and maintain your forward (inhaled) position after exhaling. This helps you to use more of your lung capacity. When you breathe deeply you get better absorption of oxygen and in this way take fewer breaths.

A deep breath is not a large breath. "Deep" means directing the normal but quick amount of air into the lower part of your lungs. Put your hand on your stomach and take a quick breath of air. If your stomach comes out a little, before your chest fills up, then you're doing it correctly.

THREE TIPS ON CORRECT RUNNING POSTURE: CHP

Here are three steps to efficient running form. These are the major aspects of improved mechanics; when mastered, they can improve any running style.

Note: *It's hard to remember all the aspects of form when you're out running. If you forget everything else about form, try to remember these three points. A friend of mine from California tells me he remembers these three by thinking CHP—California Highway Patrol—for Chest/Hips/Push:*

1. Chest Up. Lift your chest. Take a deep breath and hold that forward position as you exhale. Lydiard says to imagine you have a pulley attached to a harness around your chest. The other end of the pulley is attached to a three-story building a block away. As you run, lift your chest up and forward; it leads the way. Don't lean forward, just get your chest up and out. It will give you extended lung capacity. Even more important, this will give you an efficient and upright posture. Don't change your

shoulders or arms at all. Work only with your chest and you'll achieve better posture and lung efficiency.

2. Hips Forward. When you pull your chest up it helps pull your hips forward automatically. Before you start running, get your chest up; then put your hands on your butt and push forward. Your shoulders, head, hips, and feet should all be lined up. In this position you can extend your legs for maximum power. Lydiard contrasts this with the typical runner's position, which he calls "sitting in the bucket." When your hips are under and forward you'll feel the muscles of the calf being used and hardly any exertion in the hamstrings. You should feel light on your feet and run quieter when hips are forward.

3. Push Off by letting your ankles work automatically. When they are brought into position by a forward chest and hips, a small amount of work from the calf muscles can produce a major effect in push-off power from your feet. This "lift off" is your reward for being aligned properly.

Runners who lean slightly back as they run must overcome gravity with each step. A wear spot on the shoe heel indicates this. It's fine to land on your heel, but don't stay there. It's harmful to the knees. The knee cap is pulled tightly into the knee, grinding the cartilage against the bones. When your ankle does the work, this knee tension is reduced considerably.

If you naturally land on the heel, don't try to shift suddenly to your forefoot. After landing, shift your weight to the midfoot and let the ankle exert its leverage. Gradually make your running *an ankle reflex action*, which will give you the feeling of floating, more than pounding.

Practice These Three Tips. These three tips work together; they're not isolated factors. Try this standing up: Lift your chest and shift your hips; you should feel yourself roll off on your toes. Lining yourself up properly generates forward momentum. By running in proper alignment, you reduce wasted motion. You're directing energy and generating power in the right direction while using the momentum you've generated.

WEEKLY FORM WORK

Form work will improve your running if you practice it twice weekly, year-round. A man in his '70s taught me the value of this one summer. Dr. Miguel Dobrinski celebrated his 74th birthday with us at our Tahoe Trails running camp. He was impressively active and joined us in all our activities. But during the form sessions when accelerating or bounding, he could barely get off the ground. I didn't want to offer false hope and frankly explained to him that it was probably too late to build spring into his legs.

The following year, in our first form session, what did we see but a bouncing Dobrinski in the mountains! As he celebrated his 75th birthday, he explained that he had practiced his accelerations regularly. He had restored 30 years of bounce in one year.

FORM ACCELERATION GLIDERS

When done every 3 days or so, these little "pick-ups" will warm up your legs while they improve your running form. These are not sprints, and are not hard to do. Your mission is to play with your momen-

tum, while running with less effort. The acceleration part is easy to do on a short stretch of downhill. Simply pick up the turnover of your feet (not your stride length) on the downhill, propelled by gravity, touching lightly with your feet. As you "coast" onto flat ground, maintain that increase without any significant effort. Then let the momentum gradually decrease, back to your easy running pace for that day. Your goal is to glide very smoothly, even with a quicker turnover.

The Procedure

- Warm up with at least 10 minutes of slow jogging.
- Stop, shake shoulders, arms, head until they feel relaxed.
- Take a deep breath, exhale, and keep the forward chest orientation.
- Push hips forward with hands on butt.
- Roll off on your toes and "lift off."
- After you've established your momentum, glide for several strides (by just coasting on your momentum, and resting the running muscles).

Each of these offers you a chance to work on more efficient running form.

- Keep the legs relaxed throughout the warm-up, the gliders themselves, and afterward.
- Ease into the gliders, using downhills as the accelerations. If you don't have a downhill available, accelerate by shortening the stride, picking up the turnover rate of the legs, and then relaxing as you glide.
- Start with 3–5 gliders and increase by 1 or 2 each session to a maximum of 10 or 12.

- Two of these sessions per week will help to reinforce form improvements mechanically.
- You can use these as a warm-up before hills, speed sessions, or races. You may also do them during your recovery and maintenance runs each week.

Why? Running accelerations with good form teaches you to run faster. Through repeated outings, you get in touch with your body mechanics, and stay in touch. You instinctively become aware of inefficiencies and learn to correct them.

When? Twice a week, year-round. The idea is to set aside these periods to concentrate on form and not worry about it constantly. You needn't always be preoccupied with form. You may use the form accelerations as warm-ups for a hill workout, speed session or race; or simply put them in the middle of a normal run. A common practice is to run one on Tuesday, another on Thursday.

How Far? 50–150 yards.

How Fast? About your race pace for 5K. This is fast but not all out. Never sprint. Gradually build into this pace, hold it for 30–80 yards, then glide and ease off gradually.

Acceleration Gliders in Six Easy Steps

1. Start your warm-up by walking for 5 minutes, then walking and jogging very slowly for 5-10 minutes, and then easing into your running pace for that day. Warm down by reversing this procedure.

2. Go down! After you're warmed up, use a slight downhill segment of 20–40 running steps to get a little momentum. Be sure to keep the legs and body relaxed throughout, without increasing your stride length. As you reach the flat, coast along with the added momentum, touching the ground lightly with your feet near the surface of the road or trail. If no downhill is available, pick up your leg rhythm by shortening your stride length and gradually increasing the turnover of your feet and legs for 20–30 steps. (Turnover is simply the number of steps you take per minute.)

3. After the first few steps of the acceleration, when you feel comfortable at the faster rhythm, let the stride lengthen just a bit if you wish, but don't let it get too long. Avoid any feeling of tension or over-stretching in the back of your legs.

4. You're now up to speed, so just glide, keeping the feet low to the ground and using very little effort. At the first sign of this, reduce stride length, and touch more lightly with your feet.

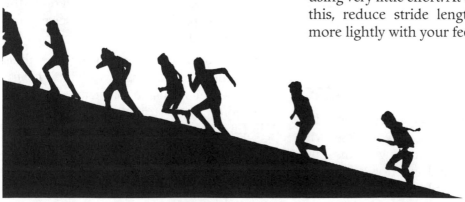

5. Continue gliding for between 10–30 steps.

6. Rest by jogging very slowly or walking between accelerations.

RUNNING FORM FOR HILLS

Making Molehills Out of Mountains. Training on hills makes running easier on any surface. Specifically, hill training will:

* Greatly strengthen lower leg muscles and quadriceps, getting you prepared for speedwork.

* Teach you rhythm — probably the most overlooked and crucial ingredient in distance racing. Good rhythm can pull you through periods of tiredness.

* Give you a good hard workout with relatively little pounding.

Erect Posture. Keep your chest out and up. Good posture will help your body mechanics, whether running up or downhill. Try not to compromise the maximum lift from each step by leaning either forward or backward as you ascend or decline. You'll get the greatest push from each step if your main elements — head, chest, hips and feet — are perpendicular to an imaginary horizontal. They are therefore lined up to best defy gravity.

Running Uphill. Hills can be a great advantage to you in a race if you understand a few principles. As your competitors struggle against the force of gravity, you can conserve energy and actually let it work for you. It may be hard to imagine when you're in the midst of a steep incline, but a hill can be a great opportunity.

* *Maintain the successful rhythm* you have established on the flat.

* *Maintain the same effort level.* Don't try to keep up the same pace on the hills as on the flat or you'll soon be worn out. A good check of this "same effort level" is your breathing.

* *Shorten your stride* and let yourself slow down gradually as you ascend. Conserve energy for the rest of the run. Keep your feet low to the ground, treading lightly.

* *Pick up the rhythm slightly* as you near the top. Some runners find a slight increase in arm rhythm helps them do this. Don't increase length or power of the arm swing, just pick up the rhythm. This helps pull you over the top and gets you ready to take advantage of gravity on the other side.

* *Think of running over the top:* You don't want to let down there.

Running Downhill. At the crest, the effort required for each step decreases. Be sensitive to this and gradually let the pace increase as gravity allows.

* *Let gravity do the work.* Gravity and increased rhythm should pull you downhill, with little energy required.

* *Don't let stride length get too long.* If it becomes too long you lose control and must expend energy to slow down. Too long a stride can pound your feet and knees unmercifully.

* *Keep your feet low to the ground, with a light touch.*

- *Experiment with your stride length* going down. Practice will show you the length that lets you take maximum advantage of gravity, yet be in control.
- *Lean slightly forward if you are going down a slight incline.*

What If You Live in Kansas? Not everyone lives where there are hills. Much of the Midwest, Texas, the East Coast along the beach, the Carolinas, Florida and Alabama is flat. One alternative — if a beach is available — is to run on the sand. (Wear your running shoes.) Warm up as you would for hills, then run 100–200 yards in sand that is neither hard-packed nor too loose. Other possibilities are highway overpasses, parking garage inclines (hopefully when there's little traffic and fumes), stadium steps, a treadmill, or running up 5–10 flights of stairs in an office building. The other rules of hill training described previously apply in all these cases.

TROUBLESHOOTING

Now that you know the principles of good running form, you'll be more sensitive to some form-related problems. We'll cover some of the most common ones here.

Shoulder Tension. If you feel this after a run, you're probably leaning too far forward or back with your head or shoulders: you're not balanced. Watch in store front windows as you run by; your hips may be too far back. Shift your hips forward, take a deep breath and maintain this forward position. Shoulder tension may also be caused by your shoulders being too high instead of relaxed, or by holding your arms too far out from your body. Whenever you feel tension building up, stop, shake your arms and shoulders and let them relax.

Tight Hamstrings. You're probably kicking too far behind yourself and not using your ankles, feet and calves enough. Shorten stride to shift the major effort to the calves and give the hamstrings a break. Lift off with your feet.

Rapid, Quick Breaths and/or Side Cramps. You're probably running too fast, especially at first. If you still can't get deep breaths when you slow down, you may be slumping your chest. Try the deep breath described above (shoulder tension) to get the chest forward. Keep it forward, breathe deeply and slowly, and the problem should go away. The ultimate solution is to use deep breathing throughout your run. *Caution:* If the problem persists, see a doctor.

Shoulder Roll. When you run by a storefront, do you see your shoulders rolling either up and down or forward and back? If so, you're probably throwing your arms across your body. Cut down on your arm swing, keeping arms low and moving forward and back. Try not to move your upper arms much.

Tight Neck. Your head may not be directly over your shoulders. If your body leans too far forward, you may be leaning your head back to compensate. Bring your chest back. Or if you run leaning too far back, your head is probably too far forward. Bring your hips forward. Check this out in store front windows also. Massage your neck after running.

A Final Note on Form

One of the great beauties of running is its free-form nature. Don't destroy this by working on form every time you run. *Most of your runs should be fun and flowing.* During those two or three times a week when you concentrate on form, focus on just that. You want each step to take you directly ahead and eliminate any excess motion and run quietly. Relax and enjoy the ride.

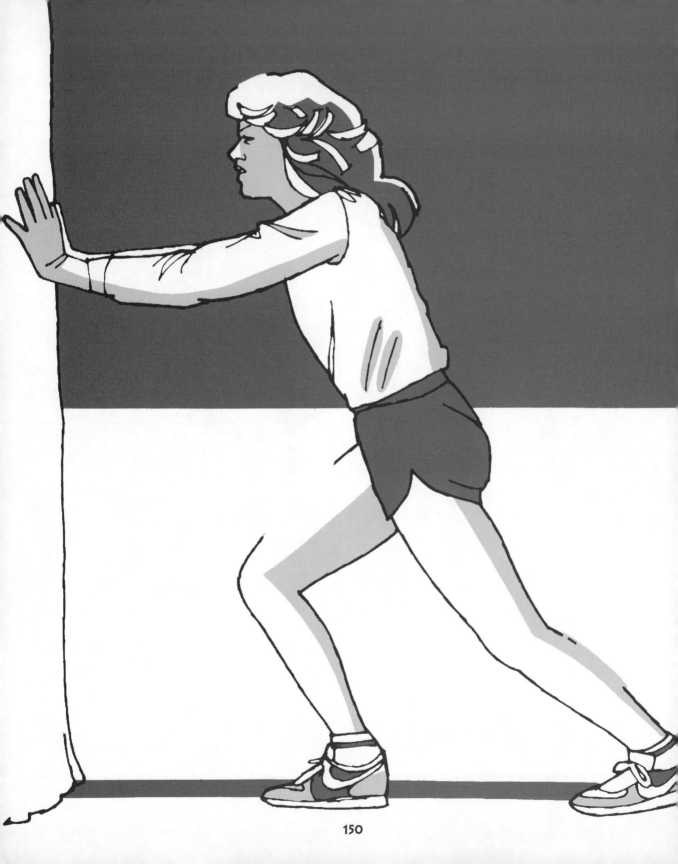

14
STRETCHING, STRENGTHENING, AND CROSS TRAINING

RELAXING AND BALANCING

STRETCHING CAN HELP—but it can also hurt! World-class athletes find that stretching regularly and properly helps them avoid tight muscles and injuries. But it's a two-edged sword. The wrong type of stretching is actually the third leading cause of runners' injuries, after too much mileage and speedwork. A survey which I've done over the last few years has shown me that among those who stretch, stretching is a leading cause of injury.

I learned about the dangers of stretching the hard way. Some years back, after reading an impressive article on the benefits of stretching, I tried to reverse the tightness of 16 non-stretching years in six months and developed a sciatic problem. Instead of gently holding a relaxed extension, I was pushing each stretch until I "felt it." The tension I was putting on my hamstring muscles was actually triggering a stretch reflex (the body's automatic protective mechanism) that shortened the muscle and caused me to become tighter each day. When the sciatica came along, I gave up stretching for a while.

Four non-stretching years later I was married. Barbara had a background in physical education and I guess she didn't look forward to spending her later years with someone who had to hobble around tightly strung like an archery bow (bent over backward). She watched me stretch and didn't hesitate to criticize. She knew that stretching had to be relaxed and told me so. With her help, I've gradually evolved the simple program of exercises that follows. I must admit that I still do not do much stretching, but Barbara keeps reminding me how it can help.

Although important in its long-term benefits, stretching will not instantly improve running. In the mid '70s many running articles claimed stretching could chase away injuries and improve speed. Since nothing could deliver all the benefits promised, unrealized hopes produced great despair as runners became injured, or failed to zoom away into the sunset.

We runners are often wishful thinkers. If a little stretching is good, then a lot must be wonderful. We think that if stretching "this far" is good, then pushing a few inches farther will turn us into fast pretzels. So stretching injuries occurred, and then multiplied. Then when the word got around that it was the third leading cause of injury, a lot of runners went to the opposite extreme and stopped stretching.

After having worked with over 100,000 average runners, I've come to believe that most runners today do not need to stretch much, if at all. Stretching has helped athletes in sports such as basketball, baseball, football, gymnastics, etc., which require the body to go through a range of motion for which humans were not designed. We were all designed to be distance runners. Our ancient ancestors had to cover thousands of miles a year to survive, and bestowed upon us all of the adaptations necessary to do the same. Distance runners, when they do it right, stay within their inherent range of motion, and often don't need to do much stretching.

Why Stretch? When runners need to stretch, due to individual needs, they avoid injury and run better. Those who have iliotibial band injury can speed up healing, and continue running (in most cases) if they stretch constantly. If you as an individual need to stretch, this chapter is for you. By understanding and fine-tuning a few simple principles, you can safely become more flexible—and you needn't spend much time doing it.

A small minority of runners find that running and other things in their lives, particularly strengthening activities, gradually tighten the muscles on the back of their legs, lower back, shoulders, and neck. While everyone should be careful about stretching out these key areas, gentle and regular flexibility exercises can reduce aches and pains in some of these cases—often with a good massage program. Those who have special problems should consult a physical therapist or other qualified expert in stretching before setting up a program. My guru in this area is the man who wrote the book on the subject (*Stretching*): Bob Anderson. I strongly recommend his book for anyone who wants to get into stretching.

No Guilt for Not Stretching: I haven't stretched in over 20 years. During that period, I haven't noticed any increase in tightness. I've only had one running injury during that period—and it was due to stepping in a hole. Many long-term runners do not stretch, with seemingly no long-term problems.

How Runners Should Stretch. Only a relaxed muscle can be extended safely and comfortably.

- *Start with a gentle massage.* By gently kneading the calf, hamstring, butt and lower back, you increase blood flow and loosen up the muscles. For about 5 minutes use your 10 magic fingers to work out any knots, but don't apply any deep penetrating pressure.

- *Gradually and slowly move into the stretch.* Back off from any tension and hold that relaxed extension for at least 10–20 seconds. If you feel the slightest pressure, pain, or the muscle starts shaking, you've gone too far. Ease back until you're relaxed again.

- Finish the stretch by slowly easing out of it.

The Principles of Stretching

- *Be regular.* Benefits come through steady, regular sessions of gentle muscle extension. Just as tightness builds up through years of standing, walking and running, so will it subside only gradually—through months of gentle extension.

- *Don't bounce.* Decades ago, runners did bouncing stretches. It was thought that a jolt to the muscle gave it the extension it needed. More recent research has shown, however, that bouncing shortens and tightens the muscles. It engages the *stretch reflex*, the body's automatic defense device against injury, which causes the muscle to tighten rather than extend.

- *Don't compete.* Don't try to stretch as far as someone else. Everyone is different in terms of flexibility. And don't try to equal your best stretch of yesterday. Some days you'll be relatively limber, others fairly tight. Just relax and move into the comfortable position that feels good that day.

When to Stretch—A New Approach

Before running? Most runners think they should stretch just before running. You see them everywhere, legs up on benches, leaning against buildings—getting ready to run. I don't recommend this. Just before running, the muscles are tight and may pull or strain easily. You are particularly at risk early in the morning when you're cold and blood flow is minimal. Pushing a cold muscle, tendon, or joint often leads to injury. Research by Dr. Ned Frederick at the Honolulu Marathon showed that runners who stretched before running had a greater tendency to be injured. The bottom line is that stretching does not warm you up for running, or reduce the chance that you will get injured during that run (unless you have a specific problem like iliotibial band that requires stretching before exercise).

After running? Stretching right after running is also a risky proposition. The muscles don't simply stop all activity when you stop running. They are still "revved up" and ready to respond for about 30 minutes; stretching may cause them to spasm. When they are working hard like this, a stretch often activates the stretch reflex—leaving you tighter than before. Many injuries are produced or aggravated when runners try to "stretch out" a muscle that has been tightened by recent exercise. This added tension actually tears the muscle fibers.

When, then? The best time to stretch is after the body is warmed up, relaxed, and when the blood is moving. Since many runners *do* stretch incorrectly, it's best to wait and stretch after warming up. Don't stretch to warm the muscles up; it won't work. Stretch in the evening, for example, or throughout the day as you have time. Many of my friends use stretching as a nice way to prepare for sleep.

Tight During a Run? Some runners will, when they become tight during a run, take extra walk breaks, or go to a "shuffle." Shuffling is running with minimum effort, as you keep your feet low to the ground with a short stride. If you think the muscle won't cramp, stop and gently massage the tight area, walk, and gently return to running.

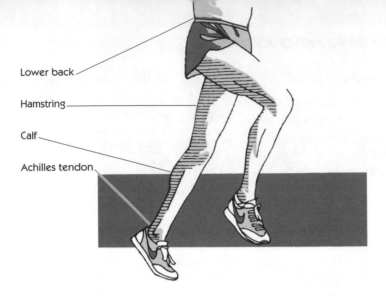

Lower back
Hamstring
Calf
Achilles tendon

Three Runners' Stretches

Three muscle groups are strengthened and tightened in running:

- Calf and Achilles (back of lower leg below knee)
- Hamstring (back of upper leg between knee and butt)
- Lower back (butt, lower back area)

To get good results, you need to stretch each group in isolation. Of the dozens of exercises for these muscle groups, we've chosen the three that have worked well for runners and that pose little injury risk. We have avoided stretches that are likely to cause injuries by their design as well as those likely to be performed incorrectly.

How to Do These Stretches. Make sure the muscles are "warm." If not, gently massage 3–5 minutes each.

- Ease into the stretching position.
- Hold each stretch at least 10–20 seconds.
- Do three times a week at first.
- Increase the length of time you hold each stretch.
- Stretch longer for any of the muscles that need it.

You can add other stretches to these basic three, depending upon your individual needs. Each session of stretching will take only 5–15 minutes, a small investment of time for such beneficial results.

Calf and Achilles Stretch. Brace your hands against a wall or pole. Extend your back leg and bend the front one. Gradually support the body weight on the back leg, keeping it *slightly* bent. This stretches the upper calf muscle. Now stop, bend the knee of the back leg more and create a slight stretch. This stretches the Achilles tendon and lower calf. Do both legs. Be careful. Stretch the muscles and tendons, don't pull them.

Hamstring Stretch. Lying on your back, loop a towel over your foot. If you don't have a towel, use pants, or a T-shirt. Don't lock the knee, but keep it slightly bent. Tighten the towel gently until you're stretching the hamstring. This is a better hamstring stretch than the familiar one you see of putting the leg up on a chair or other object, because you're less likely to overstretch. The chair puts you in a position where you can put too much stress on the hamstring. With a towel, you have the

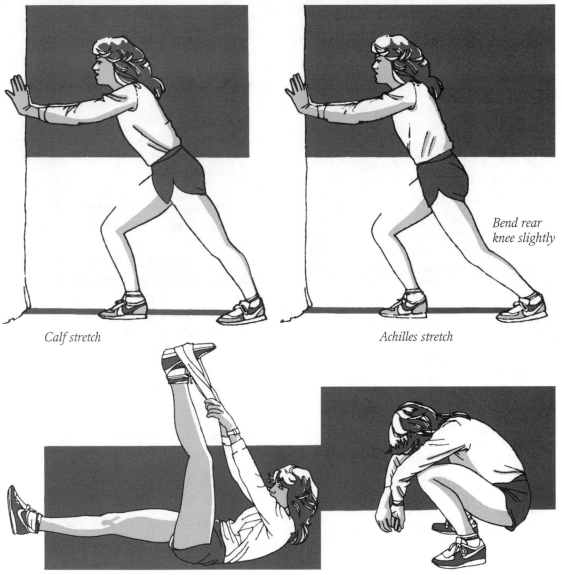

Calf stretch

Achilles stretch

Bend rear knee slightly

Hamstring stretch

Lower back stretch

flexibility to move into the exact position your muscles need. After stretching hamstrings of both legs, you can stretch your butt muscles by continuing to use the towel, bending the knee more and pulling your leg across your body.

Lower Back Stretch. Move into a squatting position. Make sure lower back is curved,

neck and back relaxed. Let your head drop forward toward a resting position on your chest. Normally, heels will rest on the ground and your Achilles tendon will get another stretch. If you are tight like I am, they'll rise; every other session, hold on to a pole or door knob and stretch with heels resting on the ground.

STRENGTHENING EXERCISES

In running, the rear leg muscles become strong, while the front leg muscles just go along for the ride. Running, except for hard sprinting, doesn't develop these front muscles much, and a strength imbalance develops between front and back.

The front muscles help balance the back ones. When they're weak, they're over-powered by forces of the rear, leading to problems in the knee, shins and lower back. Stretching will reduce tension in the back muscles, but a regular strengthening program for the front groups is needed to keep them in tone and to maintain a balanced ratio.

I believe that regular stretching and strengthening work together to produce a running body that is in tune and in touch with itself. As with stretching, the time required is not great; you need only be regular. Following are four of the best *strengthening exercises* for runners. After that we show three *potentially harmful exercises* that are often prescribed for runners. Finally, you'll read about the three postural muscle exercises I do every week.

Four Runners' Strength Exercises

To do these strengthening exercises you needn't join a gym or set one up in your basement. They can be done entirely without weights and will take only five minutes to perform. As with stretching, these exercises should be done 2–3 days a week for best results.

Stronger Quadriceps: The Stiff Leg Lift

Knee problems may develop when the quadriceps (front of thigh) muscles are not strong enough. A strong quadriceps supports the body's weight and acts to absorb the shock of landing. It also keeps the knee cap in its track by tightening the connections.

Sit on a table, bench or chair. Lift one leg at a time with knee locked and leg straight. Start with 5–10 lifts each leg and increase by 2–3 each week until you can do 40–50 with each leg. You may add some weight at this point, if you wish. *Remember, don't bend your knee.*

Stronger Shin Muscles: The Foot Lift

Shin problems or "shin splints" result from increasing mileage too suddenly, running on a hard surface or downhill, or from new shoes. *(See pp. 214–217 for a detailed description of shin problems.)* If you haven't had shin problems, you're lucky. If you have, here is an exercise that will strengthen the attachment of the tibialis anterior muscle to the shin bone.

Sit on a table or stool and hook a bucket, old purse or weights with a cloth loop over your foot. Start with one pound. Lift foot 5–10 times in two separate motions; this is an ankle motion:

- Straight up and down
- Up and toward the inside
- Remember to *lift only your foot.* Don't try to lift the whole leg as in a "stiff leg lift."

Gradually increase number of lifts to 30–50 or increase weight from one pound to 3–4. If you are one of the few runners who lands on the outside of your foot (supinates) you can strengthen the small muscles on the outside by rolling the foot up and to the outside. This will help prevent ankle turns or sprains.

Note: An alternative to the "foot lift" is the "duck walk." Walk around on your heels

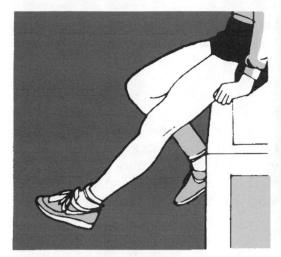

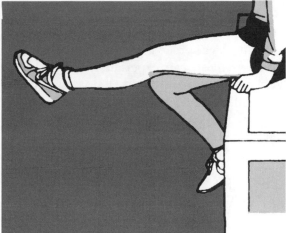

Stiff leg lift, down

Stiff leg lift, up

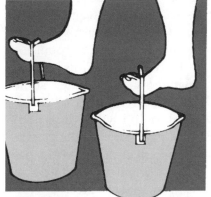

Lift straight up and down.

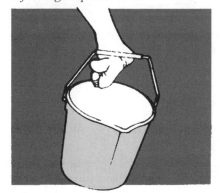

Lift up and toward inside.

for a few seconds. Every other day you could increase the time doing 3–6 of these until you can walk around for about 40–60 seconds on each. Don't do this (or any barefoot walking or running) if you have a plantar fascia injury.

Postural Strength Exercises

I've found that a bare minimum of strength training can keep the postural muscles strong and balanced. These muscles maintain the upper body in a relaxed but upright position. When neglected, they slowly weaken. Over a ten-year period, individuals gradually slump and stoop a little more. Runners notice this sooner. On long or hard runs, those with weak postural muscles will lose their form more quickly, their pace will slow, and recovery time will increase. A slumping upper body also cuts down on the efficiency of breathing and reduces oxygen absorption. After starting with about ten exercises in the late 1980s, I gradually refined them to the two that are described below. The crunch strengthens the front of the body, and arm running strengthens the muscles of the lower back, upper back, shoulders, and neck. If you're looking for beach muscles, this isn't the right program!

Arm Running

This exercise is done in the standing position with legs spread about as wide as your shoulders. You can experiment a little bit with the motion, but don't do anything that will put your back at risk. It's always safer, when using handheld weights, to keep them close to the body.

1. Stand upright and relaxed with your feet spread about the width of your shoulders or closer if shoulder-width is not comfortable.

2. Use handheld weights in both hands, choosing a weight that will give you a little challenge but is not a struggle.

3. Move the arms through the motion you'd use when running, keeping the hands close to the body.

4. Starting with two or three repetitions, increase by one rep each session until you get up to ten.

To see results, you need to do this two or three times a week. I do several sets of ten, spread throughout the day, for three days a week.

Stronger Stomach: The "Crunch"

Lower back problems can often be avoided by having strong stomach muscles, which will control the pull of a strong back and release pressure on the spine and the many nerves in that area.

Lie on your back with knees bent. Leaving feet on floor, raise shoulders and upper body slightly off the ground (by 2–4 inches). Lower slowly until you almost touch the floor and repeat. Staying within this short range will provide maximum strengthening for a variety of abdominal muscles. Going higher off the floor will not develop the muscle any better, and may cause back problems. Don't jerk yourself up as this doesn't use the stomach muscles; go slowly. Cross your arms on your chest so you won't use them for propulsion.

For years I couldn't do this exercise without hooking my feet under something. At Barbara's urging, I tried several times each night to do it without such aid and at first I couldn't get up off the ground. But the isometric effect of the effort paid off, for in about a month I could do my first one—with no help. Now I enjoy doing "the crunch" several days a week.

The "Crunch"

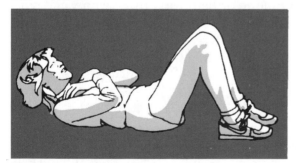

Lie on your back, knees bent.

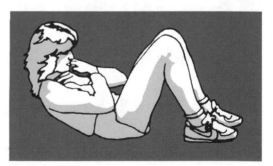

Raise head 10–12".

Foot Strength: The Toe Squincher

This is an amazing exercise for reducing or eliminating foot pain, and arch problems. *Foot pain* in the morning (which goes away as you warm up) is often caused by weak foot muscles. Running does not strengthen these muscles. A more serious problem is *plantar fasciitis*, where the pounding and weight of your body causes a strain in the strong ligament that runs from the heel to the ball of the foot. The "toe squincher" strengthens the muscles which support this ligament, helping the foot to push off with more force and support the body's weight better. It also seems to stretch the plantar tendon and balance the pulling effect of muscles that pull the tendons on the top of the foot.

Point your toes, then contract the muscles very hard for 7–10 seconds. Relax. Do this 5–10 times daily, throughout the day. Don't be surprised if the muscles cramp when you do it; this merely shows that the muscles are weak or tired and need work.

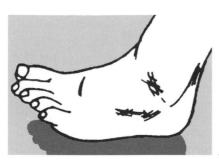

Point toes.

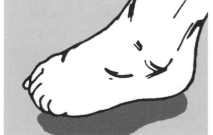

Contract.

CAUTION:
These exercises may be harmful.

The Chair Hurdle. This popular stretch puts too much pressure on the hamstring and has caused many muscle pulls. The hamstring stretch with a towel *(pp. 154–155)* does the job with less risk.

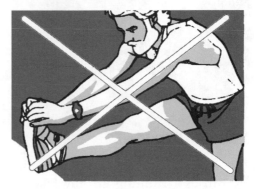

The Plow. As you bring feet and legs over your body, gravity can take you too far and put too much pressure on the neck and spine. You may do this for years and have no problems, but it's risky. The lower back stretch stretches the back gently, without risk.

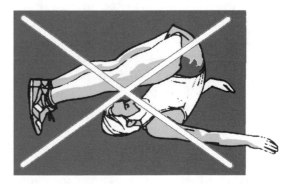

Bent-Knee Extension. Usually performed on a weight bench, you lift your leg from a 90° position to a stiff leg position with weights. This will strengthen the quads as well as the stiff leg lift, but can aggravate a knee problem. It's not worth the risk. The stiff leg lift strengthens the same muscles without the risk.

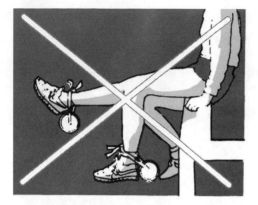

CROSS TRAINING

Because you have a great base of conditioning through running, it only takes a few minutes of another exercise to gain many specific benefits. A few minutes a week of weight exercises, for example, will bestow strength to the postural muscles, and can correct mechanical imbalances. Longer and easier sessions with a Versa-Climber or rowing machine will promote fat burning. Those who feel that running isn't enough exercise for them move on to multi-sport activities, such as triathlons. Cross training gives older runners the feeling of exertion they need on an "off" day, without the pounding on their legs and feet.

I hope that you won't get injured. But if you do, there's hope that you won't lose much conditioning through targeted cross training. Mary Decker Slaney set an American record just a few days after she came back from a non-running period of several weeks, including surgery. Performance was maintained by simulating her running workouts in the pool. I've known dozens of runners who have come back to run fast marathons (even sub-3-hour efforts) because they did significant pool running during 3–8 weeks of their vacation from running.

The best cross-training exercises are those that are targeted toward your goals. Weight training will build strength. Fat-burning exercises build up body heat, and can be continued for 45 minutes or more. Triathletes will do swimming and cycling, and runners benefit from water running and the endurance exercise machines. You must enjoy the exercises, or learn to enjoy the "glow" after doing them. The best exercises won't help you if you don't do them—and you won't do them if you hate the experience.

Fat-Burning Exercise Machines

1. Cross-country ski machines
2. Stair machines (don't do on a day of rest from running)
3. Rowing machines
4. Elliptical trainers

Easing into New Exercises

- On the first day go 5 easy minutes, rest for 20 to 30 minutes, and then go for 5 more minutes.

- You could start with two to three different exercises, alternating them and gradually increasing the session to 1 hour. To get the best effect for the marathon, it's better to use a slow continuous motion instead of quick, short bursts of high intensity for the 5K.

- During each successive session, increase each of the two segments by 3 to 5 minutes.

A Cross-Training Schedule for Triathletes (Two Workouts Each Day)

Mon	Tue*	Wed*	Thu*	Fri	Sat	Sun
Speed swim	Fun cycle	Speed cycle	Long swim	Easy cycle or off	Long	Long
Fun run	Speed run	Fun run	Fun Cycle	Easy cycle or off	Run	Cycle

*denotes days when you should rehearse race conditions for a quick transition.

- Build up to about the same duration and intensity of exercise you'd be doing if running.

- Exercise every day at first, if you wish, building up to two 30-minute sessions. You may then combine the exercise into one continuous session every other day. On the days between, you may do a different exercise routine. (See, for example, the schedule above.)

- In individual exercises or in the session as a whole, never push the muscles to the point of tiredness or loss of strength.

If you have been injured, don't do any exercise that could aggravate the injury. Plan your cross-training exercise to simulate the intensity and duration of your scheduled running session for that day. For example, if a long run is scheduled, estimate the length of the time you'd be running and spend that same amount of time running in the water, on the cross-country ski machine, and so on. As you're doing the alternative exercise, try to maintain about the same level of exertion as you would when running.

Water Running

Benefits

- Because the legs must find the most efficient mechanical path through the water, extraneous motions of the feet and legs are reduced or eliminated over time.

- The water's resistance strengthens muscles that can provide back-up strength to the primary running muscles. By alternating off and on, the main running muscles will retain their resilience longer. The smaller reserve muscles will also be able to keep you going for a little while if you overuse the main running muscles and need some help to keep running during the last few miles in the marathon.

- You get a great cardiovascular training session without any pounding. Because the prime running muscles are not being used, most injuries can heal.

Techniques

The marathon motion

Use the same running form in the water that you would use when running efficiently on land. The body should be upright, not stiff. A slight forward lean is okay, but don't lean too far. The ideal motion is a smooth one, with quick turnover. Focus on finding the most efficient path through the water. In this way you'll be cutting out mechanical inefficiencies and encouraging an efficient stride on land.

- Knees don't come up very far.

- Lower legs and feet are kicked forward.

- The whole leg is brought behind you, with the knee slightly bent.

- The back leg bends to a right angle and then returns forward.

- Arms can be moved through a range of motion similar to that of regular running. Don't exaggerate the arm-swing.

Cross-country ski motion

A strengthening exercise, the cross-country ski motion should be done in short segments of between 10 seconds and 1 minute. By weaving segments into the marathon motion, you'll increase strength in the quadriceps (front of thigh), hamstrings, butt muscles, hip flexors, and lower back.

- The legs are almost completely straight.
- The range of motion is about 20 percent longer than the range of the marathon motion.
- Move the legs like scissors through the water.

Start each segment with a short range of motion and extend it gradually. Over time, you may increase both range of motion and speed, but be careful. Remember that you're building strength and not anaerobic performance. Never extend any motion to the point that you feel you have reached your mechanical limits. And don't work so long that you're out of breath.

Sprinting

For those who have been doing speed play and don't want to risk injury while in a training program, the sprint motion can keep the speed components in good form without the risk of pounding or incurring interval-training injuries.

- Shorten your marathon motion to about half.
- Keep legs and feet directly underneath you.

- Pick up the turnover of your legs and feet so that you're going through the leg pattern about twice as fast as you go through the marathon motion.

This shouldn't be a true sprint (going all out) because you want to go at a pace that you could continue for 1 to 2 minutes. You will be huffing and puffing through the second half of each of these, as they are anaerobic. Start each sprint segment by gradually increasing the turnover. The short range of motion directly underneath you will cause your head and shoulders to rise out of the water somewhat. To keep up with the legs, the arm motion should also be a shortened version of the marathon motion.

Precautions

- Make sure that the water-running motion is within efficient mechanical range.
- If you're injured, get clearance from your doctor to make sure that you're not aggravating the injury.
- Don't over-train. Just going through an efficient water-running motion will bestow benefits. No need to push it.

Strength Training

I don't believe that you need to do any strength exercises to run long distances. If you have any doubts, look at the "toothpick" limbs of the winners of any major marathon. It's obvious that they don't spend time in the gym. The most important physics concept for running, in my opinion, is inertia. Running is easier and more fun when we spend a little energy to get moving and then fine-tune our movements to take advantage of our momentum.

I do, however, recommend a couple of strength exercises for long-term postural support. Strong and balanced postural muscles will keep you upright when you're fatigued, and improve your breathing and oxygen intake enabling you to maintain running strength and efficiency. I discovered this after my arms and shoulders were getting increasingly tired on long runs in the mid-1980s. By doing the exercises listed below, I've virtually eliminated that type of fatigue—even in marathons.

Leg Strength

Legs can be strengthened most efficiently by doing regular hill training *(see pp. 39–40)*. Running up an incline forces the leg muscles to perform against natural resistance. By doing artificial weight exercises, you can upset the natural balance that has developed between the muscle groups. Such an imbalance can cause injury. If you want to develop strength, it helps to see a strength expert. The exercises I am suggesting are those that work for me as a runner.

15
MOTIVATION

HOW TO RUN FASTER WITHOUT TRAINING

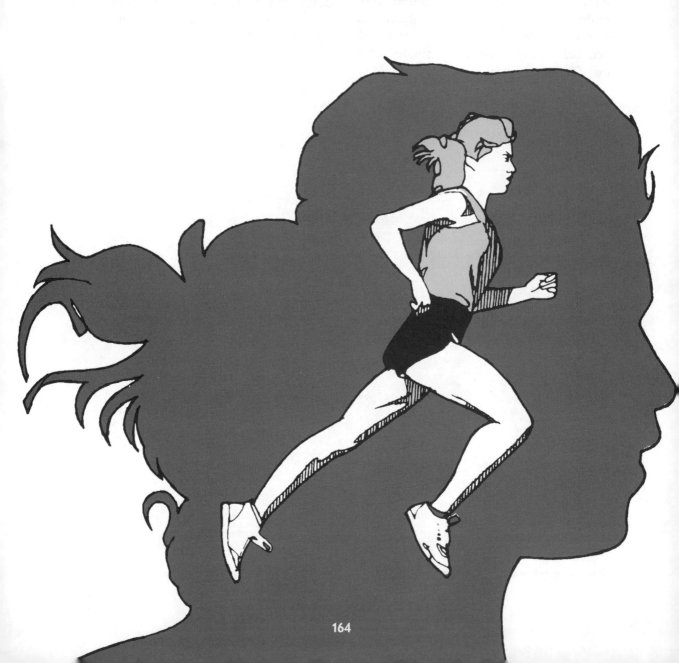

IT WAS A BRIGHT SUNNY AFTERNOON in the Munich Olympic Stadium when the world's best 800-meter runners toed the line. At the gun they sprinted for position and strategic advantage, but my friend Dave Wottle strained to stay up with the slowest runners. As the runners rounded the final turn, we could see that Dave was boxed in at the rear of the pack. Though our own sportscasters were describing his effort as an unfortunate strategy that would keep him from a medal, I knew he was lucky to be close to the next-to-last runner.

In the 1972 U.S. Olympic trials, Dave had beaten the best of the American 800-meter crop, including a Kansan named Jim Ryun. As we traveled to Norway to prepare for the games, however, Dave complained of a knee problem that wouldn't go away. After several frustrating speed sessions, which had to be quickly terminated, Dave took 2–3 weeks off to let it heal.

One day as my roommate, Doug Brown, and I were starting an easy run in the forest, we saw Wottle, full of optimism and ready to resume hard training, starting on his first run after the layoff. But when we returned from our short run, Dave was limping along, in tears. The rest had done nothing for his knee. He was certain his career was over, just as he was reaching his peak.

Trainers and coaches wanted to replace him with a healthy runner, but Wottle refused to let anyone take away his lifetime goal of running in the Olympics. He trained when the knee would let him. By the time we arrived in Munich for the first trial heats, Dave—though weakened by the prolonged layoff—was able to run enough to enter his race.

In the first qualification round he struggled to stay at the end of the pack. As he came off the final turn in last place we were ready to rush out and congratulate him for his courage in staying up with athletes who were now in much better condition. But somehow he threaded his way through the mass of bodies and finished third, qualifying for the next round. He ran two more qualifying rounds the same way, struggling to stay up, then fighting his way into the last qualifying position. We were amazed: Wottle had qualified for the 800-meter finals!

In the finals, Dave was in last place by a significant margin when he passed the half-way mark, with only one lap to go. While sportscasters in 24 languages focused on the top runners in the race, Wottle's target was the next-to-last runner, which he didn't catch until they started the final turn of the track.

Then something happened. At the toughest time of the race, when all of the other runners were slowing down due to an overly ambitious starting pace, Dave was determined not to give up even though his under-trained muscles were overfilled with the waste products of extreme exertion. His body had reached its limits, but his mind kept him going. He squeezed between two runners, stepped quickly to the outside, then the inside, and drove forward in hopes of getting out of last place. In the last few yards before the finish, a small hole opened up in the line of runners ahead—Dave slipped through, lunged at the very last moment, and broke the tape!

Dave Wottle became an Olympic medalist because he had mentally trained himself to reach his potential, whatever it was, on that day. But each of us can use this same type of power inside to get out the door on the "bad" days, to keep going, and to dig down and pull out the untapped strength.

Dave's story shows that when you get the body and mind working together, you'll find the resources inside to do anything that is realistic, and some things that are not. You'll certainly be a happier and more motivated runner than someone who runs faster but lacks this body/mind integration. Just as good teamwork can defeat a group of outstanding but not synchronized individuals, you'll be able to outperform others who may be more "capable" in the performance components, but can't get them working together.

Body, mind, and spirit only come together when you're running within yourself. Most of us are close to maximizing our physical capabilities, while using only a fraction of the potential of the other two. Running is one of the few growth experiences in life which can naturally balance all three, allowing us to reach our unique potential in speed, distance, and in life. Here are some techniques for expanding mental focus as we learn to tap into the unlimited capabilities of the human spirit.

The Mind Is Divided. The power of the mind to push the body to its potential is limited by an internal conflict. The logical side (left brain) does not communicate with the creative side (right brain). A primary mission of the analytical side is to steer you into comfort and away from stress. The more stress you generate from running and other areas, the more negative messages:

"slow down," "stop," or what is even worse, asking "why am I doing this?" If you don't have a mental strategy for dealing with this barrage of negativity, you'll start losing confidence in your ability to achieve your potential, on that day.

When you have a balance of physical and mental training, your left and right brains can work as a team: left side anticipating problems, and right side searching for resources and solutions. This puts you in control of your running, instead of reacting to one crisis after another. While the potential of our body is limited, the intuitive and creative powers of the right side are not. Not only does this side monitor our capabilities, it finds resources you didn't know that you had.

The rest of this chapter is devoted to "motivation training." You'll learn to troubleshoot motivation problems with techniques for turning a bad day into a good day. In the next chapter you'll learn three mental training techniques. First, mental rehearsal will prepare you for whatever challenge you choose, and can be applied to other areas of life. "Magic words" allow you to draw upon your past successes to create future performances. "Dirty tricks" produce surprising and significant turnarounds in motivation.

No exertion is required for this type of training. A little time spent while on your run each week will help you balance left brain and right brain, as you coordinate your body with your mind. When these elements work as a team, you'll unleash the spirit which can propel you to unexpected levels of performance.

MOTIVATION!

"A body on the couch wants to stay there. But once a body is in motion . . . it wants to continue in motion."

Everyone has days of low motivation, and periods when there's no progress. This section is dedicated to helping you push through the final few barriers when training is going well, to keep running on those days you'd like to cut the mileage short, and to get you out the door or out of bed on the really bad days.

Forward motion exercise is motivating in itself.

Many runners don't enjoy the wonderful effect of endorphins during a run because they start too fast and use all of the "pain-killers" during the run. By taking walk breaks early and often, these pain-killing relaxants and attitude-boosting hormones will make any run a better one. Don't get locked into a specific pace or a specific walk-run ratio. When you're not motivated, slow down and take more walk breaks.

It could be low blood sugar.

You may be just half an energy bar away from motivation. If your exercise time is mid-day or later, and you feel tired and unmotivated, low blood sugar is often the cause of your "exercise blues." Waiting for more than two hours to eat a balanced snack or meal (high-sugar foods don't count) will only lower your concentration and motivation. Low blood sugar is a significant stress on your system, causing the left side of your brain to unleash a stream of messages, such as the following: "You'll feel better tomorrow, take the day off"; "You have too much to do"; "The couch is waiting for you." An energy snack, with water, coffee, etc., about one hour before exercise, will often reverse the negative thoughts and get you off the couch.

Reduce the anticipated discomfort of the run.

If you're scheduled for a 4-mile continuous run, and are experiencing left-brain stress, tell that negative nagger that you're only going to go one or two miles, and will walk most of it. Most runners who do that, end up finishing a 4- or a 5-miler feeling great. If you have a race scheduled but don't feel up to it, talk yourself down to an easier time goal, or into merely running the first half of the race. With the pressure off, most racers run the whole race in a surprisingly good time.

Get a mission and write it on the calendar.

When you do this, you're more likely to be motivated on those hot, muggy days, or when snowflakes fall.

A mid-run motivation crisis is almost always the result of going too fast, for you, on that day.

The more stress you put on yourself, the more negative messages you'll receive from the left brain, which will lead to a desire to quit. Ease up, take more walk breaks, and you'll get through most of these "walls." If the weather presents you with too much heat/humidity, and/or you went too fast in the beginning or the middle of the run, it may be too late to do anything but walk. Learn from this, and back off early the next time.

Bring an energy snack with you.

Your preferred blood sugar foods can pull you out of motivational lulls. Everyone will experience a blood sugar crash after about 12–15 miles. If your blood sugar level is low when you start, energy bars, goos, etc., can boost motivation and running enjoyment in a matter of minutes. Always drink water with any of these products.

Be sure that you're not having a medical problem.

It's extremely rare, but there are a few times when you should not push through barriers. If you have or suspect a medical emergency—stress fracture, cardiovascular problem, heat disease, etc., stop immediately and get help. In fact, this is approximately a million-to-one occurrence. Even though this is an unlikely event, it's always better to be safe than sorry. If there are good reasons why your ache or pain can lead to significant health risks, it's always better to quit early and talk to a doctor.

A second level of medical alert relates to overtraining and injury. Some aches and pains are early warning signs of injuries or excessive fatigue. Experienced runners become very sensitive to the weak links, those knees, tendons, or muscles that become injured most often. By backing off early, or taking an extra day off, you may avoid weeks or months of layoff later—due to pushing through an early-stage injury.

On the very tough or fast runs

Almost every runner has at least one tough run, every month. Whether it occurs during a tour around the block, or during a 23-miler or speed session, here are my tricks for continuing:

1. *Slow down, and allow the body and mind to get a break.* Take more walk breaks as needed, take more rest between intervals in a speed session, and start back into the run slower than before. The earlier you make an adjustment, the better quality you'll be able to salvage from that workout or run—and the quicker you'll recover both physically and mentally.

2. *Break up the remaining distance into segments that you know you can do.* Take a walk break (or a shuffle break) every 3-5 minutes. You know that you can go another three minutes, right? If three minutes is too long, try one minute. Your run or race is a series of these segments, to the finish line.

3. *Use distractions.* Look ahead to the next mailbox, stop sign, fast food restaurant, water stop, etc., and tell yourself that you can take a break there. Make sure the segment is short enough so that you feel confident in getting there.

4. *In a race, focus on the person that is two people in front of you.* By looking ahead, you can be pulled past the person that is immediately in front of you. Stay mentally attached to that person, noting the outfit, the printing, the hat, etc. If you're only looking at details, you'll at least be preoccupying the left brain so that it won't zing you as badly or as often. As soon as you pass the first person, focus on the new target, two people away. See the section following, on "dirty tricks" you can play on the left brain.

5. *Use a mantra.* There are various types of words and phrases which will do more than distract you. Practice these, and

develop your own to put yourself into a positive trance. See the mantra suggestions below.

6. *Don't give up.* Remember the Dave Wottle story at the beginning of this chapter. If you respond to each thought of quitting with the internal resolve that you are going to finish, you will! Positive mental attitude alone can pull you through many difficult situations.

Mantras for Staying Motivated (to be said over and over)

Strength and Performance Mantras will connect into your hidden resources that keep you going when tired. The specific words you choose will help to make subconscious and intuitive connections with muscles, and your inner resolve. As you learn to tap into the right brain, you'll coin phrases that continue drawing on mental or spiritual resources. The following have been used when under physical and mental stress, but use these only as a primer. The best ones will be your own mantras that relate to your experiences with words that work. Action phrases not only keep you going, they help you perform as you find ways to dig deeper into your resources.

- Feet—stay light and quick, keep moving.
- My legs are strong.
- My heart is pumping better.
- There's more blood in the muscles.
- Lactic acid is going away.
- More oxygen is coming into my lungs.
- The strength is in there, I'm feeling it. I feel comfortable—I'm in control.
- I feel good—I feel strong.

Distraction Mantras start by preoccupying your left brain so that it won't send you so many negative messages. After saying these over many times, you may be able to shift into the right brain.

- I'm building a house, railroad, community, bookcase, etc.
- I feel strong like a locomotive, firehose, race car, mountain train.
- What type of novel could that person ahead of me have written?
- What type of crime could that person on the sidewalk be plotting?
- What type of movie could be staged here?
- Look at that store, car, building, sign, etc.
- Look at that person, hair, outfit, hat, T-shirt design, etc.

Vision Mantras help you feel that you're getting where you want to be.

- I can see the next mile marker.
- I can feel the pull of the finish line.
- I can feel myself being pulled along by the runners ahead.
- I can feel myself getting stronger.
- I'm pushing through the wall.
- I'm moving at the right pace to finish with strength.

Funny Mantras get you to laugh, which is a right-brain activity.

- I'm running like a clown, ballerina, football player, stooge.
- Float like an anchor, sting like a sponge.
- Where's the bounce, glide?

Running Form Mantras help you adjust to more efficient form.

- One more step, one more step
- One more block, telephone pole, stop light, etc.
- Baby steps, baby steps, baby steps
- I'm a puppet on a string.
- Feet stay low—touch lightly.
- I'm running smoothly.
- I'm running on ice.

Creative Mantras

- Talk crazy to me, right brain.
- I'm floating.
- Come to me—endorphins.
- I'm having fun.
- I'm feeling creative—I'm making adjustments.

If your goal isn't motivating any more

Having gone through more than 120 marathon training programs, I've experienced many motivation letdowns. On most of these, I've rebounded, but on a few, I didn't. Burnout and dropout are mental injuries. If you back off and adjust early, you can avoid major burnout later. Here are some adjustments to make in the middle of a training program, if you lose your drive:

1. Reduce mileage, and cut your running days to three. Walk a lot.
2. Run and walk in scenic areas, places that really motivate you to run.
3. Schedule a social run with a friend or a group of friends. Tell them that you need help. Have a good time and meet afterward for a snack or meal.
4. Have a "theme" run with friends: trivial pursuit, favorite character, best joke contest, worst joke contest, best juicy story contest.
5. Do anything necessary to add more fun to your program: after-run rewards, special outfits, or shoes after specific long runs, etc.
6. Adjust your goal event so that it is more motivating. Stay at a special hotel, get some friends to meet you there, schedule weekend activities with your family, sibling, or special friend (at events such as the Big Sur Marathon, the original course marathon in Greece, or the Disney World Marathon).
7. Sometimes it helps to choose another goal event and adjust your training accordingly.

16
MENTAL TRAINING

BEFORE ATTEMPTING something challenging like an ambitious training program, a marathon, etc., wouldn't you love to have the confidence of having already done it—without the fatigue, sweat, aches, and pains? Thanks to the wonderful world of visualization, this is now possible. Billy Mills won an Olympic gold medal by rehearsing his victory, without realizing he was doing it.

As a college athlete, Billy had not achieved his own potential; he had left something on the track. When the Marine Corps offered him a chance to continue his frustrated dream of qualifying for a U.S. Olympic team after graduation, Mills joined up, and became a member of the USMC track team.

Billy corresponded regularly with a college teammate who was training with the current world recordholder, Australia's Ron Clarke. At the end of almost every run, Billy would pick up his pace and visualize passing Clarke and breaking the finish tape.

In 1964, he unexpectedly qualified for the U.S. Olympic team in the 10K, in the shadow of America's great distance runner of the day, Jerry Lindgren. Captain Billy Mills was excited about his trip to Tokyo and proudly wore his Olympic uniform. As the starting gun fired, Mills settled into the middle of the pack where he was expected to finish. As the race progressed, however, many of the lead athletes, including Lindgren, dropped back. Mills kept going. By the final mile he was as surprised as anyone to find himself in the lead group, which included world recordholder Ron Clarke, and Mohamed Gammoudi.

As the three lead runners rounded the first curve of the last lap, Clarke was boxed in on the inside by Mills. Clarke tapped Mills on the arm to let him get out (so he'd have some room to pass the lead runner), but Mills didn't move. Clarke then burst through, shoving Mills out of the way. It was now a Clarke-Gammoudi race for the gold, with Mills too far out of position to win.

Mills fought his way back into balance, regained his stride and moved back into the inside lane, significantly behind. But coming off the final curve, Billy forgot about how bad he felt, and about how he had been pushed around. Billy saw ahead of him the same vision he had held on each run for years: Ron Clarke ahead of him, and the finish tape beyond.

Like a carbonated beverage bottle that had been shaken up, Mills built up pressure and exploded, passing Gammoudi and Clarke to hit the tape. The inner strength was there all along, but Billy had talked himself out of the competition. The daily rehearsal of this finish made his final sprint a reflex action.

MENTAL REHEARSAL

The power in Billy's rehearsal was based upon three factors: 1) it was very specific to the action he needed in the race, 2) it brought body and mind together and, above all, 3) he practiced it almost every day, it became an automatic response. By mentally touring an experience you want to have, many times in advance, you desensitize yourself to the stress of the unknown and the anticipated discomfort. This means fewer left-brain messages, but there's more going on.

Your training will introduce you to the challenges and problems which will probably occur in your event. Research on elite and almost-elite athletes has shown that most of the top athletes deal with the problems and make constant adjustments to their running. Most of the almost-elite runners (who have about the same physiological capabilities) create a distraction image that disassociates them from the experience. I don't have to tell you which group did better.

The most effective rehearsal strategy is to go over every possible challenge—even if you don't know the solution. As the left brain rehearses each problem and the negative messages that come from it, you become desensitized to this negative garbage. At the same time, the right brain gets its intuitive powers quietly working on solutions. It will do the same thing during the goal race. You'll start to have a problem and a mile or two later it has been taken care of. The right brain works 24 hours a day.

The left brain doesn't have to understand the problem or the solution. Often it doesn't even know that the problem is being solved at all—except for the lower stress level that results.

Benefits of a rehearsal

1. *Familiarity breeds success.* Mentally rehearsing a hard workout or race in advance gears up mind and body for the sequence of events. The more times you're able to rehearse, the more smoothly you'll mentally prepare for each segment and the better you'll anticipate your need for resources and adjust for success.

2. *Taking out the garbage.* The discouraging messages released under stress are reduced because you've desensitized yourself to them. In other words, there's less stress, therefore less garbage.

3. *Mind and body teamwork.* Mental rehearsals are effective during practice runs because you can edit and improve responses quickly in your mind. This doesn't get you out of doing your hard workouts, of course. Once you've had two or three runs over 15 miles, you have an experience base that will allow you to convert 15 minutes of mental rehearsal time into months of training experience.

4. *Taking control.* Instead of waiting for things to happen or taking what comes your way, rehearsal allows you to set up the steps you'll take to get through each stage and challenge of your next hard workout or race. As you anticipate problems, your right brain starts to take care of them.

5. *Creating the blueprint.* As you do the long runs, speed sessions, etc., to get ready for your goal, you draw up the plans from direct experience. The process gets easier and easier because you have the patterns in place for dealing with new problems

and old anxieties. Your greatest enemy at any point in any running challenge is not the stress. It's the internal doubt your left brain promotes and upon which it feeds. By focusing on your plan you can deal with specific actions which will give you momentum, and keep you moving toward your goal.

6. *Be creative.* As you're being realistic, unleash your creativity. Include in your rehearsal a few unexpected situations that you haven't faced yet. This will reduce your shock and stress if and when these occur in the event itself. Be sure to insert some fun rehearsal elements, such as seeing strange people along the way, talking with your fellow travelers, and noticing landmarks. Mental rehearsal will help you to enjoy your race.

Lights . . . Camera . . . Action

As if you're a stage producer getting ready for an important scene, bring on the star (you!) and watch the scene unfold, with all the lines and all the action. Then play it again, frequently, until you know the drill —even under stress. Use these thoughts for your own rehearsal, inserting other elements which customize it for you. At first you may write this down, or copy the list, but it's OK to do it from memory.

Start with a few statements which may cause you to laugh and make you feel good about your mission.

- My psychiatrist tells me that I'm okay —even if I want to do a marathon.
- I want the satisfaction of finishing with the medal around my neck.

- I enjoy the good friends I've met through training for this.
- Every mile I will slow down enough to enjoy the experience.

Focus first on the "glow of achievement."

- Sure I'm tired but I'm satisfied.
- The sense of accomplishment is unlike anything I've ever experienced.
- I've found new sources of strength inside.
- The medal around my neck symbolizes all of this, bestows a wonderful glow.
- I feel so good about myself.

Warding off the negative messages

When the left brain bothers you, diffuse the stress by saying that you're not going to push yourself:

- I have control over how I will feel—I'll go slower when in doubt.
- I have all the time in the world to finish.
- This is my day to smell the roses.

Focus on the positive effect of your training experience.

- I feel more invigorated.
- The training has improved my attitude.
- My focus is better.
- I'm positive because I'm doing something very positive for myself.
- My body is designed for forward motion and responds positively when I move.
- Natural endorphins relax me and settle me down.
- This gets the right brain connected to the body, bypassing the left brain.

Tell a joke, share a juicy story, or argue a controversial issue.

- Laughing helps engage the right brain.
- Collect a few funny thoughts and jokes that you can call up with a key word.
- Tell the joke, etc., to yourself, if necessary.

The start

Now, rehearse the start. You begin to get uneasy when the announcer calls everyone. But, as you share energy with the people around you, tell jokes, or mentally revisit some very successful experiences, you're feeling comfortable and secure. Stay with that and then, as the gun fires, gently move with the people around you. You're all in this together, moving forward toward a positive goal. It's a mass migration in which you're destined to triumph!

Challenges

It is better to know the course you will be running (study the specific course descriptions in the race flyers). But if you're unsure of the exact route, you can rehearse a generic course. It's even better to over-rehearse the challenges; if you're prepared for a more difficult experience, a less demanding one won't engage the left brain as much.

The most significant challenges will come during the last few miles, so you'll need to rehearse this segment many more times. Make a list of the possible challenges during this grand finale when the left brain is bothered by fatigue, low motivation, blisters, aches, low blood sugar, dehydration, and, again, fatigue. If you over-rehearse the difficulty of this tough part, you'll be in a better position to enjoy the end of your event.

I'm going to "gut it out."

Most of the problems, insecurities, and resulting negative messages can be managed and overcome by digging down a little deeper into your reservoir of fortitude. This source of strength comes directly from your spirit, which has the capacity to generate positive momentum continuously. By rehearsing yourself through the low points, you not only become stronger but also develop the intuitive paths that can connect you to these resources in the future: for fitness, work, personal challenges, and other areas of life.

On to the finish

And so we end where we began. The positive flow of energy toward the finish line is your destiny, pulling you past the challenges, through the doubts, and out of the depths of uncertainty itself. You've done this yourself, and you've developed a lot more than physical capabilities along the way.

REHEARSALS: 1) Getting out the door at the end of a "bad" day, and 2) Getting out of bed, when the covers feel so cozy

Here are two simple "scripts" that have helped thousands of folks get moving— and stay moving, until the endorphins start flowing. You can apply these principles to any challenging experience: 1) break up the task into a series of steps that lead to one another, 2) none of the steps are difficult, 3) rehearse the steps until you don't have to think about what to do next. This lowers your anticipated discomfort, and tells the left brain to take it easy. You'll need to adapt the following to your situation and rehearse it over and over, especially when you're going home after work each day—or the night before. The more you rehearse it, even on days when you don't need the motivation, the more likely you will move from one step to the next when you hit a low.

Scene # 1: You're driving home after a terrible work day, hungry, and your left brain has a dozen reasons why you shouldn't run.

Action:

1. Lie to the left brain, say "I'm not going to run today. I'll take it easy around the house in some comfortable clothes."

2. You arrive home, and immediately put on running shoes and clothes, telling yourself: "I'm not going to run today, just going to be comfortable around here."

3. Eat an energy snack, and drink your beverage of choice (hint: caffeine helps if you're OK with it).

4. Put on some inspirational music and read some of the affirmations in this chapter and the last one.

5. Stick your head out the door to see what the weather is doing, and just step outside.

6. Walk to the edge of the block to see what the neighbors are doing.

7. Cross the street and you're on your way!

Scene # 2: From the bed to the street

Action:

Here's another challenge for many runners: getting out of bed early enough to do the morning run. Again, you should individualize this to your own needs and situation. Concentrate only on the next step—not on running.

1. Look at your clock the night before. Tell yourself what time you will be getting up. Go through a quick mental rehearsal of yourself hearing the alarm and putting your feet on the floor. Have your clothes laid out so that you can put them on without thinking.

2. The alarm goes off. Without thinking, your feet hit the floor.

3. Without thinking, stand up and head for the kitchen.

4. Prepare your beverage of choice: coffee, tea, juice, smoothie, etc.

5. Sip your beverage and put on clothes—automatically as possible.

6. Walk out the door, not thinking about running—to test the weather.

7. Walk to the street just to see what the neighbors are doing.

8. Cross the street and you're on your way!

MAGIC WORDS

By using a few special words you can pull yourself out of the downturn of motivation and physical energy that usually happens at some point during your "hard" runs. Your magic words can turn a "bad" run into an OK and even a "good" run. Even when your conditioning and weather conditions stop you from a fast performance, the use of these words can mentally reframe any experience into a positive one.

Positive brainwashing

Magic words give you another means of taking control of your performance. You're using key words to activate internal connections that your right brain used in the past to accomplish certain goals. Take a challenge you want to overcome and think back to some experiences where you had a victory in that area. The association of experience with words trains you to connect directly to stay positive, deal with real problems, and pull the strength available when needed. But when used in a negative way, this ancient process is called "brainwashing." In either case, it is a proven and powerful method for altering attitude and behavior.

You can use my words, if you want

My three magic words are *relax, power,* and *glide*. I started using them during my competitive career to deal with three problems I encountered during difficult runs and races. Remember that the words you use become more powerful as you associate more successful experiences with them.

Relax: Usually at the end of a hard run, when I would feel my resources slipping away, I had a tendency to tense up, feeling that things were going to get worse. With the increase in negative left-brain messages due to the stress, I used to slow down and obey these messages. Now, I know that the left brain is really bluffing, making the conditions seem much worse than they really are. When I feel the first sensation of tightening, I focus on easing beyond the stress, by saying the word "relax" to myself. After years of use, the connections from hundreds of successful experiences are made once more. I now get a subtle feeling of relaxation, followed by a subtle surge of strength.

Power: When I start to slow down, the left brain tells me that my strength is almost gone, bringing on a new set of brain messages from the left side, such as "You may not finish," or "Stop now before it gets worse." By merely saying the word "power," I feel a rebuilding of my strength, with the sensation that everything is going to be all right.

Glide: During the latter stages of any long or hard run, my form gets shaky. To counter this trend, I say the word "glide" and instantly I feel smoother (even when I don't *look* any smoother). I've now associated this magic word with hundreds of runs when I started to get the "wobbles," but finished with a feeling of good form and efficiency. Now, when I say "glide," I'll receive a bit of the same sensation I felt at the end of some of my best lifetime efforts, while my pace is sometimes twice as slow.

> The words aren't magic in themselves. They come alive and make better connections as you associate each with experiences in which you overcame specific problems. The more experiences, the more magic.

When you say the magic words . . .

- You instantly feel a sense of control (at least a little).

- The words first confuse and distract the left brain, cutting off the negative messages for a while.

- A surge of confidence occurs as you apply the words.

- A series of positive memories floods the subconscious and sometimes the conscious, further cutting off the left brain.

- Sometimes this series of events will jump-start the right brain, helping you find intuitive solutions to current problems.

- You re-live (and are energized by) the past experiences during which you started to "lose it," but were able to focus on the positive, collecting all available resources.

- On a few occasions, you may set a personal record, finish an impossible run, or pass a competitor you haven't beaten before.

- More likely, you'll be able to run as fast as you were capable of running on that day.

- With each use, you become more confident and effective in using your own magic.

- This process helps to bring forth the same strengths that produced success before.

Warning: Your words will lose their magic, if you use them in a left-brain way.

Some runners can get a quick fix by using the word "power," for example, to pick up the pace for a hundred meters or so in the middle of a race. This will almost always lead to a significant slowdown at the end of the run, however, because you spent valuable resources that you needed at the end.

Dirty Tricks

A really good rehearsal (with good pace judgment) will pull you most of the way through any hard effort. By adding your magic words, you'll push forward another 1–3 miles, sometimes all the way to the finish line. But there are moments in every real running challenge, usually near the end, when the magic seems to have gone out of your words, and worse, your legs. This turns on a powerful sound system from which the left brain shouts its messages. You've probably heard most of them: "It's over. Just walk to the finish." "Slow down; it'll feel much better." "Stop now, and feel great." "Oh, do I feel bad." "I can't do it today." (And the worst one of all) "Why am I doing this?"

Everyone, even the front runners, gets these messages in races and hard runs. Blame it on the left side of your brain, whose mission is to steer you into pleasure and away from stress and discomfort. The more physical and mental stress, the more messages. By playing a few dirty tricks on this excuse-ridden "pity" center, you can regain control over your run, get on down the road, and entertain yourself. You may also find strengths you didn't know were there.

When you're tired and stressed, even the most logical runners will find that their left brains are working slowly and are therefore susceptible to being tricked. Dirty tricks are one-second ideas that distract the left side while they jump-start the right brain. As you find a series of creative images which get you into your right brain, you'll trigger other imaginative thoughts.

When you get it working, the right brain acts like a computer technician trying to connect to a damaged unit. It keeps quietly probing, hitting dead ends, and trying again until it finds the direct connections to the centers that get the job done. In addition, right-brain activity improves motivation and keeps your organism working all the way to the finish.

There's always a lot more strength inside you than your left brain gives you credit for. A dirty trick can be the catalyst that keeps you from falling apart, or pushes you to your best performance. When the tricks are tied to behaviors that attack your problems, they are even more effective. Even on the days when your goal is not possible, it's fun to play dirty tricks on the left brain. At the very least, you're more likely to be entertained all the way to the finish.

The Giant Invisible Rubber Band

When I'm passed by someone in the latter stages of a race, for example, I lasso them with a giant, invisible rubber band. For a while, he or she may continue to pull ahead of me, but I visualize how the tension is building, cutting off blood supply to the brain of that person. (I'm a great shot, looping the rubber band around the neck.) At the end of a hard effort, it takes longer for the left brain to realize the logical absurdity of my rubber band trick. By this time, I'm a half mile or so down the road. But there's more.

As the logic starts to articulate that this doesn't make sense, I laugh at myself for visualizing such an absurd concept during a race. Since laughing is a right brain activity, it gets the creative juices flowing, often spinning out a series of crazy but entertaining thoughts or images. At the same time, the right brain intuitively searches for solutions to current problems, finding hidden sources of strength and connections that got me through similar scrapes before.

Anti-Gravity Fluid

Let's say that your legs are feeling heavy, and you know that you're slowing down. Take a short walk break and slap onto your shoes some anti-gravity fluid that you have stored on your arms or forehead. Some un-right-brained folks may think that you're putting sweat on your shoes, but you know the truth. The magic powers in this substance start to work quickly, shortening your stride a little, forcing your feet to stay low to the ground, touching quickly and lightly. Not only does this trick activate the right brain, it sets in motion the running form and technique necessary to reduce pounding, restoring your tired legs.

Super Coolant

It's a hot day, you're miserable and not very close to the finish line. At the next water table, visualize that the race officials have put a special ingredient in the water which soaks heat out of your body. Take a walk break as you grab two glasses, drinking as much of one as you need (don't drink if a sloshing sound is coming from your stomach). As you pour the other cup over your head, feel the relief. Visualize thousands of molecules absorbing body heat and releasing it. Take a third cup and pour it on your shirt. Make sure that you're pouring water and not sports drinks!

You may still feel hot, but you've taken two important steps that deal directly with the problem. The walk break lowers exertion, and reduces further heat build-up. Secondly, you lose up to 70% of the body heat possible to lose through the top of your head. The evaporation process of pouring water there will maximize this heat loss. By "believing" in the magic cooling water, you'll mobilize the positive forces inside you that can keep you from overheating. Instead of letting things get worse, you'll feel more positive because you're taking actions that directly attack the problem.

Note: For more dirty tricks, see my book *Marathon—You Can Do It!*

17
WOMEN'S RUNNING

BY BARBARA GALLOWAY

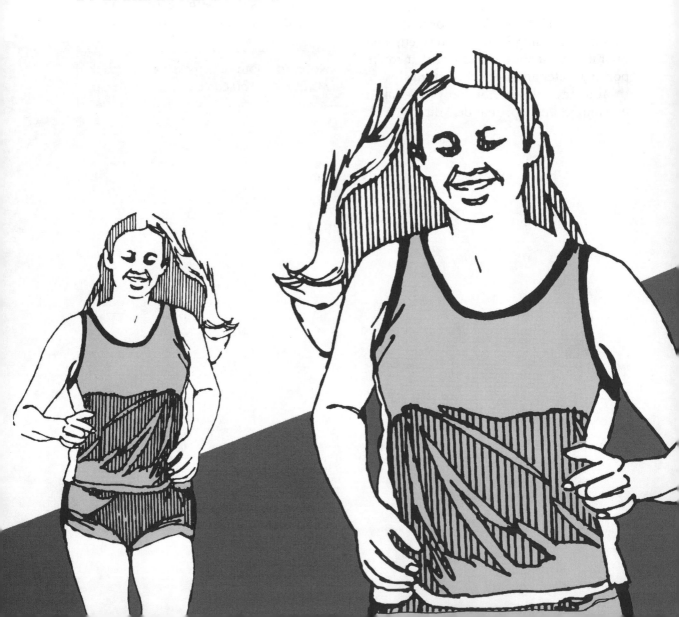

My wife Barbara has been a serious runner for years. In fact, we met at a track meet in Florida when she was on the Florida State women's track team. She has a master's degree in physical education and conducts running clinics (for women and men) during our running vacation retreats at Lake Tahoe and Athens, Greece. She's frequently asked questions about special training considerations for women and especially about running during pregnancy. As a result she's done some research and a good deal of thinking on the subject. Everything else in this book applies to runners of both sexes, but in this chapter Barbara relates what she's learned about the relation of a woman's reproductive system to running, as well as her own experiences "running with a passenger." Please keep in mind that Barbara was (is) a highly motivated runner, "addicted" to her daily runs before she became pregnant. Her experiences relate to other serious runners who become pregnant, but can also be "watered down" for any woman who wants to run while carrying a passenger.

–J.G.

TODAY, MORE WOMEN ARE STARTING to run than ever before in history. In fact, over 50% of all new runners are women, and they're sticking with it. For today's woman runner, many of whom are moms, often with full-time jobs, the bottom line is that running gives us a better attitude boost and stress release than any other activity. The daily run is a sacred time to ourselves, that women need—but seldom take.

In the '80s, I gave my first talk on women's running—and I felt awkward. All my college and graduate courses in training and physiology had told me that women respond to training the same way as men. It was difficult to find enough "women-only" information to fill a 30-minute clinic.

Two pregnancies (and two boys) later, I've learned that there are some very real differences. Although deep inside the muscle cells and throughout the cardiovascular system there is no sex discrimination, our reproductive systems cause us to face some problems men don't have to worry about.

Structural Differences in Women. Physiologists have found that a man and a woman with the same ability, exercise background and training program will have the same oxygen-carrying capacity, the same blood system development, and the same muscle cell development from training. Why, then, does the man run faster?

For one thing, men do not have the extra flexibility and width in their hips to support a developing child. Their pelvis and hips are more efficiently designed for speed and strength. Men can run faster than women with the same amount of effort. Although women can increase the size and strength of their muscles, the inherent capacity for this type of development is greater in men.

When it comes to long races, however, the scales begin to tip toward the women. At 50 miles, for example, speed and muscle are no longer an advantage and they are possibly a burden. Marathon and ultra-distance performance is based largely on the body's ability to burn fat. Women not only have an extra amount of this usually unwanted commodity, but may metabolize it more easily than men. Of course, I don't recommend these ultra-long events (over 26 miles), because they may over-use the muscles for a long, long time. The women pioneers who try them may have great success in the event, but risk long-term injuries and burnout.

Losing Weight. Running is one of the best ways to lose fat and keep it off. It's a better approach than dieting and it has the added advantage of providing a health base which will last for the rest of your life.

Through childhood many girls will have little fat on their bodies. In the teenage years, the female hormone, estrogen, begins to cause many changes, including the deposit of fat.

Men usually build fat on the outside of their muscles—and it quickly shows. Women, however, will "marble" their fat, adding deposits in the muscle itself. This kind of fat build-up doesn't show at first, because it's interspersed among the muscle cells throughout the body. But once a muscle fills up its inner storage areas, fat is stored on the hips, breasts and in thin layers over the body.

Endurance exercise stimulates fat-burning muscles to work day and night. Because these muscle cells weigh more than fat cells, you may not lose weight and may even gain some. Weight is also added because you are increasing your blood volume through exercise. At the same time, though, you are losing inches, dress sizes and unhealthy fat. To maximize fat burning, you'll need to look at both sides of this issue: the *food* in-come and the *exercise* out-go. (*See Chapter 21,* Running Off Fat, *p. 232.*)

If, for example, you have increased your exercise for several months, have gained weight, and not reduced your dress size, you need to watch your consumption of calories. The worst offender is dietary fat, the second sugar.

Don't be a slave to your scale. Weight lost in diets and fasting is mostly water. This will cause dehydration and may lead to illness. Exercise, over time, is the best way to control your weight and also produces lasting health benefits.

FOUR AREAS OF FEMALE CONCERN ABOUT EXERCISE

Whether we want to have children or not, it's natural to be concerned about how running might affect our reproductive systems. Those of us who choose to have a child are also protective of the baby and want the best conditions for its natural and healthy development.

Dr. Edwin Dale, a specialist in female reproductive physiology in Atlanta, has become an expert on the influence of exercise on women's menstrual periods and pregnancy. During the running boom in the latter part of the '70s, scores of women asked their doctors questions they couldn't answer. When the professionals consulted Dr. Dale, he discovered that the research hadn't yet been done.

Finally, Dale conducted studies of his own, working with hundreds of women and comparing notes with other specialists. According to him, there are four major areas of female concern about exercise.

Menstrual Irregularities. Though there are still a lot of questions as to why it happens, long-distance running does seem to be linked to interruption or cessation of menstrual periods in some women. Recent research indicates that a special area of the brain, the hypothalamus, closely monitors total body fat and stress and, when it perceives that the person is "'too stressed," may shut off estrogen production. When body fat in a woman falls below the level at which the hypothalamus judges she could handle a pregnancy, estrogen production stops. This could be a protective mechanism used by our ancestors during periods of famine. The good news is that there's little evidence that this loss of fertility is permanent (although it may take some time to reverse). However, don't depend upon lack of periods for birth control! Irregular or absent menses do not guarantee infertility, and many runners have been surprised to find themselves pregnant.

To women runners who are seeking to normalize menstrual activity, Dr. Dale recommends the following:

- Make sure you are getting the right balance of daily protein, grains, fat, fresh vegetables, fruits, vitamins and minerals. A diet high in complex carbohydrates and low in fat and protein is important to all runners. (A certain amount of cholesterol is necessary for estrogen production.)

- Cut back on mileage by 50% or more to reduce stress and stimulate hormone production. Cutting back one week won't be enough; it will probably be necessary to continue at a reduced rate for several months. For extra exercise, try swimming. For some reason, even world-class swimmers tend to have few menstrual problems. This may be due to lack of weight-bearing stress.

- If neither of these methods works, see your physician. He or she will investigate the case, rule out serious disease, and may prescribe hormone shots. However, most women would rather cut back on their running programs than take hormone shots, for some of the side effects can be dangerous.

Breast Support. Many women wonder if the jarring effects of running can damage the breasts. Dr. Dale reports that there is no known evidence that running causes the breasts to drop, or injures them in any way. However, most women find that some support is a lot more comfortable in a regular running program, particularly on longer runs. Many bras have lightweight elastic straps, which stretch and are not suitable for running, though they are adequate for everyday wear. Non-elastic straps, while they "support," can cut into the shoulders. Underwiring should also be avoided.

Sports bra manufacturers have come up with several bras that work well for many women. Try several different types to see which works best for you. You're looking for firm control without uncomfortable movement. Some women have found that two of the elastic type of bras work very well to reduce excess motion—although this can increase your heat build-up on hot days.

Female Organs. In spite of a few unresearched articles warning of uterine collapse due to running, there is, according to Dr. Dale, no known medical evidence for such a condition. (Of course, if there is a structural weakness in the bladder or uterus, running can make things worse.) Some women will lose urine while running, especially during hard runs or races, and this is a sign that pelvic floor strength should be improved before resuming running. *(See "Kegel" exercises, p. 188.)*

RUNNING THROUGH PREGNANCY . . . AND AFTERWARD

For all that's been written about running, there isn't much first-hand information for pregnant women. For that reason, I'll relate some of my experiences, as well as what I've learned in talking to various experts on the subject. *Please note: Much of what follows applies to experienced runners (probably addicted to exercise) who become pregnant.*

To begin with, there are three important points:

- Little is known about the effects of a mother's exercise on the fetus. Hopefully more research will be done in the near future.

- I was a runner for many years before becoming pregnant. Pregnancy is not a good time to *start* a running program; the combination of beginning running and pregnancy puts too much stress on the back, hips, knees, and other joints and muscles. If you want to begin exercising, try either a pregnancy aerobics program or swimming. If you are already running, you can probably continue doing so, modifying it as pregnancy advances—according to how you feel and what your doctor recommends.

- A woman, especially during pregnancy, has to make sure she has good pelvic floor and abdominal muscle support before even jogging. Check this out with your doctor as soon as possible. As pregnancy puts such a strain on these two muscle groups, most pregnant women runners give up jogging by the fifth month. Again, discuss this with your physician.

Conception—Thanks to a Bad Knee. Strange as it may seem, we owe both of our boys to running injuries. After four years of marriage, Jeff and I decided to have a baby, but decision and reality turned out to be two years apart. Being in good health, we assumed conception would be quick and simple. We were somewhat shocked to find my ten years of running, 17 marathons and hundreds of races might be the reasons we weren't becoming parents.

About a year before we started "trying," menstrual irregularities gave me warning signs that my reproductive system wasn't working normally. When I increased my mileage from 25 to 40 miles per week, my menses became irregular. When the weekly count went to 50 miles and beyond, they ceased entirely. For a year I waited in vain for my next period—partially happy about being relieved of the burden. As the months passed, however, I began to wonder if this might be a permanent upsetting of nature's balance and lead to future problems.

Armed with research, I was assured there was no need for concern. This was, in effect, a natural method of birth control (although certainly not foolproof). Feeling a need for fertility reassurance, I reduced my weekly mileage. My periods came back, although they were unpredictable. The cycle varied from 40–50 days and occasionally skipped entirely.

My doctors told me I may have been ovulating, even when I was missing periods. I'd participated in Dr. Dale's study of women runners, and knew that running more than 30 miles per week can reduce the secretion of reproductive hormones. For over a year we tried to conceive in vain; then a blessing came, disguised as a knee injury.

Running five marathons in six months was a mistake, compounded by my running the last three of them within three minutes of my best time. At first the knee pain was only sporadic and I could run with a dull pain some of the time. After several months, I found myself suffering with each step and was forced to cut back to 10 miles a week. My physicians now tell me that this six-week reduction allowed crucial hormones to rebuild. Finally, we had a baby on the way! Two and a half years later, during another injury "running vacation" we conceived again.

Running with a Passenger. When I first became pregnant, I was afraid I'd have to give up running. It was to be my method of coping with the mood changes and other emotional adjustments of pregnancy. But my knees still bothered me, even at only 10 miles a week, and I began to dread the coming months.

I finally stopped running altogether and enrolled in an aerobic dance class to get some exercise and burn off a few calories. Suddenly the knee pain was gone, and it didn't come back. The healing had started, undoubtedly, because of the reduced mileage. My orthopedist theorized that the sudden reduction of pain was produced by a pregnancy hormone. (It is common for pregnant women to have a reduced sensation of pain in labor due to this natural drug.) I was elated, and decided to resume my normal running.

Second thoughts were more prudent. Although I wanted to get back to my usual mileage, I was lugging around a body that was increasingly strange. Each week the weight gain was noticeable, and my center of gravity played tricks during each run. Frequent internal changes also kept me guessing.

Convinced that this was *not* the time to go for long runs or run fast, I kept all runs below those of pre-pregnancy days. What used to be a 50–60 mile week would now top out at 30 miles. As my "time" drew near, my mileage decreased.

From the sixth until the eighth month I held it to no more than 30 miles a week. From that point until birth I cut back to 18–20 miles per week, taking liberal walk breaks on the runs in the last month.

Precautionary Measures. If you're already running, you may not need to stop. If your doctor understands aerobic exercise (hopefully from current first-hand experience), ask his or her advice. If you are told not to run or exercise, and the reasons given do not seem good enough, talk to other pregnant women runners and find a specialist more familiar with exercise. It never hurts to get a second or third opinion. Many women give up their running or other exercise when there seems to be no reason to do so; they lose a wonderful source of needed relaxation, oxygen infusion, and stamina development. *Of course, you must ultimately listen to your doctor, as there are good reasons why some women should not run.*

Stay cool. If you run while pregnant, don't let your body temperature rise too high, because it can damage the fetus. If you feel too hot, walk and cool off before you continue. Drink water at every chance, as sweating is your best cooling mechanism. Avoid both extreme heat and extreme cold. Be sensible, make adjustments, and you'll usually be able to get in a run. Hot tubs and saunas should be avoided during pregnancy, especially during the early phases, because of their effects on body temperature.

Walk, you don't have to run! The psychological and physical benefits of endurance exercise are based upon keeping your pulse rate up for three half-hour sessions per week. Most pregnant women don't actually have to run to keep the pulse up. Walk briskly and if you want to run, do so for short distances.

While several studies have shown no adverse effects on the baby from *aerobic* exercise, little is known about effects on blood flow and oxygen to the baby during *anaerobic exercise. (See pp. 27–28 for definitions.)* So, when running during pregnancy, you should always be in an aerobic state—able to conduct a conversation. If you are out of breath and cannot talk, *slow down.*

Walking keeps you in shape. If you can walk for 30 minutes, three times a week, during pregnancy, you'll stay in shape and you'll feel better. Never push yourself to the point of stress. If you do run, make it fun. Walk at the first sign of any undue stress. Remember, every person is different. Don't try to match the exercise program of anyone else; make up your own. When in doubt, be conservative.

Take early precautions. If you think you may have conceived, be especially careful. These early weeks are critical for the baby.

All the "warnings" in this chapter, especially those concerning overheating and anaerobic exercise, should be heeded if there is a chance you could be pregnant. On the other hand, if you are training fairly hard during the first month, before you realize you're pregnant, there is no need for alarm.

Pay attention to your changing body. As you gain weight, your center of gravity changes. Because you're carrying such a large "package," your back may hurt and you may pull some muscles. Listen to your body and make daily adjustments in your exercise program.

How Did It Feel? I had three types of discomfort on runs. I felt sluggish when I ran. Most runners feel sluggish the first mile or two; my pregnant sluggishness lasted at least three. Miles 4–6 were often enjoyable and more than made up for the earlier discomfort. Feeling this way naturally made for a slow pace. The overall effect of the run was so good, however, that the early sluggish feelings never dampened my enthusiasm. I was invigorated afterward and felt better the rest of the day.

As the baby grew, running put more pressure and mechanical stress on the pelvic area. Ligaments do not have much flexibility, and they became tighter as I grew. Particularly pressing was the band that stretches from the iliac crest (hip bones) to the abdominal wall, which supports the uterus and the abdominal cavity. During a run this structure would get very tight and seem to "pull."

This was such a pressing and seemingly serious problem I was worried that my pregnancy-running days were just about over. I knew that many women stop running about this time (fourth month). Imagining myself at birth with sagging abdominal muscles and loose ligaments, I read all I could on the subject, consulted with doctors, and my fears were gradually calmed. I kept on running, but most women take this problem as a signal—at about the fourth or fifth month—to stop running, and substitute walking or swimming. Even though I continued to feel some pain from this tendon pressure, I have noticed no long-lasting negative effects, and it's been almost two decades.

Running During the Last Trimester. "Practice" contractions, called Braxton-Hicks contractions, may occur in the later stages of normal pregnancy. I experienced these mildly and sporadically while running in the sixth and seventh months. In the eighth and ninth months, they became increasingly harder to handle and, despite my doctor's assurances, I was sure I was going to have my baby out on the trails. The breathing exercises I learned in our natural childbirth classes helped, and of course I walked or stopped and rested while the contractions were going on.

Important note: Many doctors believe you should not run when experiencing contractions. If *sporadic* contractions occur and are not worsened by exercise, fine, but if they get worse, slow down, stop, or switch exercises.

Again, you should consult your doctor should any of these questions arise. As I said, *most women stop running before this stage of pregnancy.*

Don't get out of breath. By the seventh or eighth month the demand for oxygen increases about 10%. This makes it very easy to become anaerobic during a run, so you have to slow down and walk.

Elizabeth Noble, director of the Maternal and Child Health Center in Cambridge, Massachusetts, emphasizes the need to keep the breathing normal and avoid breathlessness. Interruption in the oxygen supply may have physiological effects on the fetus, she explains, and psychological effects as well.

Again, my romance with running isn't for everyone. Listen to your own physician—and to your own body. This is especially important if, like many women, you experience balance problems and tend to fall. It is also, of course, extremely important if you have any special health problems.

GETTING BACK INTO SHAPE AFTER THE BABY

Returning to fitness after Brennan's birth was harder than I'd expected. The reproductive part of my body required rest. But I wanted my running "mind release" more than ever to cope with the instant responsibility of caring for one who depended upon me for everything. There were some frustrating times—for about four months my body and emotions were out of balance.

You Must Rest. A body weakened by the tremendous physical drain of labor and sleep loss will not heal as fast as usual. The birth process puts a great strain on the inside and outside of one's body and it takes many weeks to recover. Rest is a prime ingredient, along with good nutrition and exercise.

Walk Before You Run. As soon as your doctor gives you the go-ahead, you can walk, 5–10 minutes at first (2–3 times a day if you feel up to it). Before you start to run again, look at the beginning running chapter, and act as if you were starting for the first time. Most women runners can begin running about 4–6 weeks after birth. Go slowly at first, even on flat surfaces, and walk before you get tired. Even if you feel great, hold back; you could overstress your body and prolong your postpartum recovery. A walking program of three 30-minute sessions a week will keep you fit and reduce stress so you can recover. There are very few women who can't walk after a few days' recovery.

Nursing and Scheduling. Since your life is going to be a lot busier after the baby is born, start organizing your day so that you include time for exercise. As a nursing mother, I found that the best running time for me, baby, and his food supply was soon after nursing. You must be responsible for your schedule. Many new mothers let their exercise go, simply because they don't focus on scheduling for it. Since your attitude (and your feeling of sanity) will be positively adjusted with almost every run, it's important for you, and your family, that you get in your run or walk.

Exercises. The abdominal muscles are stretched out of shape during pregnancy. Postpartum bent-knee curl-ups starting soon after childbirth are very important in rebuilding abdominal tone and helping to prevent back problems. Lie on your back on the floor, then raise your head, then shoulders, about 10–12 inches, then lower back down. *(See p. 158.)*

I'd also recommend "Kegel" pelvic floor exercises. Many women, especially those over 30 who have had a child, experience involuntary leakage of urine when running. The term used to describe this condition is "stress incontinence." One interim solution is to wear a sanitary pad while running. Another, better approach is to strengthen the perineal muscles that control this function. Joan Ullyot, in *Running Free*, offers a thorough description of strengthening the proper muscles. You alternate by squeezing, then releasing the " . . . muscles of the perineum, which surround the bladder neck and vagina." You can also strengthen the bladder sphincter itself by tightening, then relaxing the sphincter. When urinating, stop and start the flow; this is the sphincter muscle you're using. You can do these exercises at any time: contract hard for a second, then release completely. Do this about 10 times in a row for one exercise, then work your way up to doing 20 sets of 10.

See also *Essential Exercises for the Childbearing Year* by Elizabeth Noble (Houghton Mifflin Co., Boston, Mass., 1982), a book on health care for child-bearing women that includes information on body mechanics, posture and movement, as well as exercises. It's as valid today as when it was written.

Drink Liquids. Be very careful about dehydration. Drink plenty of water, juices or milk—small amounts (4–8 oz.) every hour rather than large amounts less frequently. Make sure your urine is always pale yellow—not darker. On a few occasions, I ran too far and had trouble nursing for an hour or so. It's better to err on the side of taking shorter runs while you're nursing.

Get Help. If the father can take time off to be with you and the baby the first week or two, it will help build a strong family relationship and a natural interdependence. Don't be shy about asking him for help. Too many mothers push the father out of the nest early. If he becomes a part of the experience and shares in the duties, he'll be more likely to identify with your problems—particularly your need to run.

Two big problems of a new mother who wants to run are finding the time, and a babysitter. Try to work this out before the birth. If the father can't help, try to find a relative, a friend, or a child-care program. Establish, early on, that you need your 30–60 minutes of exercise. Life flows better for all if an exercise-addicted mother gets her daily dose.

If You Nurse. Be extra careful when you are the baby's only source of food.

- If milk quality or quantity drops, stop running for at least three days or until milk returns to normal; also, increase fluid intake. Drink 4–6 ounces of fluid each hour you are awake.

- Try to nurse just before running.

- You need extra calories: 400–500 more than when pregnant, plus extra for running or exercising.

- Use a bra with the greatest support. Use absorbing pads to absorb "leaks."

- Fall asleep with your baby at naptime. Get as much sleep as you can.

Regain Fitness and Lose Fat. You know the old wives' tale about how you gain fat during pregnancy that you can never remove? If you're determined, you'll be gently persistent and eventually lose that weight. Don't rush. *(See* Running Off Fat, *p. 232.)*

A Final Note. In the chapter on *The Advanced Competitive Runner,* there's a section called "Too Much of a Good Thing" *(p. 135),* where hard-driving ambition and competitive instincts may push a runner beyond enjoyment and fitness to a fixation with training and/or racing. The same thing—on a different scale—can happen to a woman runner who becomes pregnant. She must avoid getting carried away by her

A Postpartum Exercise Program	
First 2–4 weeks:	Exercise the pelvic floor and abdominal muscles. Walk a little each day if you feel like it. Talk to your doctor if there are problems.
Next 4–8 weeks:	Run every other day at most. Start by jogging in short stretches as in a beginner's program. Gradually increase the amount, if you feel good.
Next 4 weeks:	Gradually ease into your normal running program. If you're a beginner, follow the beginner's plan *(pp. 000–000).*
Any time during your recovery	If you feel bad for any reason, *stop.* Don't be afraid to back off, take more rest or run less than the previous day or week. You may feel you're taking one step ahead, then one back, but small steps are better than none. Again, listen to your body!
Note: Caesarean mothers must obviously take more recovery time.	

addiction to the beneficial effects of running. Remember that the priority of pregnancy and parenthood is to put the child first, while scheduling your daily exercise.

Elizabeth Noble, author of several books on childbirth, points out that although runners may be addicted to their activity, a new dimension might be added to their lives if they could learn to "... flow with the contemplation, introspection and slowing down that naturally occurs during pregnancy. It is a time for getting in touch with the body's natural wisdom ... Women must be encouraged to take note of bodily signs and symptoms, and to trust their natural instincts."

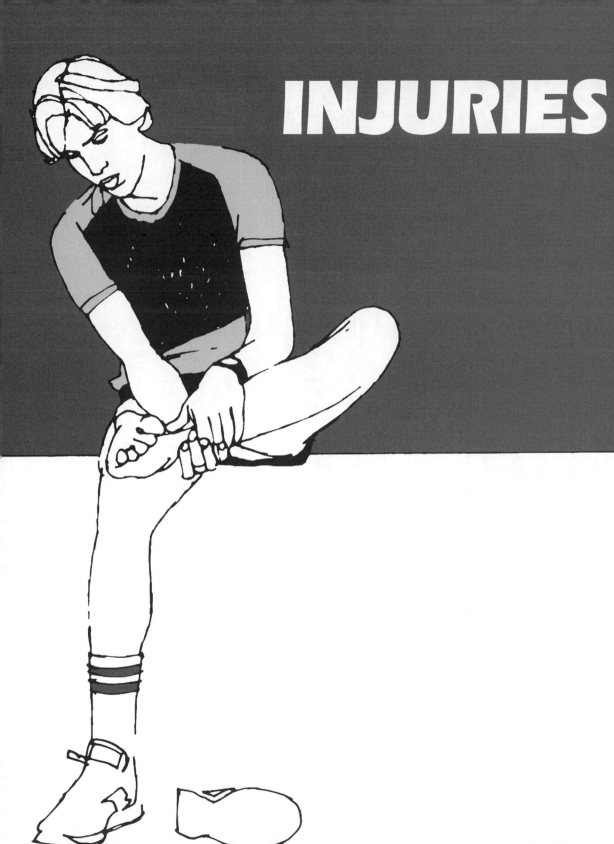

INJURIES

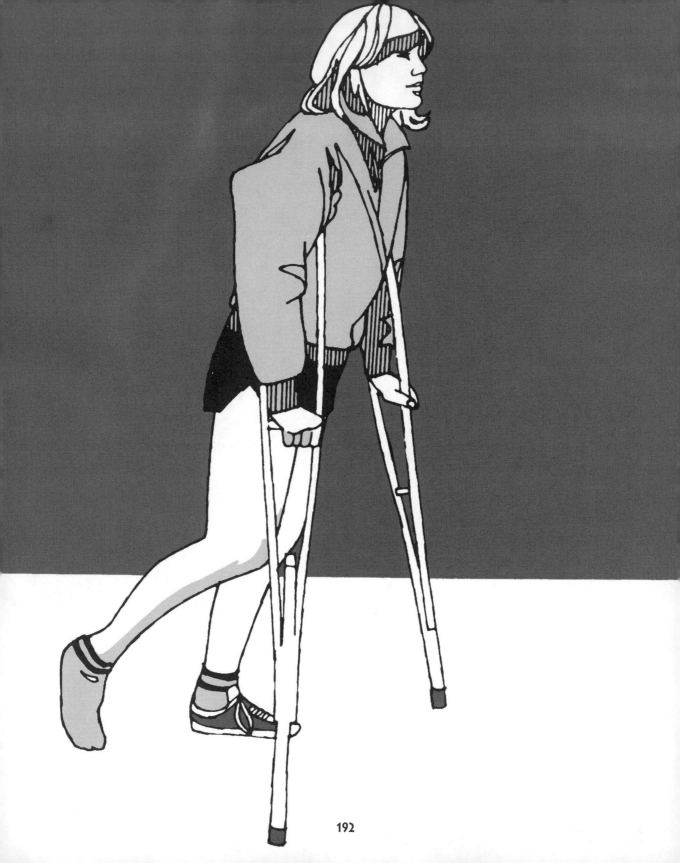

18
THE WALKING WOUNDED

LET'S FACE IT. Running is an addiction. Once you get that daily fix of aerobic exercise, improved circulation, and capillary stimulation, you feel too good to ever stop. *But* when an injury crops up and you become one of the "walking wounded," you are faced with a problem: How do you rest long enough to let it heal?

Sooner or later every runner is injured. Very few injuries last longer than 3–4 weeks; with proper care and when treated early, most injuries will be gone in a few days, with no loss of conditioning.

Note: I'm not a physician and not qualified to dispense medical advice. But having run continuously for over 4 decades, I've had just about every injury possible: strained and torn Achilles tendons, pulled muscles, shin splints, swollen knees, etc. In the process of trying to recover and get on with my addiction, I've learned some helpful things I'd like to pass along. After working with over 100,000 runners I've seen some patterns of prevention, cause, and healing. What follows in this chapter and the next is offered as advice from one runner to another and not meant to be expert medical advice. *If you are ever in doubt about any injury, see your physician.*

When Is It an Injury? Some runners have little aches and pains every day. Most of these are temporary. These everyday aches and pains indicate the breakdown of weaker tissues and gradual buildup of stronger ones. Through experience, you'll learn to tell the difference between a passing ache and an injury. Here are some helpful guidelines to help you distinguish between the two. It's an injury if it's:

- *Functional:* If it keeps you from running in a natural way
- *Continual:* If it goes on for more than a week
- *Increasing:* If it gets worse
- *Swollen:* Compare the two knees, ankles, etc., to see if one is swollen.
- *Painful:* Pain is the body's way of telling you to pay attention. Dr. Richard Schuster, a New York podiatrist, tells you it's OK to "run with annoyance, not pain." Don't use an artificial expedient such as medicine to override your body's signals and keep running.

When in doubt, consult a running doctor: either a podiatrist (who treats only foot problems and problems that radiate from the foot) or an orthopedist (who treats back, foot, leg, and other limb problems).

Take a Day Off . . . Or More. By running on an injury you aggravate the problem and geometrically increase the time needed for repair. It's always better to be conservative and take a day or two off as a safety measure when you suspect an injury. Even if there's nothing wrong, taking a few days off won't hurt your overall fitness level, and may spare you weeks or months of forced rest later.

Treating an Injury. Good medical help is the first step in treating an injury. There is a running underground which can recommend local doctors who treat runners. Talk with some long-term runners. Every injury requires special treatment and you want to find the specialist who has successfully treated the greatest number of similar problems, and who wants to get you back out on the roads.

Before You See the Doctor. Here are some guidelines for treating yourself until you can see a doctor. Be particularly sensitive to pain in the knee, Achilles tendon, heel, and bones in general. These sites can produce some long-lasting problems.

- *Stop running* for a few days. Almost all runners will benefit from the restorative effect of a few days off.

- *Learn* as much as you can. Talk to runners who may have had similar problems. Read some good books like *Listen To Your Pain* by Ben E. Benjamin, *Sure Footing* by Perry H. Julien, D.P.M., or *The Runners' Repair Manual* by Dr. Murray F. Weisenfeld and Barbara Burr.

- *Ice* the injured area. Ice helps reduce inflammation and stimulates circulation:

when blood returns to an "iced" area, it returns in abundance. The frozen ice popsicle works best: keep a few styrofoam cups of ice in your freezer; peel off the top of the foam and rub constantly on the injured area for 12–15 minutes, until it gets numb. Do this at least once a day, every day. Ice treatment is particularly helpful to tendon injuries (Achilles especially), and any injury that is close to the skin.

- *Compression.* If there's swelling, wrap the area firmly—but not so tightly that it becomes a tourniquet and cuts off blood flow. If it throbs or the color next to the compressed area changes, then it's wrapped too tight. During the day, as the swelling increases, it may be necessary to release the compression. Elevate the foot for a few minutes before, then apply the compression from the distal (away from the heart) to the proximal (close to the heart). The compression is used to pump the distal swelling back toward the heart. This and ice help prevent the pooling of blood which leaves scar tissue.

- *Elevation.* Keep the injured area higher than your head or at least off the floor as long as you can. This helps remove blood from the injury so that fresh blood can flow in greater abundance.

ICE

Remember the above three injury measures by **ICE**: **I**ce, **C**ompression, **E**levation. or **RICE**, adding the obvious element of **R**est.

- *Supplement your diet* with vitamin C, which promotes healing. Take moderate amounts, 250–500 mg three times a day. (Timed-release tablets of larger dosages are generally wasted in the intestine where absorption is low.) Calcium is also important in healing; be sure it's included in your diet.

- *Don't stretch* the injured area unless a doctor advises you to. Many injuries are actually tears in the tendons, muscles or other tissue, and stretching will only aggravate the problem.

- *Ibuprofen* reduces inflammation and kills pain and if it does not irritate the stomach, you can take several per day, preferably with meals. Ibuprofen is more effective in reducing swelling than substitutes like Tylenol. However, too much can irritate the GI tract and cause bleeding. This is rare, but it can happen, so get your doctor's approval before using any medication, even if you've used it before.

ALTERNATIVE EXERCISES: HOW TO STAY FIT AND SANE

There's a real problem when you're injured. You're used to that daily fix of oxygen and exertion. Without it you're sluggish and cranky. Sometimes, if you've stopped running enough for the healing to have started, you can do light running while the injury is healing. The secret is to stay below the threshold of further irritation of the injury.

Running, with all the pounding, is mechanically stressful and often the worst thing you can do. Luckily, most injuries will allow you to perform an alternate activity. If you can reduce the force of gravity and minimize the trauma of hitting the ground, you can let the injury heal, yet stay in shape.

We runners are spoiled. No other activity is as simple or convenient as running. Now that you're hurt, you'll have to get some equipment, or travel to a gym or pool to maintain your hard-earned fitness. It's going to be more complicated than running. Oh, the price of addiction!

When You Can't Run

Exercise effectiveness of alternatives (in simulating the cardiovascular and strengthening effects of running):

Running in swimming pool	60–100%
Cross-country ski machine	60–80%
Cycling on stationary bike	30–50%
Race walking	50–80%
Rowing machines	40–70%
Swimming	30–40%

Note: Percentages are based upon performing at approximate intensity and duration of running. Figures were arrived at by my personal experience and talking with other runners.

Before Your Start. Remember that you'll need to gradually increase the amount of any exercise that you haven't done within the past 3 weeks. Start with two sets of 3–5 minutes each. Increase by 3 minutes on each set, each alternative exercise day. Rest for at least 10 minutes between sets. You may do several types of alternative exercise during each session: 10 minutes of pool running, 5 minutes of weights, 7 minutes of cross-country ski machines, 10 minutes of pool running, and 5 minutes of rowing, for example.

You may be surprised by how quickly the body will find just the right amount of exertion in the new activity. You're used to a certain level of exercise in running, and you'll find yourself soon approximating this same amount of stress.

As in running, you'll need to do alternative exercises for about 90 minutes a week, on at least 3 days a week. You could break up the 90 minutes into as many as 9 sessions in a week, according to research done in Australia.

Running in a Swimming Pool. This exercise simulates running better than any other activity and can keep you in fine condition. Many athletes who couldn't run for 3–4 weeks have come out of the pool and run their best times ever.

Horses are taught to run this way. When you run against the resistance of water, it forces your legs and feet to find a more efficient running motion. Thus this is a good exercise even for athletes who are not injured.

- Run in thigh-deep water, about halfway between knee and hip. If this puts pressure on the injury, try deeper water where the feet can still touch bottom.
  Note: You need to run in a vertical position, rather than kick in a horizontal position.
- Use an inner tube or float and run in deep water. Some runners can do without the float and stay afloat by their

quick running movement and treading motions with the arms—but I recommend the former. If you're supported, your legs can move through a natural running motion.

Your goal is to simulate running conditions as closely as possible: Don't lift your knees, but kick your feet out in front, and pull them directly underneath you, and behind you. Stay in the water the same amount of time you'd be running. On scheduled speed days, do speedwork by moving your legs very fast and hard for the same time as for your interval distance. Simulate the workout as closely as possible. You can also build leg, butt and lower back strength by a minute or two of cross-country water running: keep your legs almost straight as you move them forward and back in a slightly longer stride than the usual running motion.

Cross-Country Skiing or Rowing Machines. This is the next-best exercise in simulating the effects of running. If you live where there's snow, you can ski cross-country. If not, you can use the ski machines available in many health clubs, which use the legs in a path similar to running. Some machines allow you to dial up the resistance, building strength in leg muscles. Rowing gives the legs a great workout, as it strengthens the back and shoulders. To maintain a base of conditioning, spend about the same amount of time you would on the roads. These two activities are excellent substitutes for running.

Race Walking. This is an activity which seldom aggravates an injury, but don't do it if there is even a *hint* of aggravation. The object is to rotate your hips and shift your legs quickly, keeping one leg on the ground at all times. This reduces the pounding of running, but uses the same muscles (plus many others). Again, you simulate your running sessions. To get the same benefits, you must cover the same amount of miles you would running. This obviously will take more time.

Recreational Walking. While you won't maintain speed when you walk, this activity will keep the legs in good shape. For maximum benefit, walk at least as many miles as you would otherwise run each week.

Cycling on an Exercycle. In fact, this "cross training" will strengthen your quadriceps, which reduces pressure on the knees. The backs of the lower legs are not worked in cycling as they are in running, and so cycling doesn't maintain your running conditioning as well as the exercises above. If you use toe clips, however, you simulate running more closely. Cycling doesn't produce the gravity stress (pounding) of running and therefore will not aggravate most injuries (although some knee problems can be significantly aggravated).

An exercycle is actually better than a real bike for several reasons: It's safer and you can maintain a steady and controlled pace without interruptions for traffic stoplights or coasting downhill. You can also do it at home, and even read a book or watch TV while working out.

You'll generate a lot of heat so it's best to have a fan or good cross breeze. As with running in the pool, simulate the long runs and speedwork on the cycle; to gain increased benefit you need to add about 20%–40% more time to each session.

Swimming. Although it's an excellent cardiovascular exercise, swimming does not keep your legs in running shape. You'll need to train about 30–60% longer, depending on how hard you swim, to roughly simulate the cardiovascular work of running.

IF YOU CAN'T EXERCISE AT ALL

You'll be surprised to learn how little conditioning you'll lose in five days of complete rest. For each week thereafter you'll lose about 25% of your fitness level. After a month you'll need to start like a beginner.

Rule of Thumb: If you were unable to do alternative exercises, you'll need at least *twice the number of weeks you took off* to gradually build back to pre-injury level.

Note: This is based on my experiences with over a hundred layoffs after injuries.

How Much Conditioning Do You Lose?

Rest Time Without Any Exercise	Estimated % of Conditioning Lost
1–5 days	0–1%
7 days	10%
14 days	35%
21 days	60%
28 days	85%
35 or more	100%

GETTING BACK ON THE ROAD

If the healing process has begun and you're responding to treatment, your doctor may let you start running before the pain is completely gone. As long as you have a solid healing effect started, you may return gently to running, but be very sensitive to the old problem. At the first sign of aggravation, back off and rest some more. Be *conservative*. It's better to take a few extra rest days than to go through the whole process again.

Even if the injured area suddenly feels 100%, it's not totally healed. You'll feel strong once enough of the cells have been healed, replaced, or supported by scar tissue. But there are still many damaged cells, and scar tissue is fragile.

Coming back requires patience and adequate rest. It may seem like you're taking one step forward and two back. Actually, you're taking one forward and two in place. This is certainly better than taking no steps forward at all.

Even if you take a long layoff, you haven't lost all the conditioning you previously gained. The strength, tone, and performance of the muscles are lost when you don't run, but the deeper cardiovascular improvements are not hard to regain. You'll need some time to recondition the exercise muscles and open up the deeper "plumbing" passages. At first it will seem like a depressing second beginning, but once you regain your conditioning base, improvement will be rapid and you'll soon be back to normal. While you're coming back, continue your alternative activities. This will give you some variety during the frustrating days of rebuilding.

STARTING BACK WORKOUTS

If you were able to do alternative exercises as often and at the same relative intensity as your running during the layoff, you should take one easy "beginner's" week and then two or three more transition weeks before resuming pre-injury workouts. If you couldn't exercise at all or did less than three days a week of alternative exercise, you'll need at least twice the number of weeks you took off to gradually build back to pre-injury levels. Here are some guidelines for both situations:

If you've had four or more days a week of alternative exercise:

- The first week, jog easy one day (with liberal walk breaks). Walk the next day.
- For 2–3 transition weeks, you can start running every other day, slower than you did before the injury, and take walk breaks whenever you feel like it. Walk every other day. Increase the length of your long run each week (only on one day) by ½–1 mile.
- For the next month, ease back into your schedule by gradually increasing the running days.
- Be sensitive to the injured area and back off at the first feeling of re-injury.

If you've had three or less days of alternative exercise:

- Set aside 30–40 minutes, three days per week. Walk, inserting short jogs of 100–300 yards, never pushing too hard. Walk until you're completely ready to run again.

- Over several weeks replace the walking with slow jogging—continue 3–4 days per week.
- For the next month, ease back into your schedule by gradually increasing the running days.
- Be sensitive to the injured area and back off at the first feeling of re-injury.

WHAT WENT WRONG?

You can actually benefit from an injury: If you analyze what went wrong, you can use this knowledge to prevent not only recurrence of the same injury, but other injuries as well. Most injuries have the same general causes: you increased total mileage too quickly; you didn't rest enough between hard days; you didn't warm up enough for a speed workout; you let the adrenalin rush of a race push you too far. I've also come to believe that dehydration and stretching before, during or immediately after running are two of the major contributing factors of injury.

Tight muscles will often be pushed into injury if you try to "stretch them out." The lack of vital fluids in the exercising cells causes them to break down sooner and it will take them longer to recover. Drinking 4–6 ounces of water during every waking hour will minimize this effect.

Once you've had to stay off the roads for a few weeks (or months) you'll be highly motivated to build some preventive measures into your training program. In some ways, the mistakes that led to the injury can be the best learning experiences of your running career.

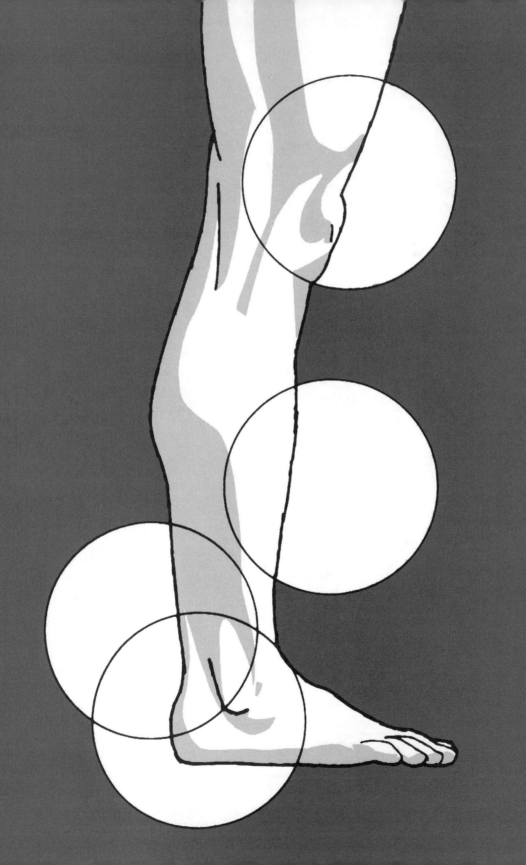

19
INJURY ANALYSIS AND TREATMENT

CONTRARY TO WHAT YOU MAY HEAR from non-runners, long-term running does not weaken or destroy your joints. Several studies have shown that runners have better joint health after 40–50 years, than non-runners. But runners often enjoy their endorphins and attitude boost so much that they ignore the early warning signs of injury until one erupts. They also come back to running too soon, aggravating the injury. Fortunately, running injuries are not degenerative in nature. The sooner you back off the stress, and treat the injury, the sooner the healing process starts.

When an injury occurs, there's no substitute for expert advice. If you get a good diagnosis in the beginning, you can avoid complications and get on the healing path. Generally your best bet is finding a doctor who: 1) has successfully treated a great number of runners with the same injury, and 2) really wants to get you back to injury-free running as soon as possible. The running underground will help you find such a person. (It's even better if the doctor is a runner, but this is certainly not a requirement.)

With a leg or foot injury, there are two types of doctors to consider: a podiatrist or an orthopedist.

Podiatrists are trained as physicians and surgeons of the foot. Leg or knee injuries are also treated by podiatrists when they relate to the foot. For example, knee problems are often caused by improper alignment of the feet and can be remedied by corrective foot devices, which a podiatrist will prescribe. Most podiatrists are fully aware of the mechanics of the entire lower extremity.

Orthopedists are M.D.'s who have taken surgical training and specialize in the bones and muscles of the body. Most are primarily surgeons and not much interested in biomechanics. However, if you can find an orthopedist who is known for treating runners and is interested in the mechanics of injuries, you'll be in good hands.

If the problem is only in the foot or has its cause there, you can see either specialist. If the problem is in the leg or foot and the *cause* is probably not in the foot, see an orthopedist.

Beware of surgery. Orthopedists are trained in surgery and are often oriented toward this form of treatment. When the knife goes in, there is a good chance that the area will not work as well as before. As a last resort you may have to let a good surgeon operate, but get several opinions and try everything else. It's also best to choose a surgeon who has successfully performed the same operation many times.

If surgery is inevitable, arthroscopy may be considered. Arthroscopy is the use of a small sterile metal tube and fiber-optic light source to look inside the body without cutting things open. It is commonly used diagnostically, and surgery can be done through the arthroscope. Arthroscopy, if used appropriately, can be helpful to the athlete by producing minimal trauma; thus a rapid return to activity is possible.

What Caused It? Think about the training components that caused the injury and make adjustments:

- stretching
- speed training
- too many miles
- too much too soon

Worn shoes are often the culprits. Check your shoes, inside and out, before you see a specialist. Another factor often overlooked is the crown of the road. Your injury may be caused by running on a surface that slants one way or another. For example, if you run against traffic, your left foot will generally be lower than your right, due to the road sloping toward the shoulder; this puts more pressure on your left knee. Avoiding these obvious problems can often start you on the road to recovery without medical treatment.

DIAGNOSIS AND TREATMENT

Note: The previous chapter shows a standard treatment and recovery program for injuries in general. Be sure to read it before you look at the following specific treatments for the four most common trouble areas: knee, Achilles, heel and shin. As stated there, this is offered as advice from one runner to another and not meant as medical treatment.

Knee Problems

The knee is the most common site of running injuries in all sports. Unlike the multi-directional ball-and-socket construction of the hip joint, the knee is a one-directional hinge joint. Four bones converge at the knee and are held together primarily by ligaments on either side and secondarily by connective tissue over the front of the knee.

The femur, or thigh bone, ends in two rounded projections with a groove between them. The patella, or kneecap, slides up and down in this groove. From the lower leg, the tibia—the full weight-bearing bone—rises and joins the femur at the knee.

On the lateral (outside) is the iliotibial band, a thick, strong fascia-tendon which combines with the collateral ligament and a muscle called the *biceps femoris* to support the knee on the outside. The weaker tendon and ligament on the inside are more prone to injury, due either to rotational stress or an outside blow to the knee.

In the front of the knee is the patella or kneecap. It is attached at the top to the quadriceps or thigh muscle. When strong, this muscle keeps the patella in its groove.

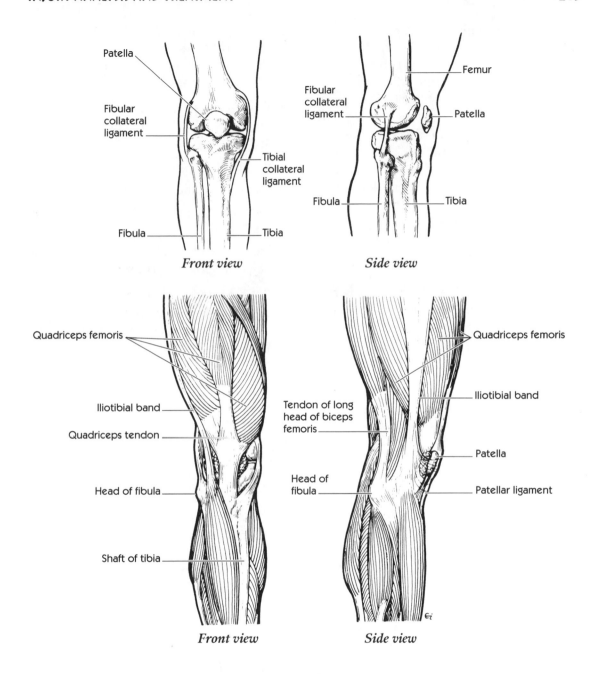

Patella

Fibular
collateral
ligament

Fibula

Tibial
collateral
ligament

Tibia

Front view

Femur

Fibular
collateral
ligament

Patella

Fibula

Tibia

Side view

Quadriceps femoris

Iliotibial band

Quadriceps tendon

Head of fibula

Shaft of tibia

Front view

Tendon of long
head of biceps
femoris

Head of
fibula

Quadriceps femoris

Iliotibial band

Patella

Patellar ligament

Side view

At the lower end of the patella, a tendon attaches and connects to the tibia.

As long as the foot is in a neutral position, the knee is aligned harmoniously between the hip and foot. The weight of the body actually helps to keep a "normal" knee in place, especially when a strong quadriceps keeps the kneecap tight and in position.

Pronation, where the foot rolls from the outside to inside, is the normal shock-absorbing mechanism in running. But when it is excessive, to the point where the arch is flat or the heel is tilted over, it causes overuse problems of the foot and leg. The knee is often forced into a weaker position on the medial side, and out of alignment. As the weight of the body comes down on the improperly aligned knee, problems arise.

Causes of Knee Injuries

Rigid-footed (see p. 247) runners tend to move their feet forward and back, with a strong pushoff, and often have problems on the outside of the knee. The *iliotibial band* is very strong and will rarely, if ever, give way. But when your running muscles get fatigued (as in a long run or a speedwork session), it

can become inflamed and irritated when the foot rolls too far to the outside or inside. *Causes* of iliotibial (outside of knee) pain are usually associated with:

- Worn-out shoes (especially mid-sole breakdown on the outside)
- Too much mileage
- Sudden increase in mileage
- Inadequate shoe cushion
- Increasing speedwork or racing too rapidly
- Not enough walk breaks from the beginning of long runs

Rigid-footed runners push and land so hard that shock may not be adequately absorbed. At first there is pressure on the bottom where the foot pushes hard. Blis-

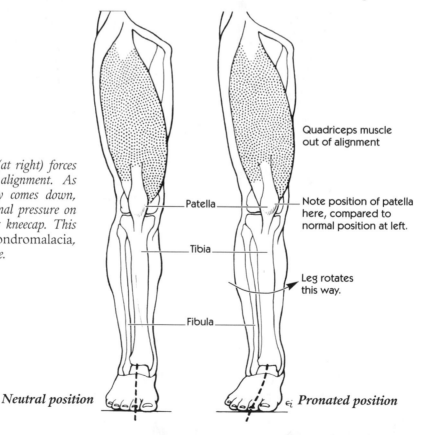

Pronated foot (at right) forces knee out of alignment. As weight of body comes down, there is abnormal pressure on cartilage under kneecap. This can lead to chondromalacia, *or runner's knee.*

Quadriceps muscle out of alignment

Patella

Note position of patella here, compared to normal position at left.

Tibia

Leg rotates this way.

Fibula

Neutral position   *Pronated position*

ters may form here, then thick callouses. Repeated abuse (especially when compensating for a sore or damaged area) will send the shock up the knee, or produce injury-producing extraneous motion.

Floppy-footed runners *(see p. 247)* tend to roll from side to side. There may be shoe wear on the outside of the heel, but also on the inside of the forefoot. Floppy-footed runners who pronate tend to have problems on the inside of the knee, or in the knee itself. Many are also coming down with iliotibial injuries. *(See section at the end of this chapter.)*

Types of Knee Injuries

Iliotibial Band Syndrome. This band of fascia on the outside of the upper leg is very strong and will rarely, if ever, give way. But when your running muscles get fatigued (as in a long run or a speedwork session), the resulting wobble can produce pain—most often on the outside or just below the outside of the knee. Pain can also be felt anywhere along the iliotibial band. This is such a common and serious injury that I have added a new section on why it happens and how to treat it at the end of this chapter. *(See pp. 217–220.)*

Runner's Knee. The first symptom is usually stiffness, especially after sitting for a long time. There's pain inside and around the knee—a general ache. This condition can occur when the (floppy) foot rolls in and puts great pressure on the inside and middle of the knee. The leg rotates and the patella often moves outside its normal path, wearing out the cartilage. As time passes, this may become *chondromalacia*—a true medical problem where the cartilage

softens and begins to disintegrate. Early *chondromalacia* is felt as a "creaky" joint, with a rough feeling under the kneecap. Joint maintenance products (with glucosamine and chondroitin, etc.) can often reduce or eliminate this problem, if you provide enough rest between runs.

Tendonitis. This is pain on the inside or outside of the knee. Tendons connect muscles to bones and they can become inflamed from a direct injury or overuse. Floppy feet tend to cause tendonitis on the inside, rigid feet on the outside.

Patella Tendonitis. This is pain and inflammation in the soft tissue just below the kneecap, or where it connects to the tibia, just below.

Plica syndrome is another, but rarer problem of pronators. It involves a pinching and folding of the membrane at the knee joint. Symptoms are similar to *chondromalacia* with pain around the joint line, either medially or laterally, but not always under the kneecap. There may be a clicking sensation, which indicates damage to the meniscus, a shock-absorbing structure inside the joint.

Treatment of Knee Injuries

- Ice massage. Keep a styrofoam cup in the freezer for this. Ice twice a day, 10–15 minutes on, 20 off, 10–15 on. Direct rubbing of ice is crucial. Merely laying on a bag of ice doesn't work.

- Don't run for at least 2–3 days to get the healing started, longer for a more advanced injury.

- When you start back, run very little at first, every other day, with lots of walking.

- No speedwork or hills for at least two weeks, or until the soreness is gone
- Knee injuries usually take more time because runners must use knees with every step.
- Even when it seems healed, continue icing, reduce mileage, and avoid speed and hills for two more weeks.
- When the problem is inside the joint, joint maintenance products (with glucosamine and chondroitin, etc.) can often reduce or eliminate this problem, if you provide enough rest between runs. The best product I've seen in this area is the Joint Maintenance Product put out by Dr. Kenneth Cooper, founder of the Aerobics Institute in Dallas, TX.

Correcting the Cause of Knee Injuries. The following steps have helped runners in the past and can be used along with advice from a good doctor:

Shoes

Rigid foot. Replace worn shoes and look for better cushioning and flexibility.

Floppy foot. Get a more stable shoe. A "board last" shoe gives more support than a "slip last" one *(see p. 246)*. Shoes with motion-control devices may help. If these measures don't do enough, ask your podiatrist about a custom orthotic which is custom-molded to your foot with the correction built in.

Foot Support. I've found that pronation problems are best treated with a firm arch support. If that isn't enough, take a foot-support system (an insole with arch support built in, and sometimes the heel "cupped") or insole, and layer it on the bottom with cork or felt. Keep adding layers under the arch until it supports your arch firmly and equalizes pressure. Many runners extend some of the build-up into the heel and forefoot (under the big toe joint) to give the foot as much support as possible and to minimize pronation. (Don't build up under the big toe joint if you have a bunion there.)

Obvious Corrections. After you figure out what happened, be wiser about whatever caused the problem. Use common sense in treatment. If your treatment makes the area hurt, for example, alter the treatment or your shoe insert.

Prevention of Knee Injuries (Before They Occur). Now that you've hurt your knee (otherwise you wouldn't be reading this) you're naturally interested in keeping it from happening again. Nothing's worse than seeing your fellow runners cruise down the roads while you're grumpily hobbling around, counting the days. However, when you do recover (and you will, believe it or not!) you have the chance to build up the appropriate muscles that will support your weight better and take pressure off this critical area.

Running strengthens the back muscles of the leg: calves and hamstrings. The longer you run, the stronger and more powerful these muscles become. Strong quadriceps are necessary to keep the kneecap in alignment, support the knee, and check the driving strength of strong back leg muscles. Running itself doesn't do much for the quadriceps. Therefore the primary exercises for preventing knee injuries are designed to strengthen the quadriceps: the stiff leg lift *(see pp. 156–157)*. (Cycling and exercycling may help to a smaller extent.

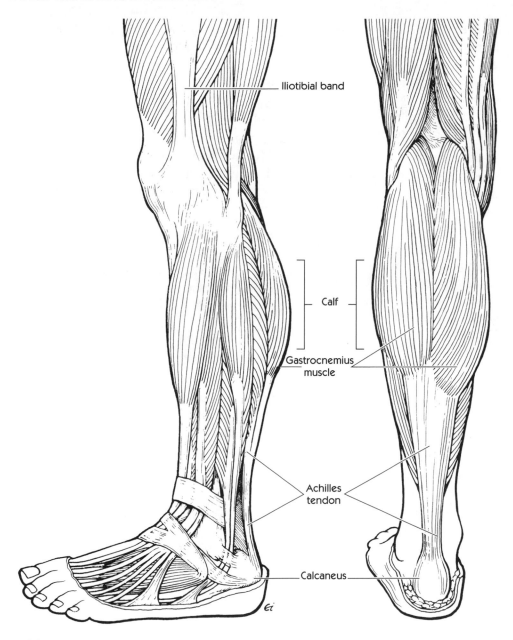

Iliotibial band

Calf

Gastrocnemius muscle

Achilles tendon

Calcaneus

Achilles Tendon Problems

Achilles was one of the greatest warriors in Greek mythology. When he was a baby, his mother immersed him in the river Styx to make him invulnerable in battle. However, she held him by the heel and this remained his one vulnerable spot. He ultimately met his end when shot by a poisoned arrow in the heel.

Most of us were not immersed in the river Styx, but are still vulnerable to Achilles problems. In several surveys of running injuries, Achilles tendon problems ranked second in occurrence to knee injuries.

They can occur in runners with both floppy and rigid foot types.

The Achilles tendon is the strongest tendon in the body. It attaches to the back of the heel bone, or *calcaneus*, rises and becomes thin behind the ankle, and then spreads out and attaches to the calf muscle group.

The Essence of Running. When the calf muscle contracts, the Achilles pulls the *calcaneus* strongly upward, lifting the rear part of the foot and preparing it for a strong "pushoff." Your power comes from this push. Other muscle groups, such as the hamstrings, are of course involved, but the calf and Achilles tendon are the workhorses.

Rigid-footed runners (especially runners with a high arch) tend to push off powerfully, using their foot like a strong lever. This stresses the Achilles throughout.

Floppy-footed runners who pronate put most of the pressure on the inside part of the Achilles tendon. The torque of pronation may also stress other areas. Hills, speedwork, and negative heel or low-heel shoes all put more pressure on the Achilles.

The Achilles tendon is covered by the *paratenon sheath.* The two are so closely attached that a problem with one is a problem with the other. Here we will consider them both as part of the same problem. The most common area of pain is in the narrowest part of the Achilles, about 1–1½″ above the calcaneus. At this point the paratenon sheath wraps over the Achilles and attaches to the ankle bone on either side.

Problems usually take two forms: tendon inflammation and tendon tears.

Inflamed Achilles. With the normal stress of running, small micro-tears occur in the tissue of the Achilles tendon. Normally they heal quickly. However, if there is too much stress and too little rest, they won't heal, will collect in an area, and produce inflammation.

Diagnosis: Compare your Achilles tendons. Inflammation is usually at the narrowest part of the tendon, at the paratenon sheath. The fluid builds between the tendon and the sheath expands. There is sometimes a cracking noise when moving the tendon, and it may be sore. (This is rare.)

Achilles Tear. When the tendon is already weakened it can be partially torn by the additional stress of speedwork, hill running, or simply stepping in a hole. A complete tear is a more serious and painful injury. This often requires surgery, but fortunately tendon tears occur in only about two percent of Achilles injuries.

Diagnosis: If you can't rise up on your toes while standing, you may have a tear. There is a lump in the lower calf area and a gap where the tendon is torn. You can feel this through the skin. If you suspect a tear, try to find a specialist who has a lot of experience with Achilles problems.

Treatment of Achilles Injuries

Inflamed Achilles

- Ice massage for 10–15 minutes at least twice a day. *(See p. 194 on icing.)*

- Use a heel lift — felt, cork, etc. (a Spenco is too soft) — in both running and street shoes to reduce tension on tendon,

- Take an anti-inflammatory medication if your doctor advises (if okay with your stomach). Be regular with it for a week or so to tell if it's effective. It reduces swelling. (To be effective, you must not miss a dosage.)

- Consult with your doctor about length of layoff.
- Don't stretch. Stretching tears out the connections and rebuilding that have taken place overnight.

Achilles Tear

- Ice massage and use heel lift as for inflamed Achilles *(see above)*.
- Don't run for at least 4–6 weeks (or length of time prescribed by doctor) to let swelling subside and healing process begin. If you stop running at an early stage, your "vacation" may be only a few weeks, but if you push the tendon too far in this state you may be out for months. Consult with your doctor. When starting

back, run every other day for another 4–6 weeks—or until things feel better and normal functioning has returned.
- Don't stretch.

Note: Beware of injections of cortisone or other steroids, for they may weaken and/or dissolve the tendon. Get several opinions before getting such a shot; it could set you back months, years, or permanently.

Plantar Fascia and Other Heel Problems

Heel pain will often indicate a problem that may last for a long time. As with other injuries, be sensitive to the problem early and avoid a long-term layoff.

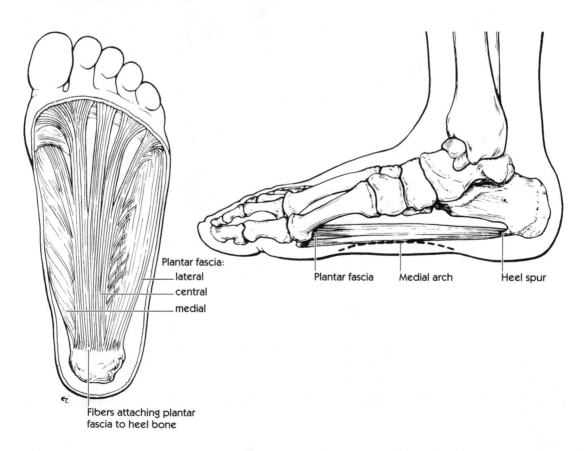

Plantar fascia:
lateral
central
medial

Fibers attaching plantar
fascia to heel bone

Plantar fascia   Medial arch   Heel spur

The *plantar fascia* (a connective tissue structure) stretches from the toes and ball of the foot, through the arch, and connects to the heel bone in three places: outside, center, and inside. Normally it helps the foot spring as it rolls forward. It also provides support for the arch of the foot. The plantar fascia helps keep the foot on track, cutting down on oscillation.

When the foot over-pronates (rolls to the inside) the plantar fascia tries to stabilize it and prevent excessive roll. In time, the inside and sometimes center connections are overstressed and pull away from their attachments.

The first sign is usually heel pain as you rise in the morning. When you walk around, the pain may subside, only to return the next morning. Inflammation and increased soreness are the results of long-term neglect and continued abuse.

A heel bone spur may develop after a long period of injury when there is no support for the heel. The plantar fascia attaches to the heel bone with small fibers. When these become irritated they become inflamed with blood containing white blood cells. Within the white blood cells are *osteoblasts* which calcify to form bone spurs and calcium deposits. The body is trying to reduce stress on that area by building a bone in the direction of stress. Unfortunately, these foreign substances cause pain and further irritation in the surrounding soft tissue.

Long-term chronic pain in the heel may be due to nerve entrapment of the calcaneal nerves which migrate through the enlarged muscle or medial arch, or by the heel spur. These nerves can be surgically cut to relieve pain. Be *very* cautious before consenting to surgery. It should be a last-resort treatment and at least two doctors should recommend it.

The Good News

Once you get the cause of the injury taken care of, and the healing started, it is possible to run while you are healing this injury. A good diagnosis can speed up the healing process greatly by focusing on targeted treatment.

Note: This information is advice given from one runner to another, and not meant to be taken as a medical consultation. Your best strategy in diagnosing and treating any injury is to see a doctor who wants to get you back out there running. He or she will keep trying various treatments until something works. If you are told that you need to stop running for a while (because it is a stress fracture, etc.), you should do just that. Ask the most experienced runners in your area for the names of doctors who specialize in your injury, who've helped other runners heal quickly. When a doctor barely listens to you, and quickly tells you to stop running, it's time for a second opinion. Sometimes even the best doctors miss something. There are times when you should talk to 2 or 3 highly recommended specialists to get the whole picture.

Where Does It Hurt?

Pain is most commonly felt on the forward inside of the heel or in center of the heel. It is usually worse early in the morning, as you hobble out of bed. It will also hurt when you've been sitting for a long time and suddenly get up. In either case, the pain often goes away as you move around, and returns after a period of being sedentary.

What Gets Injured?

When the plantar tendon gets overly fatigued, continued stress pulls and tears the connections in the center and inside the heel bone. This produces pain.

Can I Run While I Have This Injury?

Only if you get the healing started soon after the pain starts. The longer you wait, the longer it takes for the healing to get started—and the longer the recovery period will be. I've spoken with hundreds of runners who've run through their plantar fascia injuries. You want to get permission from your doctor to do this. The healing needs to have started, and you must stay below the threshold of irritation. In other words, you need to keep from further injuring the area. If running 4 miles causes increased aggravation the next morning, run no more than 2–3 miles, every other day. If it stays injured when walking 1 minute after 3 minutes of running, then run 1–2 minutes and walk 2–3 minutes. It never hurts to be more conservative in your running when injured. By running too much you'll prolong the duration of the injury. Most of the time, you don't realize what is too much until you've injured yourself. That's why it's always better to back off at the first hint.

How Does It Get Injured?

The first pain is usually a small tear of the tendon. If you take 3–4 days off from running at that point, and treat it appropriately,

it will often heal completely. Continued running with the injury will produce more damage, a build-up of scar tissue, and sometimes bone spurs. When severed connections aren't healed for months, your body tries to reconnect by extending these bone needles toward the disconnection. Over-pronation is a major cause of plantar fasciitis for those who have a floppy foot (shoe wear on the inside of the forefoot). Inadequate shoe cushion can be a primary cause for those with rigid feet (shoe wear on the outside and middle of the forefoot).

Excess foot fatigue is most often the result of the following:

- Stretching is a leading cause of Achilles injuries.

- Running faster than you should have on that day (i.e., trying to stay up with running friends that are going too fast for you). Most runners are running too fast on long runs, even though they feel fine at the beginning.

- Not slowing down the pace, from the beginning of a long run or race:
  1. when you increase the distance of the long run
  2. when it's hot and humid, or the course is hilly
  3. when your muscles are already tired
  4. when you feel the first signs of irritation of what could be an injury

- Not taking walk breaks, as you need them, from the beginning of all long runs

- Not increasing the frequency of the walk break as the long-run distance increases

- Not increasing the frequency of walk breaks when you're more tired, or feel the symptoms of injury
- Not increasing the frequency of walk breaks when the temperature and humidity are high
- Doing too many of the following within a 2–3 week period: long runs, races, fast runs:
  - Wearing the wrong pair of shoes or ones too worn out—particularly in the midsole (a shoe expert can help you determine)
  - Doing sprinting sports or too much of an activity that keeps you up on your toes (hill running, for example)
  - Not doing the maintenance training during the week, e.g., just running once between long runs, or not at all
  - Skipping a long run and trying to keep up with your group on the next long run
  - Not taking enough days off from running—especially after the first signs of injury
  - Running on a surface that is too soft or is slanted, i.e., a beach, soft grass, or a paved surface with a slant

*Treatment (**Bold** denotes the most important):*

1. Take enough time off to get the healing started (usually 3–5 days, but sometimes much more). Don't stretch!
2. **The golf-ball treatment.** Every night, sit down, take your shoe off and roll the heel on a golf ball, baseball, or softball. At first, gently roll it around the area that hurts. Gradually put more pressure on the heel as you continue to roll it, desensitizing the heel to the pressure. Roll it around for about 5 minutes.
3. **The "toe-squincher" exercise.** Point your toes and contract your foot muscles until they start to cramp. Do this 20–30 times a day. Not only will this help to support and massage the foot while it is healing. Doing this with healthy feet will help. Also consider taking vitamin C. When I have an injury of this nature, I take 500 mg of vitamin C, 3–5 times a day. Consult with a sports nutritionist for further information about vitamin C and other nutrients which can speed healing, before taking this or any supplement.
4. Get a good support for your foot. See a good running podiatrist and get a good foot support which can reduce the extra rolling of your foot. You don't necessarily need an orthotic, but get some guidance. *Note:* A hard orthotic can often aggravate the problem.
5. **Before you get out of bed, put the support in your shoe, and put the shoe on your foot.** Don't ever walk around barefooted—especially early in the morning. Most of the healing takes place when you're asleep. An unsupported foot can tear out the healing that went on overnight, prolonging the injury.
6. Ice massage. Freeze a paper cup and every night rub the ice directly on the area of pain until it gets numb (usually about 15 minutes). Be advised that there's usually no healing effect from merely applying ice in a plastic bag, towel or frozen gel pac. It helps to ice

the injury immediately after a run, but even if you miss this opportunity, ice it well at least once a day.

7. Run on a level surface. Uneven surfaces will fatigue the muscles and tendons and increase the chance of I-T band irritation. A road that is slanted can cause I-T band problems on just one run. Paved, flat surfaces are usually better than dirt or grass surfaces.

8. Get the right shoe and possibly an orthotic. Even the perfect shoe (whatever that is) will lose support from the midsole, usually without any outward sign on the shoes. To run in these shoes usually aggravates the injury. Shoe experts (such as the ones in really good running stores) can advise you in finding current shoes which can give support or cushion your feet. Over-pronated floppy feet show some shoe wear on the inside of the forefoot and benefit from motion-control shoes. You'll have to give them feedback on how the shoes feel and whether there are any discomfort areas. The shoe should be an extension of your foot without any extraordinary pressure or tension. *(For more info, see www.runinjuryfree.com.)*

9. Floppy feet which over-pronate (showing shoe wear on the inside of the forefoot) need motion-control shoes that sacrifice some cushion for stability. This type of foot can sometimes benefit from an orthotic. Try stable shoes first and if they don't control the pronation by themselves, follow your doctor's advice and try other solutions before getting an orthotic. Remember,

if you don't have a shoe that provides enough control, the foot device won't be able to do its work.

10. Rigid feet (which show wear on the outside of the forefoot) need shoes with cushion and flexibility. If the shock is not absorbed by the flex of the foot and the cushion of the shoe, the plantar tendon will take more abuse, tighten up, and increase the intensity of the injury.

11. Massage. Cross-friction massage may speed up the healing. Consult with a running massage expert and you can learn this simple technique. Massage to other muscle areas may also speed up the healing process.

For more info, see my new book *Marathon: You Can Do It!*

Heel Spur

Symptoms: Pain on forward inside or middle of heel, which unfortunately may last a long time. When massaging, you can locate the pain area and often a small lump. Bursitis is another common heel problem (often from repeated impact) that is treated the same as heel spur.

Treatment:

- Ice and use arch support as above. If you can localize the spur, cut a hole in a pad of felt and lay the hole over the spur. This supports the area around the spur and reduces pressure on it.

- The ball treatment. Every night, roll your foot over a golf ball, baseball, or softball. For the first 1–2 minutes, roll gently. As the area gets desensitized, roll a bit harder into the area of the spur. Doctors have told me that this has worn down some bone spurs enough so that they are no longer a problem. Be careful.

- Massage spur as above, 5–10 minutes a day. Start gently with thumb, gradually increase pressure until you're pushing hard directly on spur with knuckle or other firm object. Even if it hurts, it should help.

Plantar Fascia Tear (rare)

Symptoms: Sudden pain which usually keeps you from running and does not get better as day progresses. There is usually a bruise in the plantar area from bleeding and inflammation.

Treatment:

- Ice and use arch support, as above.
- See a doctor. Take 4–5 weeks off with doctor's guidance.

Stress Fracture

Symptoms: Heel hurts all day long; pain often increases as you walk or run. More pain than with other heel problems. There is often swelling and there will be pain if you squeeze the heel from side to side.

Treatment:

- Ice and use arch support.
- Walk at first, then run lightly if there is no pain.

Nerve Entrapment (happens rarely)

Symptoms: Chronic pain that has lasted more than a year may be due to pain in the nerves that migrate through the enlarged muscle on the medial arch or by the heel spur. Pain is sharp and shooting, like electric shock sensations.

Treatment:

- Try ice, arch support, massage, and do the "toe-squincher" exercise.
- If these fail, your doctor may recommend injection with a short-acting steroid or vitamin B_{12}, or surgical release of the nerve. Get a second opinion if this is the case.
- There are many dangers with injections, including the dissolving of tendon by the steroid and rupture of blood vessels or arteries by improper placement of the injection.
- Surgery has also been used for relief; releasing parts of the nerves or part of the stressed ligament connections can reduce pressure and pain. Be sure to get several opinions on either of these approaches and try to find a doctor who has handled this type of injury before.

Shin Problems

There are two types of shin problems. If you feel your lower front leg bone (*tibia*), you'll feel a flat bony area known as the shin. Just to the outside of this area is the *anterior tibialis* muscle. This muscle is used throughout the running cycle and because it receives a lot of shock, the membrane that attaches it to the bone is sometimes partially pulled away from the tibia and toothache-like pain in the area results. This most often happens when you've done too much, too soon, or changed either your shoes, the surface you've run on, or your training schedule (e.g., fartlek, intervals, etc.) without enough time to adjust to the changes. Experienced runners often have this problem after running downhill.

More recently the term *shin splint* has been used to describe an injury to the *posterior tibialis* muscle. This muscle is on the inside of the flat shin bone. It is a deep muscle and is used to stabilize the foot during weight-bearing and to push off the ground. This muscle can be stretched and strengthened in conjunction with the other calf muscles, as described in the calf and Achilles stretch *(see pp. 154–155)*. Be careful to allow this muscle to heal. Cutting back on mileage is always required.

A floppy, over-pronated foot will roll inward, forcing the shin muscles into submission and stressing one or both of them. Runners with rigid feet tend to have posterior shin problems.

Five Shin Problems. The shin bone (*tibia*) is covered by a membrane called the *periosteum*. This is a tight band of soft tissue which includes nerves and blood supply. The muscles of the shin group attach to this membrane just below the knee and near the ankle by means of tendons. When the shin group is stressed, there are five places where problems can occur: in the muscle, in the tendon, on the periosteum, on the bone itself, or in the muscle "compartments."

If you have any kind of shin problem, make sure you don't have any symptoms of the first two listed here—stress fracture or compartment syndrome—before you check out the other ones. Again, it's best to get the problem diagnosed by a doctor who is experienced in shin probems.

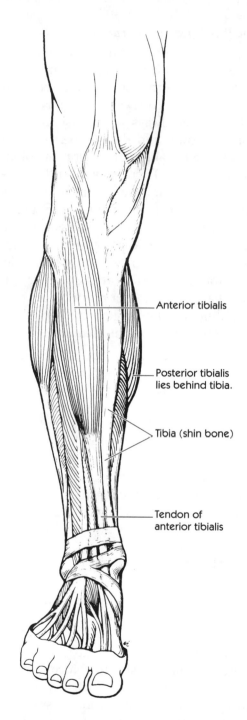

Anterior tibialis

Posterior tibialis lies behind tibia.

Tibia (shin bone)

Tendon of anterior tibialis

Bone Problems: Stress Fracture

Symptoms: Strong pulling at connection points, repeated impact, or twisting stress will sometimes produce a crack or break in the surface or cortex of the tibia bone itself. This is always a serious injury. It happens slowly and does not produce a sudden pain, although there is often throbbing pain. There may be inflammation. The best way to diagnose a stress fracture is to push with your finger at specific places on the bone. A stress fracture hurts in one specific place and does not hurt a fraction of an inch on either side. Stress fractures hurt more the farther you run. If pain remains after running, or there is numbness or tingling on the top of the foot, there is a serious medical problem.

Treatment: Bone scans can show stress fractures, but not always. Stress fractures appear on X-rays about 4–6 weeks after occurrence and last about 6 weeks—if you let the bone heal (no running or other stress). See your doctor (usually an orthopedist), who may cast the leg to keep you from overstressing the area. Try to determine what caused the fracture and consider cushioned shoes (such as air soles) or orthotics.

Muscle Compression Syndrome: Compartment Syndrome

Symptoms: Of the four muscle/bone compartments in the lower leg, most problems occur in the anterior (forward) group. The muscle has a tight band or fascia of tissue around it called a sheath. Normally the sheath expands as the muscle expands. However, when there is sudden swelling, and when the muscle is contained by bones or other muscles on two or more sides, the sheath may not be able to expand. The resulting pressure with no outlet may harm the nerve and/or blood vessels and arteries in the muscle. There may be pain or tingling in the muscle, sometimes traveling down the shin into the foot. The pain is general and usually increases dramatically as you run. The condition may come from sudden overuse, hill or speedwork, or from running too much on your toes (as in sprinting).

Treatment: This problem can be quite serious and have permanent effects if you neglect it. If you feel numbness or pain in the top of your foot, don't run through it or numb it with medications (including aspirin). If it doesn't go away after two days, see your doctor.

Muscle Stress: Myositis

Symptoms: Muscle soreness, probably inflammation. In most cases, pain seems to come from inside of upper calf muscle and eases a little as you warm up in a run.

Treatment:

- Rest: Take 3–5 days off (*no running!*) to get healing started, then try walking. If this doesn't produce pain, try some light running. Try running every other day until the injury seems to be getting better. Talk to a doctor about it and stay below the pain threshold on each run.

- Ice if there is any swelling—10 minutes, at least once a day.

- If okay with your doctor and your stomach, take anti-inflammatory medication.

- Do regular (and extremely gentle) stretching for Achilles tendon and calf muscles. (*See pp. 154–155.*)

- Strengthen shin muscle group through exercise. *(See pp. 156–157.)*
- Ask your podiatrist about a more stable shoe or orthotics.

Tendon Stress: Tendonitis

Symptoms: At the connection points, the tendons may be pulled away from the bone or otherwise injured. This usually localizes the problem at either the high or low connecting point in the leg and causes swelling. At the lower point, the problem is the posterior tibial tendon which you can see prominently when it's flexed—on the middle inside of the leg, right next to the tibia, and just above the ankle bone. If that area is sore to touch, there may also be inflammation of the toe flexor tendons which lie immediately below this tendon. Here's how to isolate the muscle group and tell if the deep posterior tibial tendons are inflamed: Sit down. Hold your foot and lift it to the inside. If it hurts, it's your posterior tibial tendon. If it hurts when you hold your foot straight and try to "claw" with your toes, then the toe flexor tendons are inflamed.

Treatment: Same as for myositis, above.

Stress on Membrane of Bone: Periostitis

Symptoms: The periosteum is the thin membrane (soft tissue) that covers the bone. Tendons attach to the periosteum rather than to the bone itself. With overstress, there can be irritation—normally at the upper and lower connection points. The pain is general in area, similar to a stress fracture, but there is no evidence of pain in a specific spot. Pain does not diminish and may even increase during a run. This may take 3–4 months to heal.

Treatment:

- Rest completely 2–4 weeks to get healing started. Confer with doctor to see when you can start running again. *(See pp. 198–199 on alternative exercises to do during this period. Running in a swimming pool is best.)*
- All other treatment same as for myositis, above.

Special Injury Report: Iliotibial Band

Note: Again, this information is advice given from one runner to another, and not meant to be taken as a medical consultation. Your best strategy in diagnosing and treating any injury is to see a doctor who wants to get you back out there running. He or she will keep trying various treatments until something works. When that type of doctor tells you that you need to stop running for a while (because it is a stress fracture, etc.), you should do just that. Ask the most experienced runners in your area for the names of medical specialists in the area of your injury, who've helped other runners heal quickly. When a doctor barely listens to you, and quickly tells you to stop running, it's time for a second opinion. Sometimes even the best doctors miss something. There are times when you should talk to 2–3 highly recommended specialists to get the whole picture.

The Good News

Almost all of the runners I've communicated with about I-T band injuries have been able to run during the recovery period, once the healing has started. Many of these folks have continued their marathon training program, after making the adjustments for the injury. Once you've determined that the healing has begun, and your training stays below the threshold that could further irritate the injury, you'll probably be able to continue your running. The first priority, however, is being conservative enough (with slower pacing, more walk breaks, and days off from running) to allow the healing to continue.

Where Does It Hurt?

Almost always on the outside of the leg, from the knee to the hip. The pain from the I-T band is most often felt on the outside of the knee, slightly below the intersection of the two leg bones. For some, pain may be centered just above that point. In rare cases it may hurt on the outside just below the hip, and occasionally the pain may radiate up and down the outside of the leg at various times. We will concentrate on the most common site, the outside of the knee.

What Gets Injured?

A strong muscle just below the hip, the tensor fascia, is connected by a long band of connective tissue that acts as a tendon, going down the outside of the leg, and connecting to the shin bone below the outside of the knee. Even when the wobbling proceeds for some time, this band of tendon tries to keep the leg from excess motion. Once the tendon itself loses its strength, and continues to be pushed

beyond its capacity, it gives way at the point of most stress. This is most commonly where the tendon connects below the knee. A bursa sac, which tries to smooth out the operation of the knee and protect the tendon from the bone, may also become irritated. Some runners strain the tendon itself, others pull away the connections below the knee, the tendon, and the bones. A second area of irritation is that just above the knee, due to the friction of the tendon repeatedly rubbing the bone slightly above the knee joint on the outside.

> **Note:** See drawings on pp. 203 and 207 for the location of the I-T band.

Can I Continue to Run with I-T Band?

Maybe. If you back off soon enough, it's often possible to run as long as you stay below the threshold of further irritation while it gets better. You will have to reduce the speed of every running segment and put more walking into your runs, more often. The longer you continue to irritate the injury, the longer it will last. Even after you start back, you must monitor the injury for the next few months. Even after the pain goes away from an injured area, there is still damage inside. One run that is done too fast (or without enough walk breaks) can bring back the damage, often worse than it was before. When in doubt, be more conservative.

How Does It Get Injured?

As long as the leg muscles are resilient, and you're not doing very much more training than you've done in the recent past, the leg system will stay in its track and adapt to slight increases. When you push your main running muscles too far, the primary running muscles get too tired to move you ahead and stay within the natural range of your foot and leg. In other words, your legs start to wobble. The further you go when wobbling, the more you will injure the area. You may not be able to pinpoint what caused the problem, but here are the most common causes:

- Running too fast, on a long run, or race, than you should have on that day (e.g., trying to stay up with running friends that are going too fast for you). It usually doesn't feel too fast. Most runners are running too fast on long runs, even though they feel fine at the beginning.

- Not slowing down the pace, from the beginning of a long run or race:
  1. when you increase the distance of the long run
  2. when it's hot and humid, or the course is hilly
  3. when your muscles are already tired
  4. when you feel the first signs of irritation of what could be an injury

- Not taking walk breaks, as you need them, from the beginning of all long runs

- Not increasing the frequency of the walk break as the long-run distance increases

- Not increasing the frequency of walk breaks when you're more tired, or feel the symptoms of injury

- Not increasing the frequency of walk breaks when the temperature and humidity are high

- Doing too many of the following within a 2–3 week period: long runs, races, fast runs:

- Wearing the wrong pair of shoes or ones that are too worn out—particularly in the midsole (a shoe expert can help you determine)

- Doing side-to-side sports: tennis, basketball, rollerblade

- Not doing the maintenance training during the week, e.g., just running once between long runs, or not at all

- Skipping a long run and trying to keep up with your friends on the next long run

- Not taking enough days off from running—especially after the first signs of injury

- Running on a surface that is too soft or is slanted, e.g., a beach, soft grass, or a paved surface with a slant

Treatment

I've spoken with hundreds of runners who've run through I-T band injury. You want to get permission from your doctor to do this. The healing needs to have started, and you must stay below the threshold of irritation. In other words, you need to keep from further injuring the area. If running 4 miles leaves it feeling worse the next day, run no more than 2–3 miles, every other day. If it stays injured when walking 1 minute after 3 minutes of running, then run 1–2 minutes and walk 2–3 minutes. It never hurts to be more conservative in your running when injured. By running too much you'll prolong the duration of the injury. Most of the time, you don't realize what is too much until you've injured yourself. That's why it's always better to back off at the first hint of pain.

1. Take enough time off to get the healing started (usually 3–5 days).

2. Take vitamin C. When I have an injury such as I-T band, I take 1000 mg of vitamin C, 3–5 times a day. Consult with a sports nutritionist for further information about vitamin C and other nutrients which can speed healing.

3. Stretch the tendon. The I-T band is one of few running injuries that is helped by stretching. Start with the stretches in Bob Anderson's book *Stretching* and experiment to find ones that reduce or eliminate the pain. You can stretch before, after, and during a run—and even in the evening, or while sitting at your desk at work. Stretching primarily reduces the tension on the tendon so that it doesn't hurt for a while. By keeping the I-T band flexible you also reduce the continued pulling on it, and may help it to heal to some extent. Experiment with different stretches for the area. The best ones are those that release the I-T band, giving you instant relief. Compare stretches with other I-T band sufferers, but very few runners will use the same stretch routine. You will find that different stretches help at different times, even on the same run.

4. Ice massage. Freeze a paper cup and every night, rub the ice directly on the area of pain until it gets numb (usually about 15 minutes). Be advised that there's usually no healing effect from merely applying ice in a plastic bag, towel, or frozen gel pac. It helps to ice the injury immediately after a run, but even if you miss this opportunity, ice it well at least once a day.

5. Run on a level surface. Uneven surfaces will fatigue the muscles and tendons and increase the chance of I-T band irritation. A road that is slanted can cause I-T band problems on one run.

6. Get the right shoe and possibly an orthotic. Even the perfect shoe (whatever that is) will lose support from the midsole, usually without any outward sign on the shoes. To run on these shoes usually aggravates the injury. Shoe experts (such as the ones in really good running stores) can advise you in finding current shoes which can give the support or cushion your foot needs. Over-pronated floppy feet show some shoe wear on the inside of the forefoot and benefit from motion-control shoes. You'll have to give them feedback on how the shoes feel and whether there are any discomfort areas. The shoe should be an extension of your foot without any extraordinary pressure or tension.

   • Floppy feet which over-pronate (showing shoe wear on the inside of the forefoot) need motion-control shoes that sacrifice some cushion for stability. This type of foot can sometimes benefit from an orthotic. Try stable shoes first and if they don't control the pronation by themselves, follow your doctor's advice and try other solutions before getting an orthotic. Remember, if you don't have a shoe that provides enough control, the foot device won't be able to do its work.

- Rigid feet (which show wear on the outside of the forefoot) need shoes with cushion and flexibility. If the shock is not absorbed by the flex of the foot and the cushion of the shoe, the I-T band will take more abuse, tighten up, and increase the intensity of the injury.

7. Massage. Cross-friction massage may speed up the healing. Consult with a running massage expert and you can learn this simple technique. Massaging other muscle areas may also speed up the healing process.

8. As a last resort, under a doctor's direction: anti-inflammatory medication and/or cortisteroid injection (i.e., cortisone) may get the healing started. Get several opinions before you agree to this, and go to the most experienced and competent doctor you can find.

CROSS TRAINING AND BALANCING

Participation in one sport to the exclusion of others can produce muscular imbalance, and often leads to specific-sport injuries. In recent years, coaches and athletes have come to appreciate the value of engaging in several activities to achieve greater muscular balance. Where running primarily works the calf and hamstring muscles, cycling builds up the quadriceps, swimming exercises the upper body, and cross-country skiing provides a superb overall body workout without the trauma of running. Here are some of the advantages of adding other sports to your training program:

Cardiovascular Training. You can increase your weekly cardiovascular training by adding other sports. If you spent the same total hours running, you'd be more likely to suffer injuries.

Variety. In the heat of the summer, swimming is an attractive alternative, as is cycling, with its built-in breeze. Exercycles, rowing machines, and indoor pools offer similar relief from winter weather. Adding other sports to your running program helps overcome periods of low motivation, and you'll return to running stimulated and refreshed.

Burning Off Fat. Those who run to lose weight become excited as mileage increases and fat decreases. Unfortunately, further mileage increases often lead to injury. Again, adding other sports can keep the fat furnaces burning and the weight under control.

Triathlons. Where the Hawaii *Ironman* is for super athletes and/or those who can train six hours a day, the scaled-down versions have become increasingly popular—especially those that can be finished in marathon time (3–4 hours) or less. If you've been running for a while, you're already trained for a third of the event. Here's a proposed schedule for starting triathlon training:

Monday:	Long cycle
Tuesday:	Speed run
Wednesday:	Long swim
Thursday:	Speed cycle/fun run
Friday:	Speed swim/fun cycle
Saturday:	Rest
Sunday:	Long run

Each activity has a long day, a speed day, and a fun day.

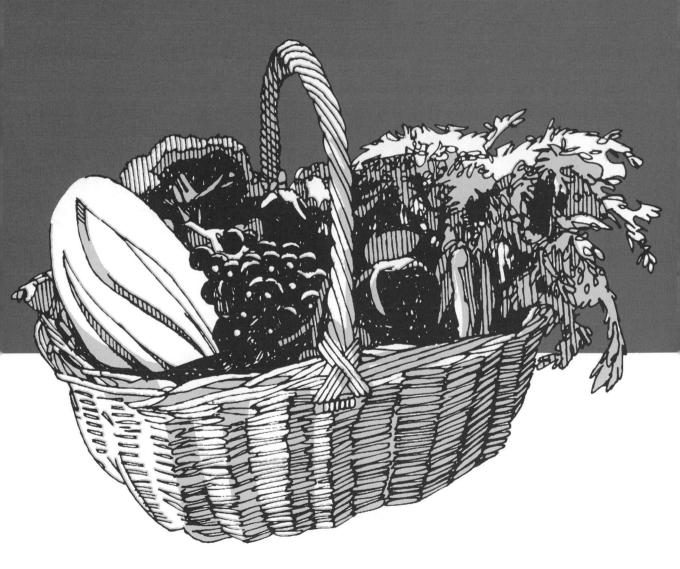

FOOD

20
FUEL

EATING FOR PERFORMANCE

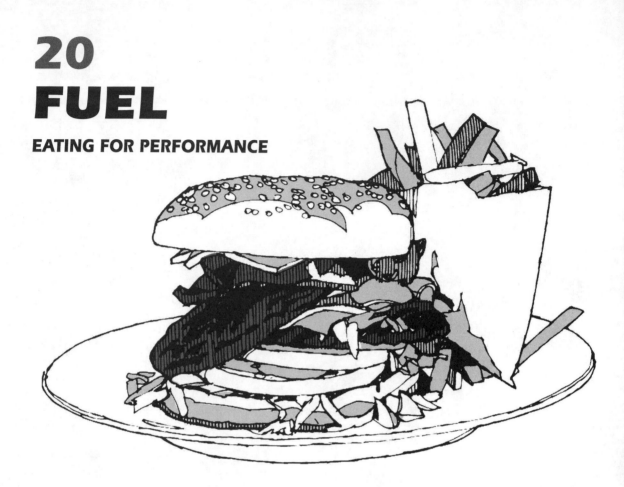

I'D LIKE TO OFFER YOU an exclusive miracle diet that could propel you beyond your goals. There are tales of such experimental approaches. In 1978, Dick Gregory prepared a special diet for one of Boston's better marathoners, Vinny Fleming. After following it for several weeks, he ran in the famous hometown marathon that year and took a special concoction at the 20-mile mark. Not only did he lower his time by several minutes, but he said he felt a great lift when he took the "brew" at 20 miles.

So far as I know, this was the only success of this mystery food, and I'm glad. I don't like hearing of "miracle foods" because they cloud the basic truth, which is that training does a lot more to improve performance than diet. It was Fleming's condition that allowed him to improve, not the drink. Given a certain level of conditioning, some diets will help a little, others will hinder a little. Diet matters more in long-term health than in an individual performance.

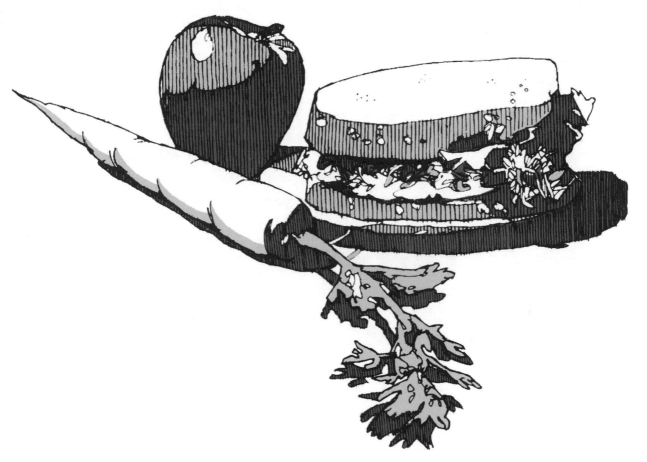

For fat-level management, you must understand the principles of your set point *(see p. 234)* and be honest with yourself. This means balancing what you want to look like with the type of eating plan you're willing to follow, not for a month or so, but as a lifestyle. Most successful dietary changes are small ones that allow you to feel good all day long so you can exercise and burn off the pounds of fat you want to lose. The fat-burning chapter *(pp. 232–242)* will detail this process, in case you have a friend who is interested in this.

The point of eating is to acquire the essential nutrients with a steady metabolic boost so that you can maintain a motivational level of blood sugar to do all of life's activities. Your energy level is greatly determined by what you eat and significantly influenced by how much and how often you eat.

225

EATING ALL DAY LONG

Yes, it's better for fat control and your energy level if you eat every 1–2 hours. Our digestion system was designed for grazing: taking in modest amounts of food all day long. Each time we eat, even small amounts, our digestive system gears up to process the nutrients and dispose of the bulk. This means that you're burning calories for an extended period beyond the eating of the snack—in order to digest the food. This increase in metabolic rate makes you feel more energetic and motivated.

The starvation reflex kicks into depositing fat when your metabolism slows down. To prevent starvation, you have an intuitive mechanism that conserves resources and adds fat to the body if you're not grazing regularly. Even if you wait 3 hours to eat, you'll increase the fat-depositing enzymes so that more of the next meal becomes fat. The longer you go without food, the more your metabolism will shut down into a fasting or low level of energy. If you're not eating enough food, "metabolism control" will cut your flow of energy so that you don't burn up your reserves. The longer you fast, the more likely you'll want to be sedentary and resist moving around. So if you're trying to exercise in the afternoon, 5 hours after your last meal or snack, your metabolism controller will probably be steering you toward the couch instead of the track or trail. *(See the next chapter for more information.)*

A small to moderate snack, 60–90 minutes before your run, will increase your metabolism significantly and can be processed efficiently.

A big meal, however, is counter-productive to exercise. As it sits in your stomach and intestines, many resources are needed (especially blood supply) and your body wants to shut down other activities. This is why you feel sleepy and unmotivated about half an hour after a big meal.

WHAT YOU EAT MAKES A DIFFERENCE

A good balance of fresh, complex carbohydrates (50–60% of the calories) along with some protein (20–25% of the calories) and a little fat (10–20% of the calories) will leave you satisfied for an extended period after eating. Too much food, too much sugar and starch, or too much fat in a meal will lead to fat accumulation.

Carbohydrates. Carbohydrates give you the energy you need in a form the body can easily use. Complex carbohydrates (such as vegetables, fruits, whole grain products, legumes, etc.) have fiber and various other nutrients neatly packaged with the energy. They keep you satisfied longer because it takes the body a longer time to process them. Simple carbohydrates (sugar, starch, etc.) are broken down so fast that you can consume a great quantity of calories without feeling satisfied. Excess calories that accumulate during a day are processed into fat if, after several hours, they haven't been used for energy.

Fat. Fat is deposited directly on your body. A little fat in each snack or meal will keep you from being hungry for a longer period. But once the fat content exceeds about 25 percent of the calories, particularly in a meal, you'll be storing significant quantities. Fat slows down digestion, so you'll be more uncomfortable if you want to run too soon after eating. The more fat you eat, the more lethargic you'll feel.

Eating fat after exercise also slows down your restocking of glycogen. A high-carbohydrate meal with 20% of the calories in protein within 30–120 minutes after a run will help you restock the vital energy supply you need for the first 15 to 30 minutes of your next exercise session. When too much fat is consumed, the glycogen is not replenished and you don't feel very good as you start each successive run.

Sugar and Starch. Sugar and starch are simple carbohydrates and are processed so quickly that you usually get hungry before you've even had a chance to burn them off. As we tend to follow our hunger pangs, meals overloaded with sugar and starch almost always lead us to consume more calories in a 24-hour period than we are burning off. Excess calories are transformed into body fat. Small quantities of simple carbohydrates are okay—especially if they are in a food that you dearly love. Don't prevent yourself from eating that piece of pizza; just enforce the one-slice rule.

Protein. Protein is the building block of our muscles. We need some each day to replace the normal wear and tear of our muscles and other tissue. By eating some protein with each of your snacks, you'll prolong your feeling of satisfaction—extending the time before you feel hungry. You can certainly eat too much protein. If your total consumption of calories during a day is more than you've burned up, the excess will be converted into fat—whether the surplus comes from carbohydrates or

protein (the fat you eat is always converted into body fat). Too much protein in the diet can cause other health problems. Most nutritionists I've interviewed have told me that a steady diet in which 30 percent or more or the calories come from protein can lead to kidney damage. Inadequate processing of protein products produces homocysteine, which damages your heart arteries.

Fiber. Fiber will also keep you from getting hungry for a while. Many types of soluble fiber, such as oat bran, coat the lining of the stomach, slowing down the release of sugars into the bloodstream. I've found that certain brands of energy bars, which have a very effective form of soluble fiber, keep me from getting hungry for about twice as long as do other energy bars with less fiber. Practically any fiber that is in a food will increase the feeling of satisfaction. The fiber in a baked potato, for example, leaves me satisfied for about three times as long as an apple even though both have the same number of calories. The fiber in grape nuts cereal fills me up for 5 times as long as does a bowl of frosted flakes with the same caloric total.

Vitamins and Minerals. I don't recommend going wild on vitamins. A variety of fresh fruits and vegetables together with sources of lean protein will usually give you more nutrients than you need, but there's more evidence each year that specific supplements help those with specific needs. If you suspect that your diet is inadequate, take a "one-a-day"-type vitamin. Some good research points to the possibility of cancer reduction if you take vitamin C (500 mg) and vitamin E (400 iu) every day. Other research shows that deficiency of the B complex can encourage heart disease through the build-up of plaque. Vitamin C definitely speeds up the healing process. Women who exercise regularly tend to be deficient in iron and sometimes in calcium.

Alcohol. Alcohol is a central nervous system depressant, and is almost certain to lower your performance if consumed within about 12 hours of exercise. The more you drink, the longer the depressing effect lasts. Alcohol also dehydrates you. It's not a good idea to drink the night before a long run, fast run, or a race.

Caffeine. Caffeine is a central nervous system stimulant that can enhance the performance and enjoyment of exercise. But a few individuals should not take it. Those, for example, who have problems with an irregular heartbeat shouldn't be drinking coffee. If you suspect that you might have problems with caffeine, check with your doctor or a sports nutritionist.

I dearly enjoy my cup of coffee before my run. It not only raises my awareness, concentration, and motivation, but also seems to get the right brain working its intuitive magic, cranking out creative thoughts. Caffeine stimulates an early breakdown of body fat into free fatty acids and triglycerides, substances that can be burned as fuel. There's also good evidence that a cup of coffee about an hour before exercise improves your endurance. But you will lose about half the water in a cup of coffee or in a diet cola. This means that only half of the fluid is available for absorption. A cup of coffee before a race is fine if you're accustomed to doing this before running, but three cups or more are not recommended.

REGULATING THE APPETITE

Over the course of a month we tend to eat the number of calories that we burn up, that rate being controlled by our internal set-point mechanism. When the mechanism senses that we're engaging the starvation reflex, it will trigger more hunger and we'll eat more calories than we're burning, producing a weight gain. By eating small meals every few hours, exercising regularly, eating complex carbohydrates, and so on, we'll tend to stay the same or burn off more calories than we've consumed. This results in fat reduction. Simple sugars and starches just slide through with no discount, producing surplus calories that are converted into body fat. Even if you eat too many calories in carbohydrates and protein, you can still go out for a walk or jog and burn them off—another way to gain control over your weight and fat level.

The best time for reloading after exercise is within 30 minutes of finishing your run. But you can still get reload benefits for the next 2 hours. Be sure to drink water or other fluids (except those containing caffeine or alcohol) during the reloading process. By drinking fluids and eating some high-quality carbohydrate snack (enhanced by adding about 20 percent protein by calorie count), you can maximize glycogen reloading and will feel better and stronger during your next run.

Fluids. The danger lies not in neglecting water entirely, but in failing to drink enough of it, regularly. Our body is mostly water; it's tucked away in various nooks and crannies. Glycogen cannot be stored without water, for example. Water cools us in hot weather through perspiration and dilation of the capillaries on the surface of the skin.

To replace the water you lose gradually throughout the day (even in cool weather), you should drink 4–6 ounces every waking hour, and include some dilute electrolyte beverages: orange, grapefruit or tomato juices or a commercial beverage such as Accelerade, which contains potassium and magnesium. Once you start running, your absorption of fluids is reduced significantly. Even if you drink gallons, your body will only absorb ounces. This means the following:

1. Regular fluid intake throughout the non-running parts of the day is your prime re-hydrating time.

2. You are going to become increasingly dehydrated the longer you run.

3. Continue to drink during the run, but don't drink excessively. Conserve fluids from the beginning by starting slower, taking walk breaks, etc.

The afternoon and evening before a race, continue drinking water and electrolyte beverages (4–6 oz. per hour) and avoid salty food. Even one salty meal at dinner can leave you significantly dehydrated at the start of the run the next morning—which means even more dehydration at the end.

As race time nears, fluids should be more dilute. During the last two hours, I drink only water; this reduces the chance of getting an upset stomach. You can't drink enough during an event to replace what you're sweating away, so, like a good camel, have some in your stomach when you start. However, continue to drink small amounts. Do not drink a large amount at one time.

During the race. Dehydration is a formidable problem during the marathon, correspondingly less so in shorter races. On a warm day, a marathon racer can lose a quart or two of water an hour through sweating. Also lost are electrolytes (ions of magnesium, potassium, sodium, calcium, etc.) that facilitate nerve transmission, and other vital functions. Most of the runners I've worked with tend to get upset stomachs from sports drinks taken during a long race like a marathon, even though they have no trouble on shorter distance races or longer training runs. The only drinks I use during a race are Accelerade and water.

Everyone is different and each runner's internal reaction to nutritive substances consumed during a race will be different. If you want to try out the electrolyte beverages, test them out on some of your long runs and races prior to your goal race, and add extra water. During the race, mix a cup of water with the sports drink you choose. You'll reduce your chance of getting stomach problems if you drink only water.

Race Nutrition Countdown. I begin my eating countdown the day before by eating small meals every 2–3 hours. On each, it's OK to eat a little protein with carbohydrates that you know will be digested easily. Your goal is to eat just enough to leave you satisfied, but not full, for 2 hours or so. Be sure to drink water or an electrolyte beverage with your snacks. That afternoon and evening I'll take water and juices regularly. If I'm hungry I'll eat only easily digestible food, such as bread, or energy bars. I'll obviously avoid fried or greasy food or other foods that are hard to digest, like peanut butter or dairy products. I'll also stay away from high-roughage items like salad, bran, etc.

The carbo-loading dinner before a race is great social fun. It's okay to eat a little, but don't overeat, and avoid salty food, particularly if the weather is predicted to be warm. Loading up too much the night before can lead to unloading during the race.

I like to wake up 3–4 hours before the race. During the first 2–3 hours I'll take 6 ounces of water or Accelerade every hour. About 60–90 minutes before the start, I usually eat an energy bar and have a cup of coffee as logistics permit. Hopefully I'll have some water with me at the start to sip, but primarily to dump on my head if the day is warm. It may look strange, but it works! (If you want to try this routine, test it out on your long runs first.)

Caffeine. There is now strong evidence that a cup of coffee an hour before a race will improve performance. This drug helps mobilize free fatty acids and triglycerides, making them available for energy utilization in the blood stream. It also helps you to wake up and get your sewage system cleaned out, avoiding the last minute lines at the "porto-johns." Too much caffeine, however, can cause dehydration and may negatively influence your heart rhythm. Be careful and try it out on several trial runs before using it in races.

THE SLOSHING RULE

When you hear sloshing in your stomach, don't drink for 30 minutes or whenever the sloshing sound goes away.

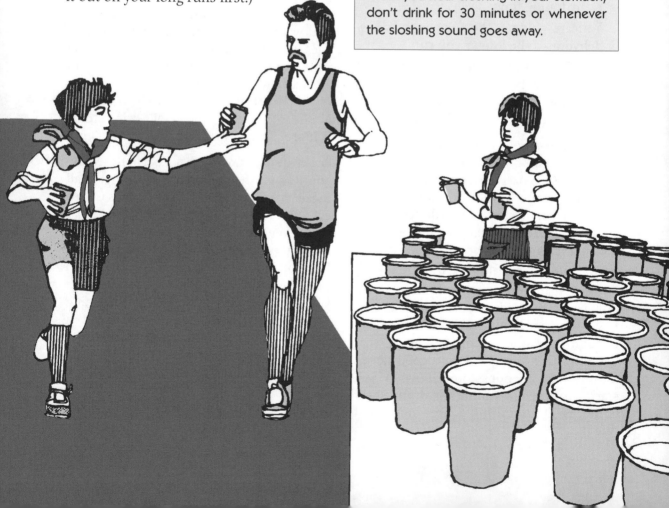

PRE-RACE DIETARY COUNTDOWN

Rules:

1. Don't try anything new.

2. Go through the same schedule and foods that worked for you in training.

3. If you hear sloshing in your stomach, you don't have to drink for the next 30 minutes.

24 hours and before: Normal balanced meals. Plenty of fluids all day long, especially electrolyte fluids (I drink Accelerade). Before marathons you can eat extra carbohydrates.

18 hours before race: Start eating small meals, every 2–3 hours. Keep drinking fluids. After lunch, cut out red meat, fried foods, dairy products, fats, nuts, and roughage.

12 hours before race: Don't overeat. Only light, digestible foods like energy bars, bread, small sandwiches, which you've tried before long runs and races. Keep drinking water and electrolyte fluids. Avoid salty foods.

4 hours and less: Water mostly, with some electrolyte fluid, in small, regular amounts. Cold water is absorbed quicker. I recommend 6 oz. every hour, 8 oz. on hot days. If you want vitamin C, take it two hours or more before the race.

During race: Drink a cup at every water station—*especially the early ones, unless you hear the sound of water sloshing in your stomach.*

Recent research has shown that consuming a snack that is 80% carbohydrate and 20% protein helps deliver energy to the muscle during exercise and restocks the energy stores afterward. I use the products "Accelerade" during exercise and "R4" afterward.

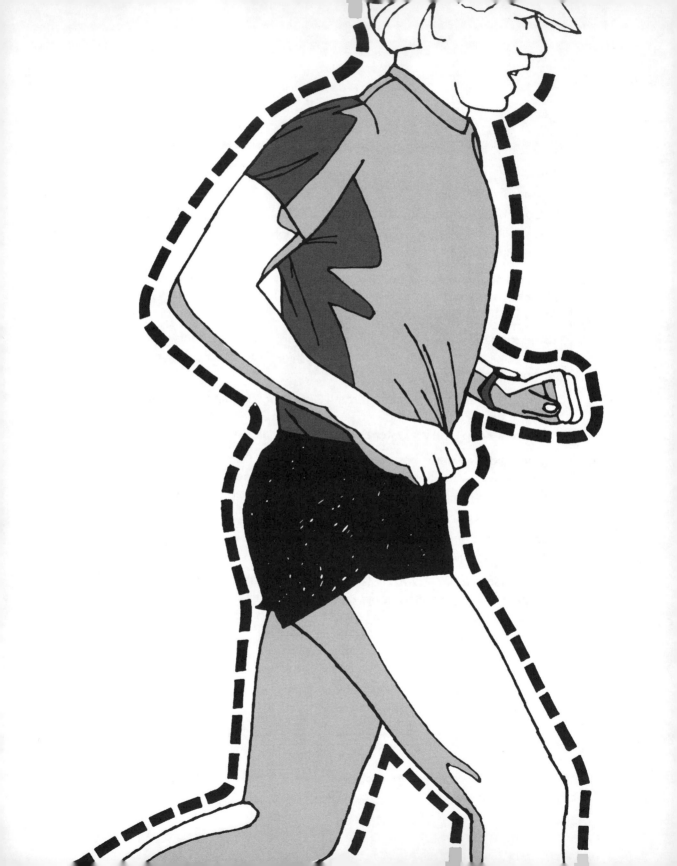

21
RUNNING OFF FAT

BY NOW JUST ABOUT EVERYONE knows that diets don't work (at least not for long). Haven't we all had friends who went on a diet, looked great for a while, and then slipped back to their old (often even greater) weight?

What *does* work, and it's becoming increasingly recognized, is exercise. And the exercise that's better than almost all the others for losing weight and keeping it off is—you guessed it—running. Running has helped me bring appetite, exercise, and food into balance. When I started running at 13, I'd guess my body fat was about 15%. After four years of running it had dropped to about 9–10%. When I started training seriously for the Olympics in 1970 it dropped again to 5–7% and has remained in that range.

Running seems to keep my body and mind in touch. I'm much more sensitive now to overeating or eating the wrong foods. My appetite shifts quickly when I increase or decrease my exercise—but this wasn't always the case. During my first 8–10 years of running, a decrease in running (due to injury) did not change my eating habits, and for a while I'd gain weight. Now, after over 40 years of regular running, my body is very sensitive and reacts quickly. If I run less, I eat less.

Lose fat—not (necessarily) weight.

Endurance exercise is probably the best method of losing fat. Not only do you burn fat as you run, you build your running muscles into fat furnaces which consume the unwanted substance at a greater rate. Muscles feed on fat, so the higher your percentage of muscle, the more fat you'll burn all day long.

What do you want to lose? Most of us who step on the scales daily will say "weight." We *can* lose weight (and health) by eating a normal or even decadent diet and dehydrating ourselves, but the fat will remain. Alcoholics often lose weight by not exercising and letting their muscles wither away.

What you obviously want to lose is fat:

- Excess baggage weighing you down every step
- Unwanted insulation keeping you hot
- An unnecessary diversion of blood and oxygen (away from exercising muscles)
- Unsightly bulges

Some people may not realize they have hidden stores of fat. Covert Bailey, author of *Fit or Fat?*, has measured thousands of people in his underwater tanks. Many are obese and don't realize it because the fat is marbled among the muscle cells. Only after most of the available fat storage spaces are filled inside the muscle tissue do these individuals begin to notice the formation of surface fat. Again, endurance activity is the best way to rid yourself of this unwanted burden and keep it off.

The scales shouldn't run or ruin your life. Muscle weighs more than fat. A weight gain when you begin an exercise program may be a *good* sign. You may be losing weight in fat as you gain muscle; without losing a pound, you'll probably lose inches.

Don't throw out the scales, however. They help you monitor dehydration. By weighing in every morning you can monitor your fluid balance. If there is a sudden two-pound drop or more, you can bet it's water and should start to replenish immediately. It takes about 35 miles of distance running to lose a pound of fat, so it's doubtful that any sudden weight loss will be fat. If you keep a record of your average weight, from month to month, the scales can tell you whether you're losing or gaining.

CHECK THE FAT

If you must check fat level, here are two ways of measuring. Calipers measure skin folds. They are quick and convenient. The other method is underwater weighing, which is generally considered to be more accurate. Here you are weighed first out of the water, and then again when submerged in a tank. You exhale as much air as possible while underwater, then the specialist takes a reading. The difference between the two weighings indicates your fat percentage, since fat floats, and lean muscle and bone sink.

Don't try to burn fat when training for a marathon or a time goal! When you're doing speed work or marathon training, you must reduce mileage between long runs to speed recovery and stay injury-free. This reduction will not burn fat off the body. If you try to diet while training for a time goal or marathon, you are likely to disrupt your metabolism, cause an inconsistent mental focus, and cause energy surges and withdrawals. Other problems encountered by those who change their diet while training hard may include stress fractures, nutritional deficiencies, and reductions in blood sugar levels. All can leave you unmotivated to exercise. It's no wonder that we see a lot of running dropouts among those who radically change their diets. After you've crossed that marathon finish line or recorded the personal record, you're free to set up a five-year plan for making nutritional changes.

In the meantime, let's look into the (unfortunately) expanding world of fat. To better understand how to take it off, we'll look first at how it goes on and the powerful biological instincts that try to keep it in storage. Then we'll focus on the long-term ways of burning it off as a lifestyle. Once you transform yourself into a fat-burning organism, you'll feel better all day long as you burn more fat.

The Set Point

Humans are lazy. With a primary mission of survival, we are programmed to build up extra fat storage as an insurance policy. For millions of years, this propensity has allowed our ancestors to survive through periods of starvation and sickness. The mechanisms of fat storage, described below, support a well-established principle called "set point," which determines how much we store. This powerful regulatory mechanism increases your appetite for weeks or months after periods of reduced calorie intake, illness, and even psychological deprivation, all of which deplete fat.

Unfortunately, it does its job too well, leaving you fatter than you were before. Understanding how the set point works as your hedge against starvation is the most important step in learning how to adjust it downward, or at least manage it, for the rest of your life.

What is fat?

When you eat a pat of butter, you might as well inject it onto your thigh or stomach: Dietary fat is deposited directly on your body. Protein and carbohydrates (even sugar) will be converted into fat only when you've consumed too many calories from those sources throughout the day. If you're trying to reduce the fat blanket, it helps to eat complex carbohydrates (baked potatoes, rice, whole grains, and vegetables) and lean sources of protein (legumes, turkey breast, nonfat dairy products, etc.).

Only body fat is used as fuel, not the fat in your diet. It is an excellent energy source, leaving a small amount of waste product, which is easily removed through the increased blood flow of exercise. While stored sugar is limited, you can't run far enough to use up your fat storage. Even a 140-pound person with the unusually low level of 2 percent body fat has hundreds of miles of fuel on board.

Fat storage differs for men and women.

Men tend to store fat on the surface of the body, often on the outside of the stomach area. Most women store fat internally at first. Thousands of pockets between muscle cells are filled up invisibly. Many young women feel that some dramatic change has occurred around the age of 30 when they suddenly start showing accumulations of fat on the outside of their bodies while maintaining the same diet and level of exercise. They've actually been storing fat inside for many years. Once the inner areas are filled, women notice a dramatic change on the outside of their thighs or stomachs, often in less than a year.

By the time humans enter their mid-20s, most have settled into an accustomed level of calorie burning and calorie consumption. Your fat level is adjusted at the percentage you've accumulated to that point. The set point is programmed to increase your fat accumulation slightly each year. Very slowly, your basal metabolism rate (the calories that are burned each day to keep you alive and doing routine activities) is reduced. But your appetite doesn't decrease very quickly, so most humans consume a few more calories than they need, each week, producing a slow increase in fat accumulation. The internal set point quickly adjusts itself to the higher level of fat which becomes the new set point. Because fat helps one survive a prolonged illness or other major interruption of good health or food intake, increased fat levels are biologically reinforced with each additional year of age.

Diets don't work!

By depriving yourself of food, you can reduce your body fat temporarily as you reduce your metabolism rate and your motivation to exercise. But, as soon as the diet is over, your set-point mechanism unleashes a starvation reflex that keeps you eating until the fat levels are slightly higher than they were before the diet. At the same time, your metabolism rate stays low to help you store fat more quickly. No matter how mentally focused you are, you'll find yourself with more fat on your frame when you mess with that very powerful survival mechanism.

By eating every 2–3 hours, you maintain a higher rate of metabolism—which burns fat. Choosing foods that take longer to digest will help you avoid the greatest compromise to a fat-burning program, overeating. The secret is to combine nutrients in your snacks that minimize the calories while maximizing the satisfaction (complex carbohydrates, protein, a little fat).

The Starvation Reflex

Over millions of years, our ancestors withstood regular famines, establishing complex and quick reactions to prepare themselves for even the possibility of food reduction. If you're getting enough food—often enough—your system doesn't feel the need to store fat. But the reflex starts into action when you've waited too long between snacks or meals on any day. The longer you wait to eat, the more you stimulate the fat-depositing enzymes. When you next eat, more of that food will be processed into fat. But that's not all of the bad news. A longer wait between meals increases your appetite, which leads to overeating—during the next meal or over the next few hours. Even if you've eaten three to five times a day but have eaten too few calories for that day's activities, you'll experience an increased appetite during the next 12 to 36 hours.

Psychological Starvation

Depriving yourself of food that you dearly love will start a psychological time bomb ticking. You can tell yourself that you'll never eat another doughnut, hamburger, french fry, and so on. You may even be able to abstain for an extended period of time.

But at some point in the future, when the food is around (and no one else is), your starvation reflex will gain the upper hand and you'll binge. Over time, the binges will lead you to consume more of that fatty food than you had deprived yourself of during the period of prohibition, and you'll experience a net gain. *Moderation is the key*.

Burning it off: Regular exercise improves disease resistance.

One of the very best and proven ways of readjusting the set point (downward) is by doing regular endurance exercise. We're not just talking about increased fat burning during exercise. The increased health benefits of regular exercise (enhanced resistance to disease, stronger heart, more efficient cardiovascular system, etc.) give intuitive signals to the body that the risk of long-term health problems has been lowered and there is less need for increased fat levels. A fit 70-year-old, for example, can often fight off disease better and quicker than can an average, not very fit, 30-year-old. Your set-point mechanism seems to have a sensor that intuitively monitors long-term trends in your body. Unfortunately, the set point is also adjusted higher in those in poor health.

Regular running and walking keeps fat off the body, burning off excess calories. Most beginning runners experience some fat burn-off, even when their weight stays the same, and particularly when their diet is not dramatically increased. If you've consumed more calories than you've burned during a given day, you can literally burn them off with an after-dinner walk or jog. This is particularly helpful if the excess calories on a given day have come from carbohydrates.

Burning fat while you sleep!

Running regularly for more than 45 minutes at a time (even with walk breaks) trains our exercising muscle cells to be fat burners at all times of the night and day. After months of regular distance running, you will have transformed a vast number of running muscle cells into fat burners that prefer fat as a fuel, even when you are sitting around all day or asleep at night. Long runs that exceed 90 minutes, when done every two to three weeks, transform the muscle cells from sugar burners to fat burners.

Sugar-burning produces waste build-up — so slow down!

Fat is the main fuel, but the body also uses another type. Glycogen is the form of sugar that is stored in the muscles for quick energy. Not only is this fuel used to get us started, but also it sustains us for the first half-hour of exercise. A small amount of it is needed even when we are running very slowly and burning mostly fat. Unfortunately, when this form of sugar is used for exercise, it leaves behind a lot of waste product, lactic acid, which causes discomfort. Running even a little too fast at the beginning depletes valuable glycogen quicker as it fills up the muscles and slows them down. This is why many runners don't feel great during the first few miles of a run. The faster the starting pace, the more uncomfortable we feel. Most of this discomfort can be eliminated with a warm-up of walking, a slow start, and more frequent or longer early walk breaks. But more waste is still produced from using up glycogen than is produced when we are burning fat.

The supply of glycogen is very limited, and it is necessary for brain function. A small amount of this fuel is burned every mile, even after you've shifted primarily into fat burning. So it's important on long runs to conserve this resource by keeping the pace slow from the beginning. When supplies run low, your body will hold back enough to keep the brain, your most crucial organ, functioning and, for the rest of your energy needs, force a breakdown of fat and protein—a very uncomfortable process. You can avoid this by gradually increasing your distance, by putting in more walk breaks from the beginning, and by running at least three days a week. *Being regular is important.*

From 15–45 minutes, your muscles start burning fat.

Your body doesn't seem to believe that you're really going out on a distance run until you keep moving forward for more than a quarter-hour. At this point, you begin to break down body fat for fuel (dietary fat is converted directly into body fat and is not burned for energy). It takes some work to break down the "excess baggage" on your body into free fatty acids and triglycerides that can keep you running mile after mile. If you continue exercising longer than about 15 minutes at a pace that is within your capacity, you start shifting into fat burning. As your exercise continues past the quarter-hour mark, you start a transition into fat burning as long as you continue to exercise at a level of exertion that is within your capacity.

After running 45 minutes, you'll be burning mostly fat.

By starting at a slow pace and taking walk breaks as needed, you can lower your exertion level enough to stay in the fat-burning zone for an extended time. This conserves glycogen for later use as you burn off the extra blanket around your stomach or thighs.

Training your muscles to burn fat

Those who are not in shape for endurance activity must train their muscles to burn fat. Beginning exercisers may have to limit their exercise to walking until they can work up to an hour or more of continuous activity. Instead of walk breaks, some completely out-of-shape beginners may need to take 1- to 2-minute "sit down" breaks every 5 to 8 minutes to stay in the fat-burning zone. After a few weeks, however, most of those novices can accomplish continuous 45- to 60-minute walks at a steady pace. At that point, they may increase the walking distance or hold the distance steady and add jogging breaks of a minute, every 3–5 minutes of walking. Some people take longer to progress. *Be patient.*

The adaptation to fat burning is more difficult for those who've done little or no exercise before. If you're in this category, do more walking and stick with it. The fat-burning process works for you the same as it does for world-class athletes. You may not notice it for a while because the changes are going on inside the muscle cells. Keep telling yourself "I'm becoming a fat-burning furnace," because you are!

Aerobic Exercise

Fast anaerobic exercise burns sugar; slow aerobic exercise burns fat. Fat in the muscle cells can be burned only when there's an adequate supply of oxygen. This is aerobic exercise: exertion that is done at an easy-enough pace so that the blood can provide all of the oxygen needed by the muscles. As soon as you increase the pace beyond your current capacity or go farther than your muscles are trained to go, the muscles can't get enough oxygen to burn fat and so they shift back to the readily available but inefficient energy source, glycogen. Your exercise is now anaerobic, meaning that the muscles aren't getting enough oxygen. The longer and faster you run anaerobically, the worse you'll feel and the sooner you'll quit because of the accumulation of lactic acid. *(For a more detailed explanation of this process, see p. 54.)*

Walk breaks and a slow pace at the start keep you in the fat-burning zone longer. If you're used to running for 5 miles (at 12 minutes per mile) with no walk breaks, try slowing down to 14–16 minutes per mile. This will reduce your level of exertion so that you can run for 6–8 miles while feeling the same way you felt after 5 miles. When you add a 1-minute walk break every 5 minutes, you can push the wall back to between 7 and 10 miles while feeling as though you covered only about half that distance. It's always better to increase your mileage gradually, so I recommend that you make this type of increase over several runs. The slower running with walk breaks will allow you to extend the distance with little or no risk of injury or over-fatigue. The extra mileage means that you are burning more calories and fat.

The continuous movement of the body during long, slow runs and walks (lasting at least 45 minutes) mobilizes an incredible number of muscle cells in the legs, back, butt, and related areas. By slowly covering several miles, three times a week, this network of muscles specializes in the work that can keep the body moving in the most efficient way. Because fat is the most efficient and abundant fuel, the muscles will adapt to become fat burners if this run is done regularly enough.

Stoking Your Fat-Burning Furnace

By slowing down enough to break the 45-minute barrier and exercise for longer periods, you show your body that you're serious about endurance. It responds by converting the formerly sugar-burning cells into fat burners. The minimum necessary is one session longer than 45 minutes per week, but the process is accelerated by exercising for more than 90 minutes once every two weeks. As the long-run distance increases significantly in a half-marathon program, you force more and more cells into the more efficient mode of fat metabolism and keep them there. To maintain the capacity of your expanding fat furnace, you'll need at least two other 30-minute sessions a week. If each of these can be increased to at least 45 minutes, you'll improve the adaptation. As always, it's better to slow down from the beginning of exercise so that you'll feel better, be more motivated to continue, and go further.

Heat build-up from regular exercise can reduce fat layer.

Running and walking elevate your core body temperature. Many experts believe that this produces a healthy "fever" that often kills off infections before they cause colds or worse. But the greater your blanket of body fat, the more heat you'll retain, which can lead to excessive fluid loss through sweating. Your body's temperature control mechanism will try to reduce this source of stress if you run regularly. After months of regular long runs, you'll slowly reduce the thickness of this "fat blanket" around you, reducing your set point, if you're not significantly increasing calorie intake. Doing heat-producing alternative exercises on non-running days, such as cross-country machine or rowing machine work, will reinforce this downward adjustment of the set point.

As more of the muscle cells adapt to fat metabolism through training, you'll be burning more fat throughout the day. Once they've run enough long runs, regularly, even sedentary office workers will burn fat while sitting in their offices or on the couch at night. Endurance-trained fat-burning cells will choose more fat as their fuel even while you are asleep. Then, in the "battle of the bulge," you'll be able to enlist as your soldiers thousands of cells gobbling fat all day and all night.

The Virtue of Patience

We Americans often want changes to occur too rapidly. If a little exercise burns x amount of fat, we are tempted to log twice as many miles to double the rate. This doesn't work. By adding too much distance too soon, you'll get tired or injured, and be forced to stop exercising or to cut back dramatically. Even worse is the possibility that you'll get mentally burned out. If you continue to run slowly and increase your total weekly mileage by no more than 10 percent, you'll reduce chances of injury and burn-out to almost nothing.

The biggest mistake runners make is to start a run too hard, too fast. This is so easy to do because it usually doesn't feel too hard, but 6 to 10 minutes later you're wishing that you were finished. By forcing yourself to start much more slowly than you want, you'll get a stream of benefits, speed your entry into the fat-burning zone, and set yourself up for more enjoyment later.

Walk breaks can help you burn off 10 pounds of fat!

To show you why it's better to go slowly, let's look at the math in the table below. Continuous running (whether slow or fast) burns about 100 calories per mile. If you're walking normally, you're burning about 50 calories per mile. Even if you're running for 2 minutes and walking for 1 minute, you're closer to the running side of the continuum, burning about 80 calories per mile. Let us suppose, then, that you're running 5 miles, four days a week. If you slowed down and took a 1-minute walk break for every 3 minutes of running, you'd feel about the same, after covering 8 miles, as you would feel if you'd run 5 miles continuously. Here's the math:

> **Run-Walk:**   8 miles (85 calories per mile = 680 calories per run) –
>
> **Continuous Run:** 5 miles (100 calories per mile = 500 calories per run)
>
> That's an increase of 180 calories per run.
>
> In one year, your walk breaks will enable you to burn off an extra 10 pounds of fat!

Priorities of Running and Fat Burning

1. Incorporating regular endurance exercise into your lifestyle
2. Building the endurance necessary to go the distance
3. Learning how to enjoy the process so you'll want to do it again
4. Staying injury-free
5. Burning fat

Unless you had nutritional problems before the program started, stick with the diet that you've been using. Certainly it's okay to divide up your food into more small meals a day and to reduce your fat intake a little, but don't make any radical changes. If you feel that you have some nutritional problems at any time, see a sports nutritionist, preferably one who has had success in working with long-distance runners. During a half-marathon program it's okay to say "I'm starting my diet later" —after the race.

A Pound a Month

Each of these can cause you to lose about a pound a month:

1. Put more walking into your first and last mile, and add a mile to the beginning and end of each run. A 4-day-a-week runner will burn almost a pound a month.

2. Eat 8–10 meals a day. The increased metabolism from eating the same food, but more frequently, can burn up to a pound a month.

3. Two-a-day runs. Add an easy 2-mile walk/run either at lunch, before breakfast, or after dinner.

A Pound a Year

Burning a little here, a little there. . . .

1. Walking up stairs instead of taking the elevator or escalator

2. Parking a quarter of a mile further away from your office each day

3. Walking half a mile at lunch

4. Taking a half-mile walk after supper.

5. Exercising on a exercycle or rowing machine for 5 minutes a day

6. Getting out of your chair or couch an extra 10 times a day

Coffee. There is some evidence that drinking coffee before exercising may help burn fat. Research on rats showed that ingestion of caffeine about an hour before endurance exercise resulted in a reduction of fat compared to rats who didn't take the drug. It is recommended that only one cup of coffee be taken about an hour before exercise.

Diets Only Work in Combination with Exercise. Most of the weight lost from diets is water. In fact, there is recent evidence that dieting without exercise will cause the dieter to actually gain weight in the long run.

Running Lean. Starvation diets are not necessary. Most runners find that their exercising allows them to eat just about what they want. The idea is to be moderate and not overeat. Calorie reduction can be a matter of taste. Gradually shift away from the fatty foods you like by acquiring a taste for similar foods with less fat.

Instead of:	Try:
Fried Foods	Foods marinated in herbs and broiled
Eggs	Egg whites
Red meat	Fish or poultry
Peanut Butter	Just a taste of it on bread or crackers
Cheese	Low-fat cottage cheese
Whole milk	Non-fat milk
Salad dressing	Small amount of oil and add apple juice (and vinegar)
Potato chips, etc.	Cut vegetables (carrots, celery, etc.), or pretzels
Mayonnaise	Fat-free mayo

Complex carbohydrates such as whole grains and vegetables will satisfy your hunger and not give you big doses of calories. In fact, some physiologists say that fats "burn in a carbohydrate flame." You need enough carbohydrates to break down the fatty acids (the body's prime source of stored fuel) into energy. Beware of additives, however; salad is wonderful low-calorie food, but 2–3 tablespoons of oil in the dressing reverses the situation. Potatoes are great low-calorie filler-uppers—but use the fat-free sour cream! (It's pretty good!)

When to eat is very important. Try eating small snacks throughout the day to avoid being ravenous at meals, which leads to overeating. When you wait a long time between meals you stimulate the fat-depositing enzymes; these little fellows take a big meal and store it in the way you want least. The longer you wait, the more enzymes are produced. Eating small amounts allows the body to burn it up as it comes in. It will also give you a steady flow of energy throughout the day—provided the snacks are not too concentrated in sugar or fat.

A slight, sensible reduction in calories, adapted gradually into your lifestyle, will allow your exercise to burn off even more calories. This sensible approach to your new healthy lifestyle can result in permanent changes: endurance exercise, a healthy diet, and a slimmer you.

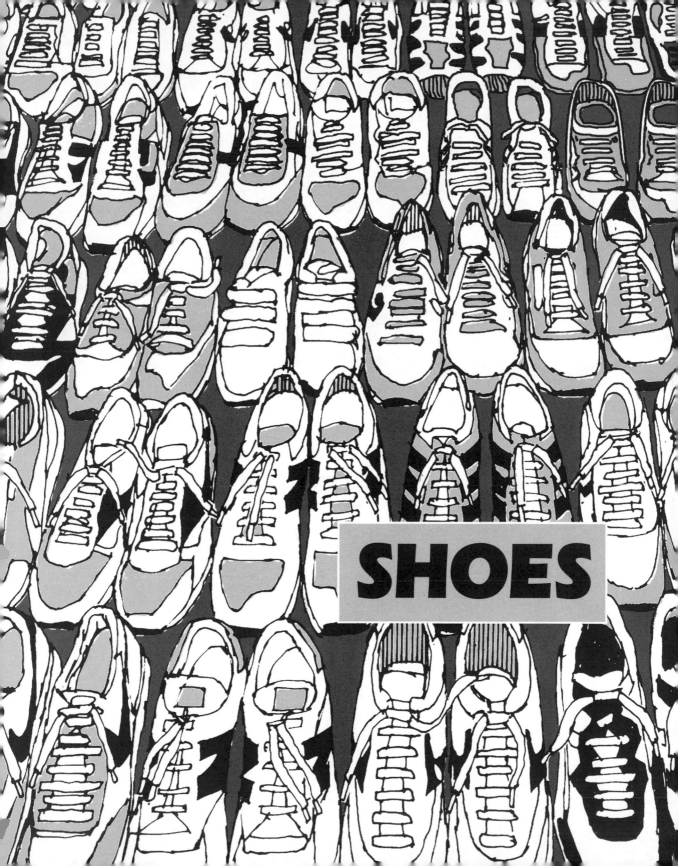

SHOES

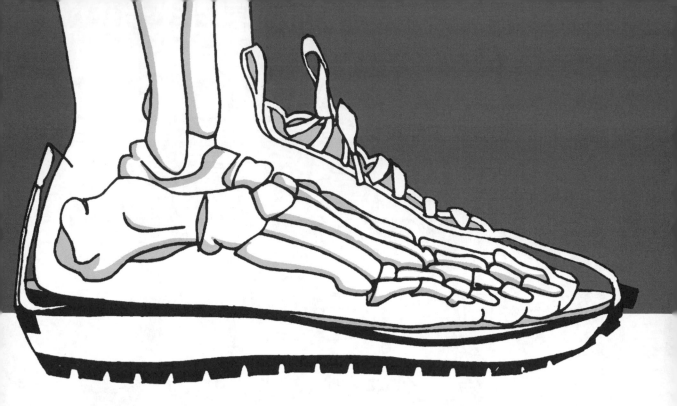

22
SHOE SECRETS

INSIDE INFORMATION ON SHOE DESIGN

LIKE THE QUEST FOR THE HOLY GRAIL, runners search for the perfect shoe. We feel that somewhere there's a perfect pair that will cure foot problems, make us run faster and lead us bounding effortlessly into the sunset. We're persuaded by ads, influenced by magazine surveys, and tempted by the shoes our friends wear.

Well, don't get your hopes too high. Although shoes have come a long way, I have yet to meet a runner who's found the perfect pair. Forty years ago the hot shoes were Converse All-Stars, regulation issue on

high school basketball teams. They were theoretically also designed for indoor running, ping-pong, volleyball, or anything the salesman could talk you into. The black cloth absorbed perspiration and salt, which would frequently rub against your feet until they were blistered or raw. There was a hard gum-rubber sole glued directly to the canvas . . . and that was it. Stability, cushioning, pronation control, and other things we now take for granted were in the realm of science fiction.

Some Running Shoe History. When I was in high school in 1960, my track coach talked about an exotic brand of shoes he'd discovered when stationed in Germany in the USAF: Adidas. My running friends and I were intrigued as we flipped through the black-and-white brochures. There were four or five shoes designed for training! It was difficult to convince our parents we needed $8 for running shoes instead of the usual $4, but we prevailed. The contrast in comfort provided by these new shoes was amazing. I was so proud I couldn't take them off. I wore them running, to class, to church, etc., much to the criticism, kidding, and olfactory discomfort of my mother and classmates.

The rapid development and innovation in running shoes since those days has been largely due to the involvement of runners in the business. In the early '60s Phillip (Buck) Knight wanted to start a running shoe import company and brought some primitive Tiger-brand models back from Japan to his coach, Bill Bowerman. Bill was a vocal critic of every shoe on the market, and these foreign shoes stimulated his pioneer spirit and inventor's ingenuity. He tore them up and improvised, then tested them on the feet of his runners, such as Kenny Moore and Geoff Hollister.

Breakfast at Bowermans. When Barbara Bowerman left for church one Sunday morning, little did she know that husband Bill had plans for her waffle iron that did not include brunch. Having worked with the overall construction of shoes for several years, Bill was now trying to find the perfect sole material—one that would offer optimal traction, cushion and better wear. Looking around in the kitchen for ideas, he spotted the waffle iron, and running shoes have not been the same since. Neither has the taste of waffles around the Bowerman household.

The rubber waffles that came out of that iron became the soles for a new generation of Oregon distance runners who found them perfect for traction on the varied terrain of cross-country surfaces. Unexpectedly, they also found that the soles improved traction and cushion on hard surfaces. Traction was best where body weight pressed the hardest, and the waffle tips were distributed liberally enough to give traction on any part of the sole.

In the process, Bowerman brought in an orthopedic specialist, Stan James, in hopes of avoiding injuries by design. The result was the Nike shoe. Word spread quickly in the running underground that some crazy runners in Oregon had finally come up with something. By 1980, Nike Inc. was selling more running shoes in America than any other company.

Today you can find a running shoe for just about any shape foot, and devices to help avoid or minimize many of running's stresses. Each wave of research spawns a new generation of shoes, which makes the previous ones practically obsolete. With all the choices available it's important that the shoes fit your own particular anatomy and running style. If not, the shoes can cause problems. The wrong shoes, for example, might cause you to tilt your foot the wrong way and cause injury, or to waste money on expensive orthopedic devices you don't need.

Our experience in fitting shoes in the Phidippides stores has shown that salespeople who are also runners can give the best advice, and help lead you through the maze of new models. The problem in many areas, however, is finding such a person—one who knows running first-hand, is up-to-date on all the available shoes, has been trained in fitting techniques and biomechanics of the running foot, and can listen to your problems and help you make a sound decision.

You'll most likely have great trouble finding such a shoe expert. Most stores—even specialty stores—just hire people at minimum wages and give them no training. The running magazines try to fill the gap, but become too technical, and their attempts to simulate running in lab tests do not work. Moreover, the mass of facts overwhelms the reader. The magazines sometimes try to clarify things by setting up a point system and rating the shoes, but this doesn't provide enough information for the individual runner. Each person needs a unique combination of features. A ranking will usually list the best shoes for a mythical "average" runner.

In this chapter I'll give you a list of important factors to consider in choosing shoes. You can then apply this information to your own running style, weight, tendencies, and aims—to find the best combination for you.

Board Last or Slip Last. It's helpful to be familiar with two basic types of shoe construction:

Board (or cement) last construction is where a piece of fiberboard material is placed between the foot and the midsole material. This provides extra support for the foot and usually reduces flexibility.

Slip last construction is where the sole and midsole material are cemented directly to the cloth upper, with no insole board. Shoes built this way tend to provide less stability, but are more flexible.

Definitions of Foot Movements. Before we begin a discussion of foot types, we'll define the basic types of foot movements:

Pronation is a normal shock-absorbing mechanism. Most runners land on the heel, then the foot rolls forward and inward with body weight on the center of the forefoot. This provides cushioning.

Over-pronation is when the runner rolls excessively to the *inside*, particularly in the forefoot. The knees and insides of the shins are stressed. This is indicated by wear on the inside of the heel, but particularly by wear on the inside of the forefoot (even when heel wear is on the outside).

Excessive supination is rolling excessively to the *outside* of the foot so that the ligaments, tendons and bones on that side are sore and strained. This is indicated by excessive wear on the outside of the sole and little wear elsewhere. This is very rare.

What Type of Foot Do You Have? The single most important factor in proper shoe selection is your foot type: *rigid* or *floppy*. The human foot is designed to be both a (rigid) lever and a (floppy) platform. This enables us to propel ourselves forward, yet at the same time adapt to varying surfaces. Many feet, because of bone structure and muscular attachments, can be described as being "hinged" predominantly one way or another: either forward and back (rigid) or side to side (floppy), with some feet having a degree of both characteristics.

The Rigid Foot

Characteristics. The rigid foot moves predominantly forward and back, with a strong push-off. Like a horse's hoof, it's an efficient lever for speed. The runner may land on the heel, but the rigid foot rolls quickly forward and gets a strong push from the forefoot. Excessive supination, sometimes seen with the rigid foot, results when feet yield too much on the outside. This may put too much stress on the bones, tendons, and ligaments on the outside of the foot.

Shoe wear. The wear pattern of a rigid foot is along the outside of the shoe, particularly on the outside and middle of the forefoot.

Shoe type needed. A rigid foot needs good flexibility and good forefront and rearfoot cushion. There is not as much need for stability as there is with a floppy foot.

The Floppy Foot

Characteristics. The floppy foot acts as if hinged from side to side. The first strike is usually on the outside (only occasionally on the inside) of the heel, but then it rolls to the inside of the forefoot. Rolling inward in this fashion can result in over-pronation and cause knee or shin problems.

Shoe wear. The wear pattern of a floppy foot is a series of spots where the foot pushes. The empty space between may show little or no wear. Of particular concern is a wear pattern on the inside of the heel or the inside of the forefoot which denotes over-pronation. Here the foot is rolling too far. The foot, knee, and hip are no longer in alignment and the knee and shin areas usually take too much stress.

Shoe type needed. A floppy foot needs support. The rear foot and especially the forefoot must have a stable platform. Shoes with a board last tend to be more stable, although a number of the stability shoes today have excellent slip-lasted platforms. Some runners need only a strong arch support. Others will need a custom orthotic to correct excess motion. If you're having problems, consult a podiatrist. Too much shoe cushion can compromise the stability of even a well-made shoe, as well as any orthopedic devices which are designed to control pronation. *Floppy feet should sacrifice cushion for stability*—there's usually a direct tradeoff.

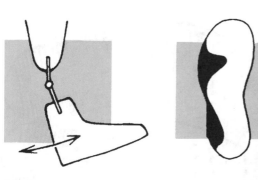

Rigid foot

Shoe wear, rigid foot

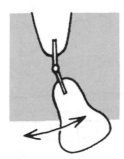

Floppy foot

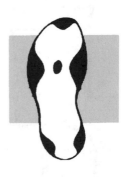

Shoe wear, floppy foot

A word on pronation. Don't assume that pronation means trouble. If you aren't having problems you'll probably get them by installing devices in your shoes. If you are a pronator and having knee or shin pain, you may benefit from correction, but get good advice first. I've seen severe pronators who don't seem to have any problems —they must have compensation mechanisms somewhere in their legs or feet.

Shoe Shape. There are two basic shoe shapes: straight and curved. Try on shoes of both types to see which is best for your foot. A straight shoe looks about the same as its mate on the bottom. A curved shoe, however, will look radically different from its partner. If your foot is curved, a straight shoe will put pressure on your big toe and toe joint. If your foot is straight, a curved shoe will put pressure on the outside and you'll probably have extra room on the inside of the forefoot. The "modified straight last" is a compromise between the two, and is the most common shape today.

Generally, the shape of the shoe should correspond to the shape of your foot. Be sure there are no areas of pressure or pain, or any feeling of binding when you flex your foot, and run in the shoe.

Shoe Fit

Expansion/contraction. Your foot will swell as you run, more so during the summer. Fit your shoes with this in mind, It's best to try shoes on in the afternoon, since feet swell during the day. You don't want your foot to slip around inside, but you don't want too much pressure on it either.

Toe room. When you run, your foot is like a pendulum. With each swing, more blood is pumped into the feet, especially the toe region, causing the toes to swell. Lack of toe room is the primary cause of toe blisters and black toenails. Generally, *1/2″ of toe room* is sufficient to avoid problems. Since one foot is usually larger than the other, fit the larger one. If you've had toe problems, look for a shoe with a rounded rather than pointed toe box.

As long as the shoe fits snugly across the middle of your foot, don't worry about 1″ of extra room at the toe. Toes want freedom like everyone else!

Heel fit. Your heel should fit snugly but not be confined. Ideally there should be a very slight give at the heel, but not enough so you feel anxiety. *The shoe should feel like an extension of your foot*, not separate from it.

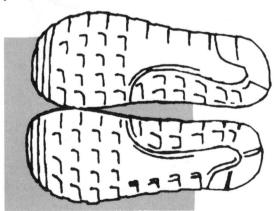

Straight shoe

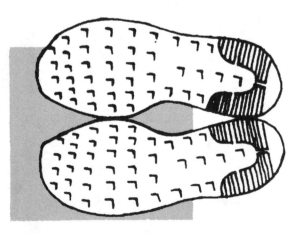

Curved shoe

Also, there should be no heel roll from side to side within the shoe.

Socks. When you try shoes on, use socks of the same thickness as those you'll be running in.

Take a Test Ride. Be sure to walk around in the shoes as much as possible. This tells you how the shoe responds to your feet in motion. Some stores do not let you run in the shoes—but you really should. This is the only way to tell how the shoe fits and works. Look around for a store that allows this.

Cushion. If you run on a golf course all the time, you'll need very little cushion in your shoes. Most of us, however, have to deal with the shock from pavement every step of the way—at least in many of our runs and races. If our shoes don't absorb the shock, it gets passed up the line—to feet, knees, hips and to crucial muscles and tendons. Remember the two foot types, and their differing requirements:

- *The rigid foot* needs cushion and flexibility, especially in the forefoot.
- *The floppy foot* needs stability, and only enough cushion to take the edge off road shock. Too much cushion can allow excessive pronation.

Note: Floppy feet that need more cushion can benefit from a good insole, such as that provided by the Spenco company.

Over-pronators. Beware of soft shoes. Too much cushion will allow your foot to keep on rolling as it pronates. This problem increases with the vertical layers of midsole material in the shoe. You want adequate shock absorption until the foot reaches a flat, stable resistance. Then the foot will either get a little push from the shoe, or at least be able to make its own force as it pushes off.

Too much cushion causes instability. In addition to magnifying pronation problems, it causes you to waste energy with each step. If you run in the shoes before buying them, you'll feel the cushion in action.

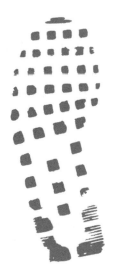

Creative Lacing

Cutting heel slippage:

You can get a tighter heel fit by tightening the top laces. To avoid pinching the foot, use the stirrup lace method. This distributes pressure over four, rather than two, holes.

Relieving lace pressure:

Popularized by Arthur Lydiard, this eliminates pressure on the top of the foot from laces crossing under the border. It takes a while to learn, but is a secure, comfortable system.

Releasing spot pressure:

If you have spots on the top of your foot that are under pressure, just skip the eyelets that go across that area. This relieves pressure there and allows you to tighten other areas.

More toe room:

This lacing system, suggested by Harry Hlavac, D.P.M., makes your toe area more of a "tent." By pulling tightly on the short (straight) lace, you'll increase the amount of toe room and reduce pressure on the toes.

Isolating individual laces:

If one area of your foot needs to be loosely laced while others remain tight, just loop lace around lace hole.

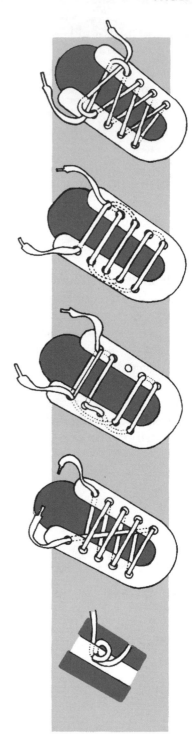

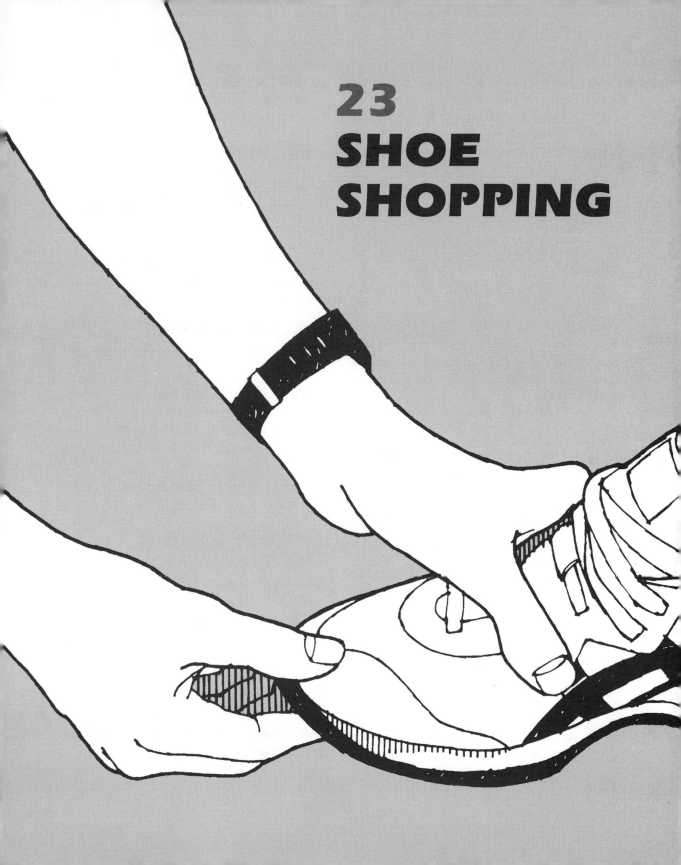

23
SHOE SHOPPING

SOME SHOE COMPANIES invest millions in research while others opt for big advertising budgets . . . and some do both! This makes it difficult to tell the help from the hype. How do you sift through the gleam of new designs, the claims for spectacular features, the hundreds of shoes in running stores?

It helps to find a store staffed by runners who are trained in fitting. The ideal advisor will listen to you, offer several choices, and watch you run in the shoes until you find the right one. However, you're the one who has to make the final decision; even the best salesperson can't get inside the shoe with you and feel how it fits. Also—unfortunately—a lot of stores either don't have good advisors or may try to sell you any shoe—whether it's right or not—just to make the sale.

SHOE SELECTION CHECKLIST

Here are some key questions to consider in making the right shoe choice. Copy this and take it into the store with you.

How Many Miles a Week Do You Run?

☐ *Under 20:* Practically any of the better-brand shoes—Adidas, Asics, Brooks, Etonic, Nike, Saucony, etc.—will do. These shoes shouldn't break down for a long time. Unless you have some diagnosed foot problems, you don't need an expensive pair.

☐ *20–50:* Most running shoes are designed for people in this group. As your mileage increases, look for better quality.

☐ *Over 50:* You need a sturdy shoe, designed for the way you run and for your foot type.

On What Surfaces Do You Run?

☐ *Grass or dirt:* You don't need much cushion, but should look for traction, stability, and protection from rocks.

☐ *Pavement:* Adequate cushion. Remember, when you gain cushion, you lose stability. If you pronate excessively, you must strike a balance, but should choose on the side of stability.

Is Your Foot Floppy or Rigid?

(To determine which type you are, see pp. 246–247.)

☐ *Floppy:* Stable platform, less cushion, sometimes pronation-control devices (often built into shoes). Look for a shoe with a board last (or at least a stable platform). *(See p. 247.)*

☐ *Rigid:* Flexible, cushioned shoe. Look for a slip-lasted shoe. *(See p. 247.)*

Is Your Foot Straight or Curved?

(See p. 000.)

☐ *Straight:* If a curved shoe puts pressure on the outside of your foot and there's extra room on the inside, you have a straight foot.

☐ *Curved:* If a straight shoe causes pressure on your toe and joint, you have a curved foot.

In general, the shoe should be an extension of your foot—no points of pressure or pain.

INJURIES THAT INFLUENCE SHOE CHOICE

If you've had shoe-related injuries, it's best to get medical advice. The trouble is, things keep changing so fast in the shoe market that podiatrists and orthopedists can't possibly test out all the new shoes and haven't the time to follow up on how the old shoes hold up over time. So it pays to know some basic principles yourself about what to look for.

Through the years I've found that some problems can be helped by certain types of shoes. In the Phidippides stores we've helped thousands of runners select their shoes.

The following is offered, not as medical advice, but from one runner to another:

Knee Problems or Shin Problems

- *Rigid foot:* More cushion and flexibility. If your ankle turns or twists frequently, look for a shoe that's stable and strong on the outside throughout.
- *Floppy foot:* Strong platform, board last (or similar) construction with little or moderate cushion. Strong heel construction.

Achilles Problems. Higher heel lift, heel counter that fits your heel well, but does not pull on the tendon when shoe flexes. For this reason, limited flexibility is also needed. Shoe should have excellent rearfoot stability.

Plantar Fasciitis (Heel Pain). More stability through board last (at least a flat platform that doesn't buckle from side to side). Heel counter must be secured to midsole very well and should fit your heel with no room to roll.

Shin Splints. Stable platform, moderate cushion

OTHER SHOE TIPS

Breaking in Shoes. I'm amazed at how many people go out and run 10–12 miles the first day in a new pair of shoes and then complain about blisters. Walk around the first day or two. Wear the shoes during your normal daily activities if you can (or around the house at night), so they will begin conforming to your feet. At first, run only a mile or two, then gradually increase. After about seven days they should be broken in.

Breaking Down Shoes. Several areas of the shoe will break down simultaneously. Each step destroys the individual separation of air bubbles and breaks down the midsole, causing it to flatten. As it compresses, you lose cushion and support. This happens so gradually you may not notice it until you compare it to a new shoe.

The upper part of the shoe stretches and weakens at stress points. As this happens, the foot loses its support laterally. This is particularly a problem for pronators. With less support there is more likelihood of injury. As the materials fatigue, the foot is allowed to roll more and more. Monitor this slow breakdown by trying out new shoes and comparing the cushion and support at periodic intervals.

Alternating Shoes. Shoes last longer if you let them rest and dry out between runs. Thus it's good to have two pairs. When one pair has been used for half of its "life," get a new pair and start alternating. However, it's not good to alternate between a brand-new pair and a worn-out pair, as this can cause injuries.

Ned Frederick, physiologist and director of research at Nike, recommends that when you find a shoe that works well, buy two pairs. This ensures that you'll have another pair of the same model (before it's superseded by a newer and different design). It also gives you a reference point: you keep one pair in the closet and run in them only once a week. By directly comparing these to the other, everyday pair you'll gradually break in the new pair, and you'll know when the old pair should be designated for "lawn mowing" only.

What's That Smell? Three friends were traveling in Greece and, after checking into their hotel, took a run. After dinner later that night, when they opened the door to their room, they were met with such a horrendous odor they quickly shut it and called the management. The proprietor was apologetic and called the fumigators. All were convinced that an animal must have crawled into the room and died. After several minutes inside, one of the fumigators emerged, holding at arm's length a well-seasoned pair of running shoes belonging to the Americans.

Shoes have materials and glue that react differently to perspiration. Wash with soap and water and a stiff brush. A light soaking in baking soda will help the inner odor, but board-lasted shoes will often buckle after soaking. After washing, lightly squeeze the water out and put them to dry in a warm place, with paper inside them. Saddle soap will keep the leather parts soft.

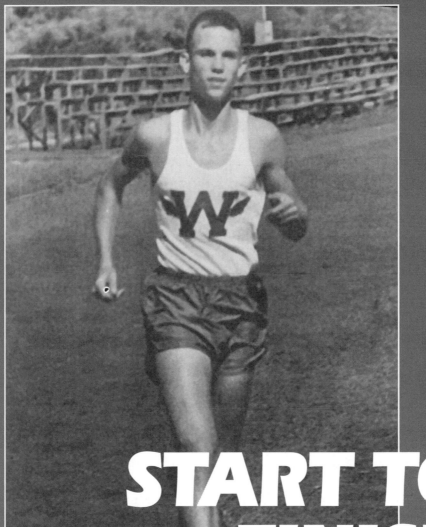

START TO FINISH

24 SHOULD KIDS RUN?

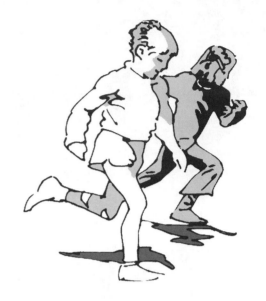

The Benefits. The earlier a child starts running, the better the cardiovascular foundation for later years. Such a development gives the child a head start in long-term health benefits and in competition, should it follow. At each stage, the heart, lungs, and circulatory system are strengthened and the effects are multiplied through the growing years. However, the most important ingredients are fun and success. If a child feels good about running, he or she is likely to continue.

Our two children, Brennan and Westin, were competitive in various sports teams except for running, until they were 13. Both ran on low-key junior high teams and competed in track and cross-country in high school. They are enjoying running in their post-scholastic years more than ever, and are fired up about improving their times each year.

The Dangers. For more than two decades I've pursued the issue of possible damage that endurance running might do to joints, bones, or vital parts of a growing body. According to several orthopedists that I stay in touch with, there is no evidence of any long-term damage when children train using sensible programs, even very rigorous

ones. If you are in doubt you should contact your pediatrician or family physician.

But one of the real dangers for young runners is psychological burnout. Most child running stars or top high school athletes never reach their running potential because of the "too far, too fast, too soon" syndrome. Well-meaning but over-zealous parents or coaches naturally want to get children involved in healthy activity and may influence them to train too hard, and race too often. Many kids wil push themselves into burnout unknowingly. Without the sense of pace and restraint bestowed by maturity they are driven until they become bored, disillusioned or discouraged.

The Real Goals. I became addicted to running at age 13, probably because I had not experienced the pressure of competition or the gut-wrenching fatigue of speed work and racing before. My goals were relaxation and the good feelings from exercise. If kids can appreciate these internal rewards, they will probably be on the road to a lifetime fitness program. There's also a lot of fun in low-key competition, trips and running friendships. It's important that the main goals of running be the psychological and health benefits and that victories, times, and trophies not become ends in themselves.

If you "hold 'em back," they'll want to continue. When kids are restrained slightly, their desire builds inside. Carefully monitor your child's program and hold back slightly on a regular basis—not letting youthful enthusiasm run unchecked.

Racing. Informal competition is OK for most kids, but I feel that children's racing teams, with intense speedwork and regimented competition, are not right in early years. An occasional road race, fun run, or school field day can provide informal competition without great pressure. Marathon training and age-group racing are often too intense and likely to produce early burnout. Marathons can be run throughout one's life, so there's no need to rush into them.

A RECOMMENDED PROGRAM

One through five years: Encourage running and all types of vigorous activity. Take the child to an occasional race, say things like "Someday when you grow up, you may want to run in a race like this . . ." Talk about some of the health benefits.

5–11 years: If the child shows an interest in running, you can provide encouragement.

Run along with him or her and talk about the health benefits. Never force, push, or extend the run too far; at the same time, don't let the child push too hard—save that desire for the next time. Use road races or fun runs as rewards for regular exercising. Soccer is a great sport that develops teamwork while children learn and practice running technique.

11–12 years: If there is a junior high running program and your child wants to participate, monitor it. Two to three workouts a week and three to four races a season are reasonable. Avoid intense interval work and high mileage. Running in local races could be based on practicing three times per week.

13–18 years: Encourage other activities along with running—studies, music, dating, work on the school yearbook, etc. Now the young runner can start training seriously as long as it doesn't get out of control. Avoid high mileage (above 40–50 miles a week), intense speedwork, and races every weekend. At 16–18, a physically mature and talented runner could try national competition—if ready. (I don't believe in national competition for kids under age 16. Let it be a mystery how they stack up against their age-group peers. A few local races for kids this age are plenty.)

18 and older: You are now an advisor. He or she can decide when to run a marathon, how hard to train, whether to enter national competition, etc. The rules of sensible training, adequate rest, planning, etc., as outlined earlier in the book, now apply.

Note: A growing number of college admission offices are looking favorably at kids that participate on high school cross-country teams. An official from an elite university explained: "You know at least three important things about high school cross-country runners: they're not in it for the glory, they are disciplined, and they're not afraid of hard work. People with those traits do well at our institution." In fact, the cross-country runners tend to be among the best student athletes and leaders, at most high schools.

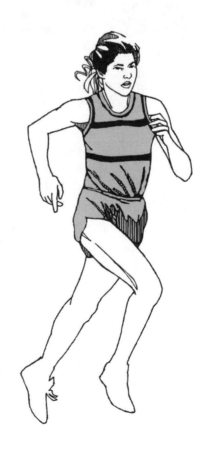

25 RUNNING AFTER 40

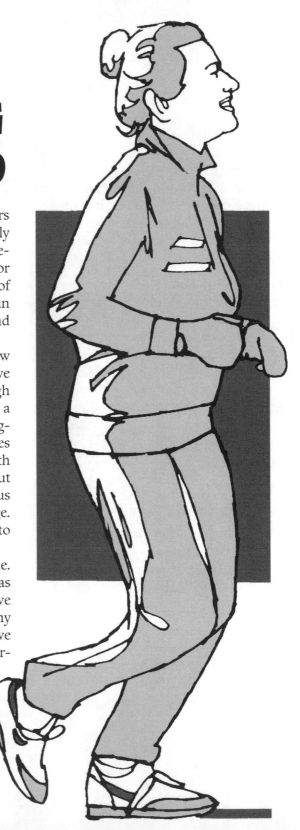

WE HAVE NO CONTROL over time. Like stars speeding through space, we head certainly toward the end of life as if it were a mysterious black hole, not knowing when or where we might enter it. Running is one of those significant distractions that can make our passage more interesting and stimulating.

Although we can't predict exactly how long we'll live, there's growing evidence we can affect the aging process. Through healthy living habits, we not only have a better chance of living longer, we can significantly improve the quality of our lives while we're here. Having now worked with at least 100,000 runners who were about 40 or older, I've noticed that most of us become more introspective as we age. Running gives us a very positive way to enjoy our inward discovery.

For a fit person, age is hardly an issue. While my muscles don't feel as good as they did even 10 years ago, I can still have a wonderful run if I check my ego (and my watch) at the door. I've come to believe that the quality of life is primarily determined by two factors: vitality and attitude. Running maintains both at the highest possible level.

Sure, runners notice the aging process: a little slower starting in the morning, a few more aches and pains now and then, slower healing of injuries. As I edit this book I'm 56, having long passed the 40-year "wall." I've made a few alterations to my running, such as running slower, and I enjoy running more now than ever. I've not noticed any more aches and pains than I did in my 30s and have only had one running injury in the past 20 years that kept me away from running for more than two days (a two-week injury vacation due to stepping in a hole). Not only is there abundant life beyond 40, your body and mind work better if you run (and walk) regularly.

Slower Recovery Time. It's a fact that our recovery time slows down a little bit, each year. I've found that by taking more days off per week, most runners can reduce leg fatigue, maintain weekly mileage, and enjoy their running more as they get older. If you want to exercise on the non-running days, walk or choose another cross-training mode.

Suggested Number of Running Days per Week by Age

40–50	Four running days per week
51–60	Run every other day
61–70	Three running days per week
71+	2–3 days of running, with cross training

Slower Pace on Easy Days. I seemed to "hit the age wall" within a year of turning 40, so slowed down my pace and reduced weekly mileage from 60 to 35 per week. After two years of this, my legs had not only recovered completely, they were asking for more exercise. I continued to start all of my runs at 3–4 minutes per mile slower than I could run for that same distance.

After a mile or two, I will sometimes increase the pace slightly. On most days, however, I just relax and enjoy the endorphins as I go slowly. I'm back up to running 60–65 miles a week, injury-free.

Walk Breaks Speed Recovery. Of all the training innovations for older runners, walk breaks offer the most, in maintaining fresh legs. Read the section on walk breaks. They allow runners in their 70s to cover as many miles as they did in their 30s without injury or excess fatigue. I take walk breaks on almost every run.

Walk-Break Frequency by Age

40–49	Walk for 1 min. every 4–10 min.
50–59	Walk for 1–2 min. every 4–8 min.
60–69	Walk for 1–2 min. every 3–6 min.
70–75	Walk for 2 min. every 3–6 min.
76+	Walk for 2–3 min. every 3–4 min.

A Mid-life U-Turn. Cathy Troisi came to one of my running retreats full of excitement and apprehension. She wanted to raise money for a charity by running a marathon, but had never done any regular exercise in her life, at the age of 47. When I told her that she would have to take liberal walk breaks every minute or two, the light bulb came on. She knew she could do that.

Six months later she called, full of excitement, having finished her first marathon in 6 hours. She had run 2 minutes and walked 2 minutes. She had already entered her next one a few months later. During the next few years, I started to feel guilty from having inspired her to obsession: 6 marathons a year, then 12 a year, running 4½ minutes and walking 1 minute.

Eight years after she started, Cathy e-mailed me the exciting news that she had just run a 4:13 marathon, running 2 minutes and walking 1 minute. Since she is now doing about 20 marathon (or longer) events a year, Cathy has found that the 2:1 ratio allows her to recover much quicker. She has yet to suffer an injury.

Running Every Other Day. Just before he turned 60, the late Dr. George Sheehan changed his "running week" from six days to three. Many of us figured that the good doctor was losing interest—until, at 62, he ran his fastest marathon ever. George's schedule was to run ten miles every other day. He told me that this helped him maintain condition better than running 5–6 miles *every* day. He added long runs when he geared up for a marathon.

Jack Foster, who took up running at 33 and ran a 2:11 marathon at age 41, celebrated his 50th birthday in 1982 by running just over 2:20 in the marathon. This was incredible in itself, but even more so when you consider that he had also shifted to a three-day running week.

You won't run as fast as Foster (he's the best in the world for his age), but the same principles apply to all runners as they pass the master's checkpoint. Scientists have known for years that the longer runs are better for the system. You might consider running longer three days per week and resting more in between. This allows time for other adult (or childish) pursuits.

Running After 60. Mavis Lindgren grew up in rural Canada and had a series of childhood illnesses. Her parents moved west to British Columbia to be near hospitals which might be necessary to save their little girl's life. In her teens she contracted tuberculosis; after a struggle she defeated it, but it left her weak and sickly for most of her adult life. In her 50s she caught a series of infections which led to a three-year lung infection. Doctors then told her —this was 30 years ago—that this sickness would be her last. How right they were!

Instead of dying, Mavis held onto life for another few years and was barely able to join her husband Carl as he began a walking program. Although doctors had told her to avoid exercise all her life, she started to jog along with Carl; at first she could only go 2–3 yards. She kept at it, and suprisingly, a year later was jogging about a mile.

Until she was 85, Mavis not only ran marathons, but set records for her age group. She's lively and energetic, and the woman that couldn't resist infection for over 50 years didn't even get a cold for over 25 years.

All in the Family. I've watched a young boy without much obvious talent work his way to become one of the nation's top collegiate distance runners. I've seen housewives become world-class marathoners and old friend Frank Shorter, Olympic champion. But the person who has inspired me the most isn't an Olympian, a world recordholder or a national champion. Instead it's a man who was my hero when I was a young boy, a man who started to run when he was 52.

At that age, Elliott realized that over half of his high school football teammates had died of degenerative diseases. At 200 pounds, he was a heavy fat eater and non-exerciser whose doctor had told him he had to exercise if he was to survive. This former high school all-state football player just *knew* that 30 years of inactivity shouldn't prevent him from running circles around the slow joggers he saw in the park outside his office. Reality, however, was harsh; when he began his exercise program, he couldn't make it to the first telephone pole.

Each day Elliott pushed himself to that next telephone pole. After 4–5 months, he could run a mile or so. Running helped the weight come off and as it melted, running became easier and less painful. At first, walking was rough on his ego, but he found that interspersing the running with walks helped increase his endurance with reduced stress. He had to leave his competitive days behind and learn that running could be fun.

Elliott kept up with his telephone pole course and soon found he could run a 5K, then a 10K. He wasn't interested in form at first, but as it improved he found he could go farther. As he learned to run efficiently he realized that his 8-minute miles felt similar to the 5-minute miles of his college track days. He had made the transition by listening to his body.

Slowly his body remembered how to run. In 1978 he qualified for the Boston Marathon, 45 pounds lighter than when he'd started. Then a few days before his 59th birthday, Elliott ran the Callaway Gardens (Georgia) Marathon in 2:59!

This is an exciting story for me, for Elliott Galloway is my dad. What's inspired me most is the daily discipline and positive health style which has made Dad younger than he was 40 years ago. My greatest running experience is doing the entire 1996 Boston Marathon with my dad. While he was one of my most difficult runners to convert to walk breaks, he is still covering 30–40 miles a week because he is taking them regularly. My dad is again my hero. I hope that I can be like him, when I grow up.

None of us has firm control over the thin thread of life from which we're suspended. As we watch the seconds tick off on the great clock of our lifetimes, we can choose either to accept the deterioration that comes from neglect, or take control of our health and lives. There are thousands of stories like my dad's, each a significant act of courage. Each person that's done it now has a psychological edge in the battle of passing years. You don't have to just sit there and let things get worse as you get older. The choice is yours.

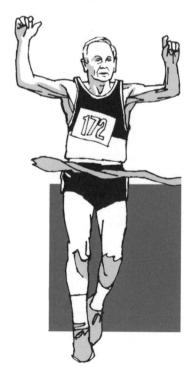

PERFORMANCE TIPS FOR THE 40+ CROWD

- **Run twice a day** (except for long runs). This reduces the pounding of a continuous run.
- **Acceleration gliders** *(see p. 145–147)* will keep a lot of your speed, without the wear and tear of speedwork.
  - 4–8 accelerations every running day, if desired
  - 2–6 accelerations every running day, if desired
  - 2–6 accelerations twice a week
  - 2–3 accelerations 1–2 times a week
- **Long run pace:** at least 3 min./mi. slower than goal pace for the longest race you plan to run in the next 3–5 months
- **Cross Training:** You can maintain conditioning, while reducing running days per week, by increasing cross training, especially water running and cross-country ski machines.

It's the Little Things

Because of the slower recovery rate, the small violations of overtraining will produce greater risk of injury, excess fatigue, and loss of running fun:

- *Junk miles:* Older runners are better off not running at all on a short mileage day. You can add those miles to various running days throughout the week, if desired.
- *Starting too fast:* The leg muscles of older runners take a lot longer to recover when going even 10 seconds per mile too fast.

- *Over-striding:* Many runners suffer a longer recovery time when they lengthen their stride even an inch at the end of a hard run. Older runners will ache more and will ache longer when they do this.
- *Over-stretching:* When older runners push a stretch too far, even on one stretch they can produce an injury that can last for months, due to slow recovery.
- *Over-exertion:* Keeping on just a mile or two past your fatigue point can leave the legs feeling like they don't want to run, for weeks. When in doubt, stop early.

Big Runners

Most runners gain weight, each decade. This extra burden increases the recovery time even longer. It's always better to err on the side of taking more walk breaks, and fewer days per week, if you want to keep resilient legs as the decades go by.

Age	Fitness Level	Pounds Overweight	Your legs feel like you are:
20–29	very fit	10–20	30–39
20–29	average	10–20	35–45
20–29	unfit	10–20	40–50
20–29	very fit	over 20	35–45
20–29	average	over 20	40–50
20–29	unfit	over 20	45–55
30–39	very fit	10–20	40–49
30–39	average	10–20	45–55
30–39	unfit	10–20	50–60
30–39	very fit	over 20	45–55
30–39	average	over 20	50–60
30–39	unfit	over 20	55–65
40–49	very fit	10–20	50–60
40–49	average	10–20	55–65
40–49	unfit	10–20	60–70
40–49	very fit	over 20	55–65
40–49	average	over 20	60–70
40–49	unfit	over 20	65–75
50–59	very fit	10–20	60–69
50–59	average	10–20	65–75
50–59	unfit	10–20	70–80
50–59	very fit	over 20	65–75
50–59	average	over 20	70–80
50–59	unfit	over 20	75–85

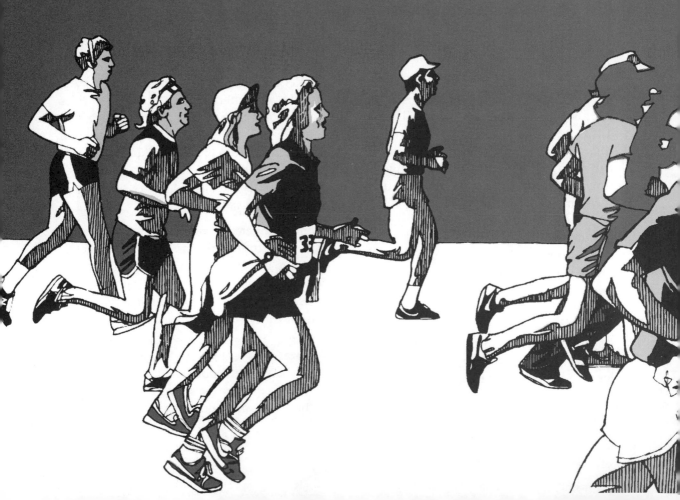

APPENDICES

PREDICTING RACE PERFORMANCE

THIS CHART WILL HELP YOU PREDICT a future race performance based upon a past race at another distance. The figures are reprinted from *Computerized Running Training Programs* by James B. Gardner and J. Gerry Purdy and are based upon what the authors call a *normal performance curve*, which enables one to "... predict a performance at one distance based on a performance at another distance ... It does not predict an exact competitive performance, since there are many tactical, psychological and environmental factors which affect each performance. ..."

One of the questions that arises in considering such a chart is, "Doesn't each runner tend to excel at a certain distance?" Your best distance may be a 10K and therefore your marathon time shown on the chart will not be up to the "equivalent" time shown on the same line. Or your best race may be a marathon ..., etc. Gardner and Purdy continue: "It should be noted that a performance in an event that is not the runner's specialty will typically be at a lower performance level than his performances in his own event. Yet the normal performance curve still applies. ..." They also point out that the athlete must be trained for the event in which he is competing in order to score at a near-equal level to his other events.

From a shorter distance to a longer one: If you predict your marathon time from a shorter race and fall short, you have the speed, but not the endurance, for the longer race. To remedy this, alter your program so you run longer (and possibly less frequently) and increase the number of repetitions in your speed sessions to 13. When predicting from a 5K to a marathon, you must rely on ideal conditions in the latter (which I've never experienced in over 120 marathons). Even on a cool day, you should add 10–20 minutes when you are predicting performance in the 26.2-mile event.

Remember that performance times will be slower when the temperature rises above 55° F. If your 5K time predicts a certain time to 10K, for example, you will need to go slower from the beginning of the race, if the temperature is expected to rise to 80 degrees. *(See p. 63 for performance adjustment recommendations.)*

From a longer distance to a shorter one: If your 10K time is not as good as predicted by your marathon or half-marathon time, you have the endurance, but not the speed. *(See Chapter 8,* Speed, *and Chapter 12,* The Advanced Competitive Runner.*)*

> **Note:** In altering your program, do so carefully and *gradually.* Be sensitive to how your body feels if you deviate from the 10K or marathon charts.

5km	8km	10km	15km	20km	25km	30km	Marathon	50km
12:58	21:23	27:09	41:50	56:50	1:12:05	1:27:32	2:06:18	2:31:43
13:02	21:30	27:17	42:05	57:09	1:12:29	1:28:02	2:07:02	2:32:35
13:06	21:38	27:27	42:20	57:29	1:12:54	1:28:32	2:07:45	2:33:28
13:11	21:45	27:36	42:30	57:49	1:13:19	1:29:30	2:08:30	2:34:21
13:15	21:52	27:45	42:45	58:08	1:13:44	1:29:54	2:09:14	2:35:15
13:20	22:00	27:55	43:00	58:29	1:14:10	1:30:05	2:10:00	2:36:10
13:24	22:08	28:04	43:20	58:29	1:14:36	1:30:36	2:10:46	2:37:05
13:29	22:15	28:14	43:30	59:09	1:15:02	1:31:08	2:11:32	2:38:01
13:33	22:22	28:24	43:45	59:30	1:15:28	1:31:41	2:12:19	2:38:58
13:38	22:30	28:34	44:00	59:51	1:15:55	1:32:13	2:13:06	2:39:55
13:43	22:38	28:44	44:20	1:00:13	1:16:22	1:32:46	2:13:54	9:40:53
13:48	22:45	28:54	44:35	1:00:34	1:16:50	1:33:20	2:14:43	2:41:51
13:52	22:52	29:04	44:50	1:00:56	1:17:18	1:33:54	2:15:32	2:42:51
13:57	23:02	29:15	45:05	1:01:18	1:17:46	1:34:28	2:16:22	2:43:51
14:02	23:10	29:25	45:20	1:01:41	1:18:14	1:35:03	2:17:12	2:44:52
14:07	23:20	29:36	45:40	1:02:03	1:18:43	1:35:38	2:18:04	2:45:53
14:12	23:28	29:47	45:56	1:02:26	1:19:12	1:36:14	2:18:55	2:46:56
14:17	23:35	29:57	46:13	1:02:49	1:19:42	1:36:50	2:19:48	2:47:59
14:23	23:45	30:08	46:30	1:03:13	1:20:12	1:37:26	2:20:41	2:49:03
14:28	23:53	30:20	46:47	1:03:37	1:20:42	1:38:03	2:21:34	2:50:08
14:33	24:00	30:31	47:05	1:04:01	1:21:13	1:38:40	2:22:29	2:51:13
14:39	24:10	30:42	47:23	1:04:25	1:21:44	1:39:28	2:23:24	2:52:20
14:44	24:20	30:54	47:41	1:04:50	1:22:15	1:39:57	2:24:20	2:53:27
14:50	24:30	31:06	47:59	1:05:15	1:22:47	1:40:36	2:25:10	2:54:35
14:55	24:40	31:18	48:18	1:05:40	1:23:20	1:41:15	2:26:13	2:55:44
15:01	24:48	31:30	48:36	1:06:06	1:23:52	1:41:55	2:27:11	2:56:54
15:07	24:58	31:43	48:55	1:06:32	1:24:25	1:42:35	2:28:10	2:58:05
15:12	25:08	31:55	49:15	1:06:58	1:24:59	1:43:16	2:29:10	2:59:17
15:18	25:17	32:07	49:34	1:07:25	1:25:33	1:43:58	2:30:10	3:00:30
15:24	25:27	32:20	49:54	1:07:52	1:26:08	1:44:40	2:31:11	3:01:44
15:30	25:37	32:33	50:14	1:08:19	1:26:42	1:45:22	2:32:13	3:02:59
15:36	25:48	32:46	50:34	1:08:47	1:27:18	1:46:06	2:33:16	3:04:15
15:43	25:58	32:59	50:55	1:09:15	1:27:54	1:46:50	2:34:20	3:05:32
15:49	26:09	33:12	51:16	1:09:44	1:28:30	1:47:34	2:35:25	3:06:50
15:55	26:19	33:26	51:37	1:10:13	1:29:07	1:48:19	2:36:30	3:08:09
16:02	26:30	33:40	51:58	1:10:42	1:29:45	1:49:05	2:37:37	3:09:29
16:08	26:41	33:54	52:20	1:11:12	1:30:23	1:49:51	2:38:44	3:10:51
16:15	26:52	34:08	52:42	1:11:42	1:31:01	1:50:38	2:39:53	3:12:13
16:22	27:03	34:23	53:05	1:12:13	1:31:40	1:51:26	2:41:02	3:13:37
16:28	27:15	34:37	53:27	1:12:44	1:32:20	1:52:14	2:42:13	3:15:02

5km	8km	10km	15km	20km	25km	30km	Marathon	50km
16:35	27:26	34:52	53:50	1:13:15	1:33:00	1:53:03	2:43:24	3:16:28
16:42	27:38	35:07	54:14	1:13:47	1:33:41	1:53:53	2:44:37	3:17:56
16:49	27:50	35:22	54:37	1:14:20	1:34:22	1:54:43	2:45:50	3:19:25
16:57	28:02	35:37	55:01	1:14:53	1:35:04	1:55:35	2:47:05	3:20:55
17:04	28:14	35:53	55:26	1:15:26	1:35:47	1:56:27	2:48:21	3:22:27
17:11	28:27	36:01	55:51	1:16:00	1:36:30	1:57:19	2:49:38	3:24:00
17:19	28:39	36:25	56:16	1:16:35	1:37:14	1:58:13	2:50:56	3:25:34
17:27	28:52	36:41	56:41	1:17:10	1:37:59	1:59:08	2:52:15	3:27:10
17:34	29:05	36:58	57:07	1:17:45	1:38:44	2:00:03	2:53:36	3:28:48
17:42	29:18	37:14	57:33	1:18:21	1:39:30	2:00:59	2:54:58	3:30:27
17:50	29:32	37:31	58:00	1:18:58	1:40:17	2:01:56	2:56:21	3:32:01
17:58	29:45	37:49	58:27	1:19:35	1:41:04	2:02:54	2:57:45	3:33:49
18:07	29:59	38:06	58:55	1:20:13	1:41:52	2:03:53	2:59:11	3:35:33
18:15	30:13	38:24	59:21	1:20:51	1:42:41	2:04:53	3:00:39	3:37:19
18:23	30:27	38:43	59:51	1:21:30	1:43:31	2:05:53	3:02:07	3:39:06
18:32	30:42	39:01	1:00:20	1:22:10	1:44:22	2:06:55	3:03:37	3:40:55
18:41	30:56	39:20	1:00:49	1:22:50	1:45:13	2:07:58	3:05:09	3:42:46
18:50	31:11	39:39	1:01:19	1:23:31	1:46:05	2:09:02	3:06:42	3:44:38
18:59	31:26	39:58	1:01:50	1:24:12	1:46:58	2:10:07	3:08:17	3:46:33
19:08	31:42	40:18	1:02:20	1:24:55	1:47:52	2:11:13	3:09:53	3:48:30
19:17	31:57	40:38	1:02:52	1:25:38	1:48:47	2:12:20	3:11:32	3:50:28
19:27	32:13	40:58	1:03:24	1:26:21	1:49:43	2:13:28	3:13:11	3:52:29
19:36	32:30	41:19	1:03:56	1:27:06	1:50:40	2:14:38	3:14:53	3:54:32
19:46	32:46	41:40	1:04:29	1:27:51	1:51:38	2:15:48	3:16:36	3:56:37
19:56	33:03	42:02	1:05:03	1:28:37	1:52:37	2:17:00	3:18:21	3:58:44
20:06	33:20	42:23	1:05:37	1:29:24	1:53:37	2:18:14	3:20:08	4:00:53
20:17	33:37	42:46	1:06:11	1:30:12	1:54:38	2:19:28	3:21:57	4:03:05
20:27	33:55	43:08	1:06:47	1:31:00	1:55:40	2:20:44	3:23:48	4:05:19
20:38	34:13	43:31	1:07:23	1:31:50	1:56:43	2:22:01	3:25:41	4:07:36
20:49	34:31	43:55	1:07:59	1:32:40	1:57:47	2:23:20	3:27:36	4:09:56

5km	8km	10km	15km	20km	25km	30km	Marathon	50km
21:00	34:50	44:18	1:08:37	1:33:31	1:58:53	2:24:40	3:29:34	4:12:18
21:11	35:08	44:43	1:09:15	1:34:24	2:00:00	2:26:02	3:31:33	4:14:42
21:22	35:28	45:07	1:09:53	1:35:17	2:01:08	2:27:25	3:33:35	4:17:10
21:34	35:47	45:32	1:10:33	1:36:11	2:02:17	2:28:50	3:35:39	4:19:40
21:46	36:07	45:58	1:11:13	1:37:06	2:03:28	2:30:16	3:37:46	4:22:14
21:58	36:28	46:24	1:11:54	1:38:02	2:04:40	2:31:44	3:39:55	4:24:50
22:10	36:48	46:51	1:12:36	1:39:00	2:05:53	2:33:14	3:42:06	4:27:30
22:23	37:10	47:18	1:13:18	1:39:58	2:07:08	2:34:46	3:44:21	4:30:12
22:36	37:31	47:46	1:14:02	1:40:58	2:08:25	2:36:20	3:46:38	4:32:59
22:49	37:53	48:14	1:14:46	1:41:59	2:09:43	2:37:55	3:48:58	4:35:48
23:02	38:16	48:42	1:15:31	1:43:01	2:11:02	2:39:32	3:51:21	4:38:41
23:15	38:38	49:12	1:16:17	1:44:05	2:12:23	2:41:12	3:53:46	4:41:38
23:29	39:02	49:42	1:17:04	1:45:09	2:13:46	2:42:53	3:56:15	4:44:39
23:43	39:26	50:12	1:17:52	1:46:15	2:15:11	2:44:37	3:58:47	4:47:43
23:58	39:50	50:43	1:18:41	1:47:23	2:16:37	2:46:23	4:01:23	4:50:51
24:12	40:15	51:15	1:19:31	1:48:32	2:18:06	2:48:11	4:04:02	4:54:04
24:27	40:40	51:48	1:20:22	1:49:42	2:19:36	2:50:02	4:06:44	4:57:21
24:43	41:06	52:21	1:21:15	1:50:54	2:21:08	2:51:55	4:09:30	5:00:42
24:58	41:32	52:55	1:22:08	1:52:08	2:22:42	2:53:50	4:12:20	5:04:08
25:14	41:59	53:29	1:23:02	1:53:23	2:24:19	2:55:48	4:15:13	5:07:39
25:30	42:27	54:05	1:23:58	1:54:40	2:25:58	2:57:49	4:18:11	5:11:15
25:47	42:55	54:41	1:24:55	1:55:59	2:27:38	2:59:53	4:21:13	5:14:56
26:04	43:24	55:18	1:25:54	1:57:19	2:29:22	3:02:00	4:24:19	5:18:42
26:21	43:53	55:56	1:26:53	1:58:41	2:31:07	3:04:09	4:27:29	5:22:33
26:39	44:23	56:35	1:27:54	2:00:06	2:32:55	3:06:22	4:30:45	5:26:30
26:57	44:54	57:14	1:28:57	2:01:32	2:34:46	3:08:38	4:34:05	5:30:33
27:16	45:26	57:55	1:30:01	2:03:00	2:36:40	3:10:57	4:37:30	5:34:43
27:35	45:58	58:36	1:31:06	2:04:31	2:38:36	3:13:20	4:41:00	5:38:58
27:54	46:31	59:19	1:32:14	2:06:04	2:40:35	3:15:46	4:44:36	5:43:20
28:14	47:05	1:00:02	1:33:23	2:07:39	2:42:38	3:18:16	4:48:17	5:47:49

RACE PACE CHART

This chart will help you plan your race by giving you key check points along the way. During a race it gets increasingly difficult to do the mental arithmetic needed to tell if you're on pace at each mile marker. If you write these checkpoint times on your hand or arm in indelible ink, it should help you to stay on pace. This chart can also be used after a race to tell your actual pace. **Note:** mi= miles, km= kilometers.

Minutes per mile	Times for the following distances: 2mi	3mi	5km	4mi	5mi	6mi	10km	7mi	8mi	9mi	15km
4:50	9:40	14:30	15:01	19:20	24:10	29:00	30:02	33:50	38:40	43:30	45:03
5:00	10:00	15:00	15:32	20:00	25:00	30:00	31:04	35:00	40:00	45:00	46:36
5:10	10:20	15:30	16:03	20:40	25:50	31:00	32:06	36:10	41:20	46:30	48:09
5:20	10:40	16:00	16:34	21:20	26:40	32:00	33:08	37:20	42:40	48:00	49:42
5:30	11:00	16:30	17:05	22:00	27:30	33:00	34:10	38:30	44:00	49:30	51:15
5:40	11:20	17:00	17:36	22:40	28:20	34:00	35:12	39:40	45:20	51:00	52:48
5:50	11:40	17:30	18:07	23:20	29:10	35:00	36:14	40:50	46:40	52:30	54:21
6:00	12:00	18:00	18:39	24:00	30:00	36:00	37:17	42:00	48:00	54:00	55:56
6:10	12:20	18:30	19:10	24:40	30:50	37:00	38:19	43:10	49:20	55:30	57:29
6:20	12:40	19:00	19:41	25:20	31:40	38:00	39:22	44:20	50:40	57:00	59:03
6:30	13:00	19:30	20:12	26:00	32:30	39:00	40:24	45:30	52:00	58:30	1:00:36
6:40	13:20	20:00	20:43	26:40	33:20	40:00	41:26	46:40	53:20	1:00:00	1:02:09
6:50	13:40	20:30	21:14	27:20	34:10	41:00	42:28	47:50	54:40	1:01:30	1:03:42
7:00	14:00	21:00	21:45	28:00	35:00	42:00	43:30	49:00	56:00	1:03:00	1:05:15
7:10	14:20	21:30	22:16	28:40	35:50	43:00	44:32	50:10	57:20	1:04:30	1:06:48
7:20	14:40	22:00	22:47	29:20	36:40	44:00	45:34	51:20	58:40	1:06:00	1:08:21
7:30	15:00	22:30	23:18	30:00	37:30	45:00	46:36	52:30	1:00:00	1:07:30	1:09:54
7:40	15:20	23:00	23:49	30:40	38:20	46:00	47:38	53:40	1:01:20	1:09:00	1:11:27
7:50	15:40	23:30	24:20	31:20	39:10	47:00	48:40	54:50	1:02:40	1:10:30	1:13:00
8:00	16:00	24:00	24:51	32:00	40:00	48:00	49:42	56:00	1:04:00	1:12:00	1:14:33
8:10	16:20	24:30	25:22	32:40	40:50	49:00	50:44	57:10	1:05:20	1:13:30	1:16:06
8:20	16:40	25:00	25:53	33:20	41:40	50:00	51:46	58:20	1:06:40	1:15:00	1:17:39
8:30	17:00	25:30	26:24	34:00	42:30	51:00	52:48	59:30	1:08:00	1:16:30	1:19:12
8:40	17:20	26:00	26:55	34:40	43:20	52:00	53:50	1:00:40	1:09:20	1:18:00	1:20:45
8:50	17:40	26:30	27:26	35:20	44:10	53:00	54:52	1:01:50	1:10:40	1:19:30	1:22:18
9:00	18:00	27:00	27:57	36:00	45:00	54:00	55:54	1:03:00	1:12:00	1:21:00	1:23:51
9:10	18:20	27:30	28:28	36:40	45:50	55:00	56:56	1:04:10	1:13:20	1:22:30	1:25:24
9:20	18:40	28:00	28:59	37:20	46:40	56:00	57:58	1:05:20	1:14:40	1:24:00	1:26:57
9:30	19:00	28:30	29:30	38:00	47:30	57:00	59:00	1:06:30	1:16:00	1:25:30	1:28:30
9:40	19:20	29:00	30:01	38:40	48:20	58:00	1:00:02	1:07:40	1:17:20	1:27:00	1:30:03
9:50	19:40	29:30	30:32	39:20	49:10	59:00	1:01:04	1:08:50	1:18:40	1:28:30	1:31:36
10:00	20:00	30:00	31:04	40:00	50:00	60:00	1:02:08	1:10:00	1:20:00	1:30:00	1:33:12

Distance Equivalents:

1 kilometer = .6214 miles	25K = 15.54 miles
10K = 6.21 miles	30K = 18.64 miles
15K = 9.32 miles	Half-marathon = 13.1 miles (21.1 km)
20K = 12.43 miles	Marathon = 26 miles, 385 yards

Minutes per mile	Times for the following distances: 10mi	20km	Half-marathon	15mi	25km	30km	20mi	Marathon	50km
4:50	48:20	1:00:04	1:03:52	1:12:30	1:15:05	1:30:06	1:36:40	2:07:44	2:30:10
5:00	50:00	1:02:08	1:05:33	1:15:00	1:17:40	1:33:12	1:40:00	2:11:06	2:35:20
5:10	51:40	1:04:12	1:07:58	1:17:30	1:20:15	1:36:18	1:43:20	2:15:28	2:40:30
5:20	53:20	1:06:16	1:08:55	1:20:00	1:22:50	1:39:24	1:46:40	2:19:50	2:45:30
5:30	55:00	1:08:20	1:12:06	1:22:30	1:25:25	1:42:30	1:50:00	2:24:12	2:50:50
5:40	56:40	1:10:24	1:14:17	1:25:00	1:28:00	1:45:36	1:53:20	2:28:34	2:56:00
5:50	58:20	1:12:28	1:16:28	1:27:30	1:30:35	1:48:42	1:56:40	2:32:56	3:00:17
6:00	1:00:00	1:14:33	1:18:39	1:30:00	1:33:10	1:51:48	2:00:00	2:37:19	3:06:20
6:10	1:01:40	1:16:38	1:20:50	1:32:30	1:35:45	1:54:54	2:03:20	2:41:41	3:11:30
6:20	1:03:20	1:18:43	1:23:01	1:35:00	1:38:20	1:58:00	2:06:40	2:46:03	3:16:40
6:30	1:05:00	1:20:47	1:25:13	1:37:30	1:40:55	2:01:06	2:10:00	2:50:25	3:21:50
6:40	1:06:40	1:22:52	1:27:23	1:40:00	1:43:30	2:04:12	2:13:20	2:54:47	3:17:00
6:50	1:08:20	1:24:56	1:29:34	1:42:30	1:46:05	2:07:24	2:16:40	2:59:09	3:22:10
7:00	1:10:00	1:27:00	1:31:32	1:45:00	1:48:40	2:10:30	2:20:00	3:03:03	3:37:20
7:10	1:11:40	1:29:04	1:33:57	1:47:30	1:51:15	2:13:36	2:23:20	3:07:55	3:42:30
7:20	1:13:20	1:31:08	1:36:08	1:50:00	1:53:50	2:16:42	2:26:40	3:12:17	3:47:40
7:30	1:15:00	1:33:12	1:38:20	1:52:30	1:56:25	2:19:48	2:30:00	3:16:39	3:52:50
7:40	1:16:40	1:35:16	1:40:30	1:55:00	1:59:00	2:22:54	2:33:20	3:21:01	3:58:00
7:50	1:18:20	1:37:20	1:42:42	1:57:30	2:01:35	2:26:00	2:36:40	3:25:23	4:03:10
8:00	1:20:00	1:39:24	1:44:52	2:00:00	2:04:10	2:29:06	2:40:00	3:29:45	4:08:20
8:10	1:21:40	1:41:28	1:47:02	2:02:30	2:06:45	2:32:12	2:43:20	3:34:07	4:13:30
8:20	1:23:20	1:43:32	1:49:15	2:05:00	2:09:20	2:35:18	2:46:40	3:38:29	4:18:40
8:30	1:25:00	1:45:36	1:51:25	2:07:30	2:11:55	2:38:24	2:50:00	3:42:51	4:23:50
8:40	1:26:40	1:47:40	1:53:07	2:10:00	2:14:30	2:41:30	2:53:20	3:47:13	4:29:00
8:50	1:28:20	1:49:44	1:55:18	2:12:30	2:17:05	2:44:36	2:56:40	3:51:35	4:34:10
9:00	1:30:00	1:51:48	1:58:00	2:15:00	2:19:40	2:47:42	3:00:00	3:56:00	4:39:20
9:10	1:31:40	1:53:52	2:00:11	2:17:30	2:22:15	2:50:48	3:03:20	4:00:19	4:44:30
9:20	1:33:20	1:55:56	2:02:22	2:20:00	2:24:50	2:53:54	3:06:40	4:04:41	4:49:00
9:30	1:35:00	1:58:00	2:04:33	2:22:30	2:27:25	2:57:00	3:10:00	4:09:03	4:54:50
9:40	1:36:40	2:00:04	2:06:44	2:25:00	2:30:00	3:00:06	3:13:20	4:13:25	5:00:00
9:50	1:38:20	2:02:08	2:08:55	2:27:30	2:32:35	3:03:12	3:16:40	4:17:50	5:05:10
10:00	1:40:00	2:04:16	2:11:07	2:30:00	2:35:20	3:06:24	3:20:00	4:22:12	5:10:40

ABOUT THE AUTHOR

In the 1970s, Jeff Galloway was one of a group of young American runners who would change distance running forever. Jeff and his running buddies — Frank Shorter, Bill Rodgers, Steve Prefontaine, Don Kardong, Amby Burfoot, Kenny Moore and others — captured the attention of a new generation of fitness-minded Americans, and the running boom was born. What had been a sport for the few became an activity for the millions.

Jeff was born in Raleigh, North Carolina, started running in high school, and was very "average" until his senior year, when he became state champion in the 2-mile. He attended Wesleyan University and was All-American in cross-country and track. In preparing for the 1972 Olympics, Jeff, along with Frank Shorter and Jack Bacheler, spent two months training in the mountains at Vail, Colorado, and all three made the Olympic team that year. Jeff, according to runner/writer Joe Henderson "... should have been an Olympic marathoner, but instead made the team in the 10K and then helped friend Jack Bacheler make it in the longer distance."

In 1973 Jeff set an American record in the 10-mile. He won the first Atlanta Marathon at age 18, and was the first winner of Atlanta's Peachtree Road Race in 1970. In the mid-'70s he began to follow a training program that emphasized more rest and less weekly mileage, coupled with a long run every other week. At age 35 he ran the Houston-Tenneco Marathon in 2:16.

Jeff Galloway's Competitive Career

High school:	1-mile: 4:28;
	2-mile: 9:48
College:	1-mile: 4:12;
	2-mile: 9:06;
	3-mile: 14:10
Other times:	6-mile: 27:21
	10K: 28:29
	10-mile: 47:49
	(U.S. record, 1973)

Jeff met his wife Barbara at a track meet in Florida. Barbara was on the Florida State women's track team. They were married in 1976. Barbara runs practically every day and has competed in over 40 marathons. Her best 10K time is 41:50 and marathon time, 3:18.

Jeff is now on the road over half the time. Because of his busy schedule, he often runs 2–5 miles, two or three times per day. He generally totals about 60 miles a week. He has currently run over 120 marathons, at the rate of 3–4 per year. Every ten years he returns to the site of his first victory, Atlanta, and tries to beat his time of 2:56 as an 18-year-old. So far he's been successful. In 1993, at age 48, he ran just under 2:51.

Jeff and Barbara live with their sons Brennan and Westin in Atlanta, Georgia. Like their parents, both boys are (naturally!) runners.

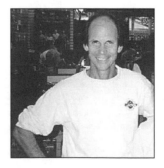

INDEX

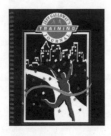

JEFF GALLOWAY'S TRAINING JOURNAL

This spiral-bound training tool leads you through the process of setting up a training program, step by step. Not only can you set up and record your progress for a year at a time, you'll be able to analyze the data in tables: logs for shoes, injuries, speed sessions. Graphs for morning pulse will help you monitor overtraining.

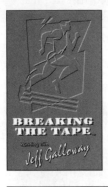

"BREAKING THE TAPE"

In two 30-minute VHS videotapes and a 30-minute motivational audiocassette, Jeff Galloway talks you through the world of running information. The first 30-minute segment includes tips on nutrition, stretching, choosing the right shoes, running injury-free, and cross training. Tape Two covers form, pacing, peaking, setting realistic goals, building an interval speedwork plan for the 5K and 10K, and Jeff's six-month marathon training program. This is great for individual instruction or for group clinics and exercise reinforcement.

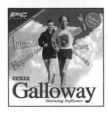

GALLOWAY'S TRAINING SOFTWARE

Based on the techniques Jeff uses in his marathon programs across the country, this program will set you on the path to success, whatever your goals!

The Galloway Plan creates exciting training programs for all ability levels from beginner on up. The plan sets up a detailed training schedule for you based on:

• Your running history and experience
• Your race distance (marathon or half-marathon)
• Your personal goals (race goal time, train to finish, fat burning)
• Your race date

Week by week, throughout your training, Jeff is there on your computer screen to monitor your progress, adjust the training schedule, and give you tips and training advice that will keep you motivated each day, right up to your race. Whatever your running experience, Jeff's program can give you the best program for your special situation.

For more information or to place an order, call 1-800-200-2771 or go to www.RunInjuryFree.com

JEFF GALLOWAY'S FITNESS VACATIONS

Lake Tahoe

Imagine yourself on a hike or a run along a crystal-clear lake, surrounded by beautiful mountains, with an endless series of trails and other recreational opportunities. Even when the temperature goes above 85°, you'll be comfortable in the 10–30 percent humidity. Jeff has been having camps on the North Shore of Lake Tahoe for 21 years.

After a morning run along scenic paths in national forests or on the Truckee River bike path, you'll have breakfast. Jeff and staff will then present seminars on the topics listed below. Most afternoons are spent hiking in beautiful mountain areas.

You'll meet inspiring and friendly experts such as stretching expert Bob Anderson, Sister Marion Irvine (a humorous and inspiring nun who qualified for the Olympic trials at age 50), Joe Henderson (running's most prolific writer), Dr. Gary Moran (physiologist and expert in biomechanics and strength training), Dr. David Hannaford (sports podiatrist specializing in running injuries), and John Bingham ("The Penguin" from *Runner's World*). Visit www.RunInjuryFree.com for this year's dates and staff.

Swiss Alps

Join Jeff Galloway for a delightful running tour of the Swiss Alps and run or walk a 30K trail event. During 11 days, you'll stay in the beautiful alpine resort town of Davos. The Swiss Alps is a fairytale area of sparkling lakes and lush green valleys surrounded by rugged peaks. Besides excursions to scenic Swiss towns, we'll spend a day in Zurich, and you'll have an option to visit Lucerne.

For more information, call 1–303–755–2888 or email: apostolos@athensmarathon.com

Typical Camp Schedule:

7:00	Group run/walk/stroll
8:00	Breakfast
9:00–12:00	Clinic Sessions
12:00	Lunch
1:00–6:00	Hiking, Sightseeing, Exploring
6:00	Dinner
After dinner	Philosophizing and storytelling

Clinic Sessions:

- Nutrition • Mental Strength • Stretching
- Getting Better as We Get Older
- Motivation • Water Running • Cross Training
- Marathon Training • Running Faster
- Fat Burning • Strengthening

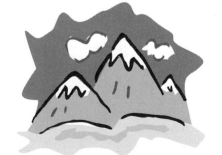

Call 1-800-200-2771, ext. 10 for more information.
www.RunInjuryFree.com

THE *RUN INJURY FREE* NEWSLETTER

Stay in touch with the latest running ideas and concepts with Jeff's free monthly email newsletter. Training, fat burning, marathon gatherings, and runner feedback.

To sign up for this FREE newsletter, call 1-800-200-2771 or go to www.RunInjuryFree.com

JEFF'S COLUMN IN *RUNNER'S WORLD*

Read Jeff Galloway's monthly column in Runner's World magazine (www.runnersworld.com).

GALLOWAY'S MARATHON TRAINING GROUPS IN 32 MAJOR CITIES
Getting to the finish line injury-free

The group guides you, encourages you, and supports you during your 6-month marathon training program. There are currently groups in the following cities:

Atlanta	Daytona	Louisville	Sacramento
Augusta	Denver	Macon	Salem
Austin	Fort Collins	Miami	San Francisco
Bethesda	Fort Worth	Nashville	Sarasota
Boulder	Greenville	New Orleans	Tampa
Charlotte	Gwinnet	New York	Tucson
Chicago	Hampton Roads	Northern Virgina	In Canada:
Cincinatti	Hartford	Orlando	Ft. McMurray
Columbus, GA	Houston	Raleigh/Durham	
Dallas	Jacksonville	Richmond	

Not in a city near you? No problem.

Join our Individual Training Program.

Enjoy the guidance of a trained Virtual Group Leader.

For more information:
  www.RunInjuryFree.com
  1-800-200-2771, ext. 12

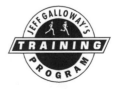

MORE WORLD-CLASS FITNESS BOOKS
FROM SHELTER PUBLICATIONS

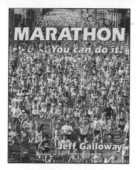

Marathon
You Can Do It!
by Jeff Galloway

Jeff Galloway's revolutionary new book outlines the way for just about anyone to run a marathon.

- 11 training programs for every type (and speed) of runner
- Jeff's unique "walk breaks" that eliminate injuries
- Up-to-date advice on staying motivated, nutrition, and burning fat

"If I can do it, anybody can. It really works!"
—Rosemary Shannon (age 52)

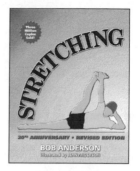

Stretching
20th Anniversary Revised Edition
by Bob Anderson

One of the world's most popular fitness books, now revised.

- 3½ million copies sold, in 23 languages
- Stretching routines for all sports (including running and everyday activities)
- New hand and wrist stretches for carpal tunnel problems

"A must-read for anyone who wants to stay supple for life."
—*The Washington Post*

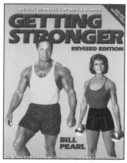

Getting Stronger
2nd Edition
by Bill Pearl

A revised edition of the best-seller on weight training. Of special interest to runners are off-season and in-season weight training programs for distance running and new rehab exercises for knees.

- 550,000 copies sold
- 80 one-page training programs
- General conditioning, sports training, and bodybuilding

"A must for anyone serious about fitness."
—*Newsday*

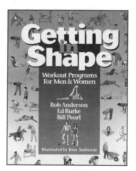

Getting in Shape:
Workout Programs for Men and Women
by Bob Anderson, Bill Pearl, and Ed Burke

A unique workout book for anyone who wants to get back in shape.

- Stretching, weightlifting, and cardiovascular training
- 3-point programs

"An all-in-one book by masters from each corner of the fitness triangle."
—*Dallas Morning News*

CREDITS

Editor (this edition)
Robert Lewandowski

Editor (first edition)
Lloyd Kahn

Production Manager
Rick Gordon

Graphics Production
Robert Lewandowski

Book Design
Rick Gordon, David Wills, Robert Lewandowski

Line Drawing Illustrations
Richard Golueke, Edna Indritz, David Wills

Proofreading
Robert Grenier

Printing
Courier Companies, Inc., Stoughton, MA, USA

Production Hardware
Macintosh G3/400 computer, Agfa Arcus II scanner

Production Software
QuarkXPress, Adobe Photoshop, Nisus Writer, Microsoft Word

Typefaces
Guardi, ITC Kabel, and Lithos

Paper
60 lb. Williamsburg Offset

Special thanks to the following people, who helped with this book in one way or another:

Bob and Jean Anderson, Don Baxter, M.D., Debbie Beckman, Rich Benyo, David Betta, John Cantwell, M.D., Tom Conklin, David L. Costill, Ph.D., Dianne Etheridge, Ed Fox, E. C. Frederick, Ph.D., Barbara Worral Galloway, Brennan Galloway, Westin Galloway, Teresa Gibreal, Patty Harris, David Hannaford, D.P.M., Joe Henderson, Perry Julien, D.P.M., Michele Langevin, Arthur Lydiard, Allan McDonald, M.D., Carol Miller, Irving Miller, D.P.M., Stanley Newell, D.P.M., John Pagliano, D.P.M., Michael L. Pollock, Ph.D., Gerry Purdy, Richard Quiñones, Laura Riley, Kirk Rosenbach, Victoria Seahorn, Greg Sheats, George Sheehan, M.D., Chris Twiggs, Diana Twiggs, M.D., Don Weiner.